Re-engineering Affordable Care Policy in China

T0298582

Presenting a comprehensive examination of China's medical care system, this book tackles issues of policymaking, organization, management and financing in the context of the provision of affordable care in China.

Making use of extensive field investigations, interviews and a thorough analysis of documents, this book examines the re-structuring of the medical care system, spanning more than three and half decades from 1979 to the present day. Assessing the difficulties of regulatory control in the health care sector, it also explores theoretical alternatives, including post-Weberian constructs of uncertainty and control, as well as franchise and asymmetric information in market transactions. Ultimately, it argues that patient medical care has become less and less affordable amid shrinking government subsidies, breakdowns of public insurances and increases in user charges, especially between the mid-1990s and mid-2000s. Whilst the government took decades to re-organize the public hospital system and rebuild public insurances, it faced a dilemma of enforcing both low-cost medical care and maintaining revenue flow to public hospitals through marketization.

Re-engineering Affordable Care Policy in China provides extensive discussion of the policymaking process as well as detailed analysis of policy contents. As such, it will be invaluable to students and scholars of Chinese social policy and public administration, as well as Chinese Studies more generally.

Peter Nan-shong Lee is Professor Emeritus at the Department of Political Science at National Chung Cheng University, Taiwan.

Routledge Contemporary China Series

193 China's Regions in an Era of Globalization
Tim Summers

194 China's Climate-Energy Policy
Domestic and International Impacts
Edited by Akihisa Mori

195 Western Bankers in China
Institutional change and corporate governance
Jane Nolan

196 Xinjiang in the Twenty-First Century
Islam, Ethnicity and Resistance
Michael Dillon

197 China Studies in the Philippines
Intellectual Paths and the Formation of a Field
Edited by Tina S. Clemente and Chih-yu Shih

198 Innovative and Creative Industries in Hong Kong
A Global City in China and Asia
Grace L K Leung

199 Illicit Industries and China's Shadow Economy
Challenges and Prospects for Global Governance and Human Security
Edited Victor Teo and Sungwon Yoon

200 Re-engineering Affordable Care Policy in China
Is Marketization a Solution?
Peter Nan-shong Lee

For more information about this series, please visit: https://www.routledge.com/Routledge-Contemporary-China-Series/book-series/SE0768

Re-engineering Affordable Care Policy in China

Is Marketization a Solution?

Peter Nan-shong Lee

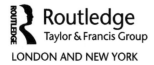

Routledge
Taylor & Francis Group

LONDON AND NEW YORK

First published 2019 by Routledge

2 Park Square, Milton Park, Abingdon, Oxfordshire OX14 4RN

52 Vanderbilt Avenue, New York, NY 10017

Routledge is an imprint of the Taylor & Francis Group, an informa business

First issued in paperback 2020

British Library Cataloguing in Publication Data
A catalogue record for this book is available from the British Library

Library of Congress Cataloging-in-Publication Data
Names: Lee, Peter N. S., 1940- author.
Title: Re-engineering affordable care policy in China : is marketization a
    solution? / Peter Nan-shong Lee.
Description: Abingdon, Oxon ; New York, NY : Routledge, 2019. |
    Series: Routledge contemporary China series ; 200 |
    Includes bibliographical references and index.
Identifiers: LCCN 2018035008| ISBN 9781138542365 (hardback) |
    ISBN 9781351009041 (ebook) | ISBN 9781351009027 (epub) |
    ISBN 9781351009010 (mobipocket encrypted) |
    ISBN 9781351009034 (Adobe reader)
Subjects: LCSH: Medical policy--China. | Health care reform--China. |
    Medical care--China--Marketing.
Classification: LCC RA395.C53 L44 2019 | DDC 362.10951--dc23
LC record available at https://lccn.loc.gov/2018035008

ISBN: 978-1-138-54236-5 (hbk)
ISBN: 978-0-367-66333-9 (pbk)

Typeset in Times New Roman
by Taylor & Francis Books

Contents

List of illustrations   vii
Preface   viii
Acknowledgements   xi
List of Abbreviations   xiii

PART I
Issues and concepts   1

1   Introduction   3

2   Repackaging health care service and paths to reform   26

PART II
Rebuilding the state in the health care sector   51

3   Institutional framework and managerial mechanisms   53

4   Financing Medical Care Services   75

5   Re-inventing medical care insurances   98

6   Price control amid the rise of regulated markets   121

PART III
Re-making China's medical care delivery   145

7   Learning from the enterprise style of management   147

8   Franchising of medical care services and unintended policy
    consequences   167

9   Drug franchising and financial management   189

10 Regulatory control in expanding drug markets   208

PART IV
Conclusion 233

11 Review and assessment 235

Index 245

Illustrations

Figures

2.1 Paths to the Reform: De-regulation of market and property rights
    restructuring   36
3.1 The supervisory and managerial system of public hospitals in
    China   58
4.1 The trend of total health expenditure in GDP, 1978–2012   79
4.2 Percentages of medical care expenditure in GDP, 1978–2012   80

Tables

1.1 Command-oriented management vs. transaction-oriented
    management   17
2.1 Classification of benefits and entitlements of health care service in
    China   29
6.1 Average medical care expenses in China: outpatients and
    inpatients, 1990–2008   134

Preface

This book is concerned with re-engineering affordable care policy in China that represents a long and exceedingly complex process lasting for a time span of nearly four decades from 1979 to the present. This preface will briefly introduce main issues of this book as well as the author's intellectual and theoretical concerns. For sure, it is an enormous task for top policymakers to make the transformation of health care system, covering a nation of 34 provincial jurisdictions, 334 municipalities and more than 2,000 counties. The system consists of 954,389 health care institutes of various types, including 14,328 hospitals, coupled with 21,979 hospital beds, serving a population of 1,400 million people. It embraces a total of 8.61 million of medical personnel, including 2.66 million doctors, and 2.44 million nurses. The total spending of heath care amounts to 2,426,878 million RMB, about 5.15 percent of GNP in the year of 2011.

Starting from the early 1950s, sovereign planners endeavored to provide affordable care to the Chinese people through two approaches, namely, public providers and public insurances. Through the first approach, public providers (often public hospitals) rendered health care services at a low price and were heavily subsidized by the government. Public insurances, the second approach, shouldered a considerable portion of financial burden of enrollees, including Public Financed Medical Care (PFMC) for public personnel, Labor Insurance Medical Care (LIMC) for staff and workers in the state-owned enterprises (SOEs), and Rural Cooperative Medical Care (RCMC) for the peasants. In one way or others, people enjoyed health care benefits for the first 30 years of the PRC. At the beginning of economic reform, the government started to rebuild health care facilities, restore the proper medical care services, and improve management of public hospitals in order to meet the medical demands of the people who had just recovered from economic stagnation and political turmoil. Some issues of health care services emerged gradually, and the government, with different policy agendas, tackled one issue at one time throughout health care reforms.

Focusing on the public hospital system, the government had to deal with the acute shortage of funding and meager pay for medical personnel by choosing the marketization option, namely, introducing user charges at the providing unit level, during the early years of the reform era. While proven to be effective in fulfilling revenue targets and improving resource management at the providing unit level, user charges worked against the government's low price-policy of medical care, posing such as a thorny issue of regulatory control, especially price control. User charges bring in good revenue to public hospitals, as new drugs and advanced medical devices are lucrative. While many patients complained about high charges, many other patients found it affordable in the midst of stronger purchasing power, the increase of compensation and rapid improvement of living standards. Re-inventing public insurance has been another challenge in order to alleviate the financial burden of the patient. Beginning in 1994, it took about one and half decades for remaking Basic Medical Care Insurances (BMCI) for the employed population in urban areas, but a shorter time span for the introduction of New Rural Cooperative Medical Care Insurance (NRCMCI) for the peasantry, and Urban Resident Medical Care Insurance (URMCI) for the unemployed, retired and marginal sectors of urban population. A full cycle of re-engineering endeavor has completed as all these public insurances were put into implementation during the early 2010s.

Taking advantage of extensive field investigations, interviews and a thorough analysis of documents, the study is intended, from the perspective of public policy and management, to fill gaps regarding the re-structuring of the medical care system from 1979 to the present. Centering on the policy concern of affordable care, the study addresses re-engineering health care provision at the micro and macro level during economic reform, building upon contributions by authors, experts, and health care economists in their articles and reports about reforms in the provision of curative care services. At the micro level, main tasks of re-engineering were devoted to inaugurating user charges and franchise funding, budgetary reform and accountability systems, performance appraisal and incentive schemes. At the macro level, sovereign planners undertook major re-structuring work with regard to allocation of health care resources through institutional means, public financing, public insurances and regulatory measures. To deal with the discrepancies between policy goals and implementation, moreover, the study tries to analyze unintended policy outcomes in the process of policy implementation, covering issues related to revenue-maximizing behaviors, exorbitant charges, over-provision, abuse of prescription drugs, weakening of public and preventive care, and inequality in health care resource allocation.

Highlighting the differences between the private and public sector, theoretically speaking, the study tackles the issues of policymaking, organization, management, and financing with reference to the provision of affordable care in China. The study will start with a discussion on Graham Allison's early book first published in 1971 that borrows the analyses of policymaking, organization, management from the private sector to apply them to the public sector on the basis of the case of Cuban missile crisis. Further to the Allison's theoretical construct, it will examine various China scholars' endeavors to analyze the Chinese experiences of policymaking, organization, management (including financing) in the public sector in the light of business/industrial management.

To be discussed further, some theoretical highlights of the book are as follows. First, the study will also shed light on top Chinese policymakers' search for new combinations of policy tools falling between the state and markets, while identifying and analyzing their relative strengths and weaknesses. On the basis of a survey of learning from business/industrial management, the study conducts a dialogue with authors on new public management (NPM) from the early 1990s to the early 2010s . Instead of being confined to a simple dichotomy between state and market, the proposed study tries to answer the question: how can either the state or markets be better consolidated in the public sector? And in which type of services? In what kind of policy/program? In which functional area in the health care sector? And if they each either fail or succeed, why? Second, the study will examine the pros and cons regarding the application of franchising to the health care sector. Within the centrally planned economy (CPE), franchising is part of financial strategy for economic development. It was used effectively as a revenue tool in the industrial sector in the Chinese case as well. As sovereign planners insist to make public hospitals and public insurances as two main pillars of health care system, they intend to rely heavily on franchise funding through the introduction of user charges to deal with funding issues in the realm of curative care services, prescription drugs and modern devices. How successful they have been? This study will try to evaluate the case. Last but not least, the book tries to account for the issue of compliance and non-compliance with special reference to subsidized public hospitals which play conflicting role in serving as vehicles in implementation of low-price policy and in generating revenue to improve the rate of self-sufficiency. To explain the phenomena of irregularities, the study endeavors to discuss and assess various theoretical alternatives, for example, the post-Weberian constructs such as uncertainty and control within organization as well as franchise and asymmetric information in market transactions.

Acknowledgements

Upon completing this book manuscript, the author cannot help but reflect on the long intellectual journey with regards to his research on reengineering affordable care policy in China. Although the author basically travelled by himself in climbing up one mountain after another, he was encouraged and supported in one way or others by many friends without them the author could not have reached his destination. In theoretical terms, the author is intellectually indebted to numerous brilliant scholars and authors of master class, who enable him to stand on their shoulders to examine the most challenging theoretical issues of the latest centuries. The author has duly noted them throughout the chapters of the book. When dealing with concrete research work, however, the author would like to take this opportunity to register his gratitude and appreciation to academic institutes and academic friends whose assistances are most helpful along the way to bring the research project to fruition.

In fact, before any researcher outside China can make sense out of an exceedingly complex and enormous scale system of health care, including delivery, insurance and drug, it is essential to have some feel how the system works. One needs to know how participants, such as patients, doctors and nurses, hospital directors and management, insurance executive agencies, and government officials and policymakers interact with one another and how do they perceive, understand and interpret their interactions in subjectively meaningful ways. This research project began with field study in China earlier on, supported by University Grants Committee of Hong Kong Government. Focusing on interpretative schemes, the author was able to conduct extensive interviews, including more than 60 interviewees, as individuals or panels, and complete surveys of two cities, namely, Guangzhou and Shanghai. Subsequently, the author conducted a follow-up research to cover the case of Xiamen, that was funded by National Science Commission in Taiwan. The author conducted in depth and through archival research in Universities Services Centre for China Studies at the Chinese University of Hong Kong, without its rich and quality collection this book volume could not have possibly been completed.

Thanks are due to Guangzhou Academy of Social Science and Shanghai Academy of Social Science, making possible of several field investigations, many interviews and surveys. Special appreciation is reserved to Li Jiangtao, Cai Guoxuan and Tong Xiaoping at Guangzhou Academy of Social Science, who lent the author very much needed help in the study of medical care issues in China in general and in Guangzhou in particular. Wu Susong of Shanghai Academy of Social Science provided him much assistance to conduct research on Shanghai case in some detail, allowing him to have some close look at medical care delivery and insurances in Shanghai. Several scholars were very kind by granting him audience on a series of challenges of health care reform. In time the sequence of meeting, they include Professor Li Jiangfan of Nanhua Technology University, Professor Hu Suyun, Shanghai Academy of Social Science, Professor Gu Xin, Beijing University and Professor Du Lexun, Harbin Medical University. Moreover, much appreciation is reserved to Ms. Chen Weichi, Mr. Edward Lee, Professor Liu Chaolung, and Professor Steve Ching for their assistance as well as advice in making figures and tables in this book volume.

During the process of write-up, Ms. Veronica Tanihara read the first draft of book manuscript carefully and suggested many revisions. The author greatly benefits from Professor Timothy Guile who read the second draft first from the angle of a layman, and then from the vantage of an academician, resulting in considerable work of re-organizing and re-writing chapter by chapter, section by section, and paragraph by paragraph. The author would like to register his appreciation to entire editorial team of Routledge who did a very proficient job, making the entire volume look nice and neat, and above all, much better than he could imagine originally.

List of Abbreviations

BMCI	Basic Medical Care Insurance
CCP	Chinese Communist Party
CPE	centrally planned economy
CRSW	Congress of Representatives of Staff and Workers
CTORM	comprehensive trade-wide oriented residential management
CT	computerized tomography
COE	collective-owned enterprise
CURS	comprehensive undertaking responsibility system
DRS	director's responsibility System
ESM	enterprise style of Management
EM	economic management
ECT	electronic convulsive therapy
FUS	financial undertaking system
GDP	gross domestic product
GNP	gross national product
GMP	good manufacturing practices
GSP	good storage practices
LMCES	large medical care expenditure subsidy
MRI	magnetic resonance imaginary
MCSPP	medical care subsidy to public personnel
MOF	Ministry of Finance
MOH	Ministry of Health
MLSS	Ministry of Labor and Social Security
NRCMCI	New Rural Cooperative Medical Care Insurance
NPM	New Public Management
OPP	out of pocket payment
PA	personal account
PRC	People's Republic of China
RHCP	regional health care planning
RSS	revenue-sharing system
RCMC	Rural Cooperative Medical Care
SGBPM	State General Bureau of Pharmacy Management

STRC	State Institutional Reform Commission
SRDC	State Reform and Development Commission
SEMCI	supplementary enterprise medical care insurance
SMCI	supplementary medical care insurance
TUs	Trade Unions
UPS	unified planning system
URS	undertaking responsibility system
URBMCI	Urban Resident Basic Medical Care Insurance
USFA	unified social funding account
WHO	World Health Organization
W/R differentials	Wholesale/retail differentials

Part I
Issues and concepts

1 Introduction

The study is concerned with the re-engineering of affordable health care policy in China, addressing the question of how sovereign planners adopted policy tools at both macro and micro levels within the Party-state hierarchy in order to make low price, essential medical care available to all during the era of economic reform. At the macro level, sovereign planners took advantage of policy tools inherited from the centrally planned economy (CPE) built prior to 1979, in restructuring the ways of allocation of health care resources (e.g., through institutional means, public financing, public insurances and regulatory measures). At the micro level, main tasks of re-engineering were devoted to inaugurating user charges, budgetary reform and accountability systems, and performance appraisal and incentive schemes. What are the designs and characteristics of these policy tools? How effective are they? What are their limitations and weaknesses? These are issues to be tackled throughout this book.

In conceptual and theoretical terms, one needs to treat the provision of affordable care during the economic reform era in a dynamic rather than static sense. One cannot hold the engineering endeavor constant for it has experienced rapid changes not only on the demand side but also supply side of health care services. As the Chinese people started to leave austerity of the pre-reform period behind and have a first taste of improvement of compensation packages and stronger purchasing power, consumers' durables (such as mechanical refrigerators, washing machines, etc.), and modern bath and toilet facilities have found their way into households, coupled with electricity and running water. Accordingly, their appetite for more welfare and better health care have been enhanced, reflecting on the demand side, for example, for the new mixes and enriched contents of health care, different types of service for the aging population, changing profile of illness, new categories of care induced by medical science and technology, new drugs, and advanced medical devices. On the supply side, relative weight among various funding sources have drastically shifted, for example, the fluctuation of the government subsidies, disintegration and rebuilding of public insurances, and steady increase of user charges, all registering on the changing balance of health care between the public sector and non-public sector in the post-Communist society.

Besides, the enforcement of low-price policy goes hand in hand with the introduction of franchise funding and new regulatory tools, shaping and affecting the quality and quantity of health care made available to patients in the midst of expansion of health care markets.

As a whole, this study provides a broad, systematic and in-depth treatment of issues of policymaking, organization, management, and financing of affordable health care in China, building upon evidence-based research by health care economists in their articles and reports about reforms in the delivery of curative care services for nearly three decades (Gu, Bloom, Tang et al. 1993; Hsiao 1995; Liu, 1995; Ho 1995; World Bank 1997; Bloom and Gu 1997; Ma 2008; Ng 2008; Yip & Mahal 2008; Yip & Hsiao 2008; Tam 2010). Nevertheless, this study will take one step forward beyond the contributions of these health care economists. It is intended, from the perspective of public policy and management, to fill gaps regarding the re-engineering of affordable health care policy during the economic reform by taking advantage of extensive field investigations, interviews and a thorough analysis of documentary material.

Highlighting the differences between the private and public sector, theoretically speaking, the book tackles issues of public management, and public financing with reference to the provision of low price, essential medical care to all in China. Focusing on the Chinese experiences, the study will try to make a critical assessment on the use and abuse of business/industrial management in the public sector. To deal with the discrepancies between policy goals and implementation, moreover, the study endeavors to analyze unintended policy outcomes in policymaking process, covering issues related to revenue-maximizing behaviors, "exorbitant" charges, over-provision, abuses of prescription drugs, weakening of public and preventive care, and inequality in health care resource allocation.

The book will also try to shed light on top Chinese policymakers' search for new combinations of policy tools falling in between the state and markets, while examining their relative strengths and weaknesses. On the basis of a survey of learning from business/industrial management, the study will conduct a dialogue with authors on new public management (NPM) (Rainey 1991; Massey 1993; Hughes 1998; Pollitt & Bouckaert 2011). Instead of being confined to a simple dichotomy between state and markets, the study endeavors to answer the question: how can either the state or markets, as policy tools, be better consolidated in the public sector? And in which type of services? In what kind of policy/program? In which functional area in the health care sector? And if they each either fail or succeed, why?

The theme and overview

The theme of the volume concerns re-engineering affordable health care policy during the economic reform in China. Heavily relying on a state-oriented approach, the early phase was devoted to the task of streamlining in the name of "economic management," and rebuilding hospitals and medical care facilities in urban areas and rural counties in aftermath of Mao's era (Chapter 7) (Peng, Cai & Zhou 1992: 3–14). In the subsequent phases, they began to adopt a market-oriented approach—marketization (often taken "commercialization") of services, featuring user charges, budgetary reform, and financial accountability in the name of "undertaking responsibility system" (URS) during 1985 and 1988 (Chapters 7 and 8) (Ho 1995; World Bank, 1997: 17–25; Zhonggongzhongyang & Guowuyuan 2009; Du et al. 2009). User charges quickly assumed an increasingly large role among several funding sources at the health care provider level, as medical devices and drug sale expanded their share in the medical care markets from the late 1980s (Chapters 8, 9 and 10). Meanwhile, the rapid expansion of market economy, public finance reforms, and breakdowns of conventional public insurance programs inadvertently resulted in dwindling shares of the government subsidies and insurance payments to providing units and ordinary patients (Chapters 4 and 5). Consequently, the balance of funding among three main sources (i.e., government subsidies, insurance payments and user charges) at the providing unit level was drastically upset, and it was not restored gradually until after the early 2000s (See Chapter 4). It is deemed theoretically meaningful to address the changing balance among these three funding sources and explore alternatives to account for such a long-term trend.

Furthermore, marketization moved to higher gear with two steps: first, through opening up of enterprise-managed health care facilities to community, and second, in a more substantive way, by inaugurating property rights reform through the separation between public hospitals and non-public hospitals (through an exercise of so-called "classification" of hospitals) starting in 2000 (Chapters 2 and 3). It promised growth of profit-oriented, non-public hospitals, which is built on the private ownership. However, in spite of "classification," the governments at central and local levels seemed reluctant to make full use of non-public hospitals to allocate health care resources. Nor did they intend to lift the restrictions over non-public hospitals (e.g., limiting their participation in public insurance programs) quickly. As a consequence, public hospitals have still dominated health care market throughout China. Another re-engineering attempt of delivery was initiated in 2009, focusing on the experiment of corporatization of public hospitals (Chapter 2). Overall, these market-oriented reforms have brought China's health care provision forward to a parallel structure between profit-oriented hospitals and non-profit-oriented hospitals, a feature commonly found in various advanced countries such as Great Britain, Germany, and the USA.

At the conceptual and theoretical level, the book represents an endeavor to assess how far business/industrial management can be transplanted to the public sector by focusing on two analytical dimensions: policymaking process and management. In the West, the study of public administration has borrowed heavily from business/industrial management since the early 1980s, but its intellectual root can be traced back to the early 20th century (Henry 1989:

20–50; Hughes, 1998: 22–80; Pollitt & Bouckaert 2011: 6–22). In reviewing the long history of its intellectual journey, authors note that while academics advocated the similar theoretical theme at several historical junctures, practitioners made repeated attempts to introduce business/industrial management to the public sector. As theory-building endeavor has moved ahead, practical experience has further accumulated (Massey 1993; Ferlie, et al.: 1–29; Pollitt & Bouckaert 2011). However, empirical research has fallen behind, especially studies covering non-Western countries. Taking advantage of an in-depth research on health care in China, the study proposes to re-examine this century long movement of "learning from business/industrial management," and tries to answer to what extent, on what issues and in which functional areas business/industrial management is found applicable to the health care sector.

To tackle the policymaking dimension, the study tries to highlight such features as the exercise of mandatory power, plurality of policy actors, multiple policy goals, and cost of information. And most importantly, it endeavors to portray how policymaking in the public sector differs from that in the non-public sector. In dealing with the management dimension, furthermore, arguments and debates converged on the choice of the state, the markets or often a mix of both in order to find and design the best policy tools for allocating health care resources and making the best effort to cure the illnesses of great multitude of people throughout the country.

These re-engineering efforts will be examined in light of the latest academic trends in the field of public management. As the new public management (NPM) found an inroad into the domain of public administration starting in the early 1980s, some authors, with much enthusiasm and optimism, promised that the "market paradigm" might be able to supplant the conventional public administration, and they often argued in terms of a simple dichotomy between state and market (Hughes 1998: 52–80). From an alternative perspective, however, this study will examine the role of the state and markets, respectively, regarding the merits and demerits of each on the basis of an empirical investigation in the medical care delivery system in China, rather than indulge in the controversy of the substitutability of one for the other. Do markets fare better than the state in terms of revenue and resource management in medical care in the Chinese case? Are markets more likely to consolidate in a type of performance that is measurable, and the type of service the cost of which is attributable and retrievable? Is it true in China that the state tends to be effective in setting and implementing policy goals involving social utility—the type of service the cost of which is, by and large, not attributable to and retrievable from users, and the performance of which is less quantifiable and measurable? These are questions to be addressed in this volume.

This volume will be devoted to an analysis of salient issues of affordable care in the policy cycle from policymaking, implementation, and management to policy outcomes and feedback, but the main focus will be implementation and management. From the perspective of public management, this study will deal with issues in the macro management of medical care, focusing on process, mechanisms, and interrelation among key programs (e.g., differential-quota appropriation, supplementary insurance, collective bidding for procurement of drugs, etc.) in China's medical care system. It will also analyze so-called "output linkages" from the state to society in the forms of state subsidized and public insurance funded curative services, coupled with analyses of its instrumental and technical dimension (e.g., user charges, performance appraisal, retained revenue, wholesale/retail differentials in pricing schemes, etc.) whenever it is found pertinent.

This volume consists of several parts. Part I has two chapters. An introductory discussion is given here in Chapter 1. Chapter 2 addresses the restructuring of both the demand side and supply side of health care in China. The former deals with the repackaging and reclassifying of health care services that determines medical care benefits and entitlements made available to users, highlighting the challenges in adopting appropriate operational definitions for essential health care, including essential curative care. And the latter focuses on the paths of evolution of the state and markets in health care, examining various combinations of policy tools in the allocation of health care resources to various sectors of the people. Part II consists of four chapters, mainly examining the application of policy tools at the macro level, for example, institutional designs, public finance, public insurances and regulatory control. Chapter 3 addresses on the issues of institutional restructuring and rebuilding within the Party-state hierarchy in light of its policy implications in health care resource allocation, coupled with installation of planning and managerial apparatus at the municipal, provincial and central level. Chapter 4 examines financing in the health care sector during the economic reform, focusing on the issue of the changing balance among three major funding sources (i.e. government subsidies, public insurances and user charges). It will also analyze the government's changing role in the controversy of "load shedding" of various echelons of the government, in addition to an analysis of the trends of state "retreat" and "advance" in public finance. Chapter 5 is concerned with a discussion on the disintegration and rebuilding of public insurances as well as some broad financial implications on health care delivery. Chapter 6 deals with the government's regulatory control, especially price control, over the providing unit in order to fulfill the ideal of affordable care, accompanying with discussion on the thorny issue of controlling revenue-maximizing behavior at the providing unit level.

During the early years of the economic reform, the re-engineering efforts focused on transplanting the "enterprise style of management" (ESM) at the providing unit level, including accountability systems, incentive schemes, and performance appraisals. This effort was soon followed by the adoption of a franchise funding policy anchored in the introduction of user charges and budgetary reform, starting in 1985, and expanded further in 1989 and beyond. Part III provides an extensive, in-depth treatment on restructuring health care delivery, featuring the commercialization of curative care services together with medical devices and pharmaceuticals. It will first tackle the issues pertaining to inaugurating ESM marked by a brand of "bandwagon" phenomenon manifested in the policy episode of "undertaking responsibility system" (URS) in Chapter 7, as the building of ESM was made a pre-requisite to budgetary reform and revenue retention schemes. Chapter 8 will be devoted to the introduction of user charges in the delivery of curative care services. In view of increasing weight of franchise funding from pharmaceuticals and medical devices, the government's price control intensified its strains considerably with providing units. Chapter 9 will make a close examination on the role and behaviors of the providing unit and medical personnel in the sales of pharmaceuticals and medical devices, while Chapter 10 provides an analysis of the growth of drug markets, regulatory control, and unanticipated policy outcomes, highlighting irregularities in pricing game in "new drugs," substitutable drugs and over-prescriptions as well as the formation of pockets of vested interests in the three-way collaboration among the drug industry, providing units and medical personnel. The book will be concluded with a revisiting and discussion on overall features of re-engineering endeavors in Chapter 11.

The policymaking role of the state

The book will be devoted to a discussion of the significant roles of both the state and markets in the allocation, deployment, organizing and managing of health care resources in the transition from CPE to a mixed economy in China. Overall, the study is intended to examine alternative policy tools which are often taken as the state or markets or a combination of both. In a conceptual term, either state or markets represents a system, embracing several closely related functional components in the public policy circle from policymaking, coordinating, organizing and managing to outcomes and feedback. In a broad sense, "state" here refers to the system of command-oriented activities while "market" is concerned with transaction-oriented processes.[1] In 1977, Lindblom borrowed from concepts and theories derived from the database of business/industrial management, and treated the state and market as two alternative systems in coordinating policies for the allocation of resources in the public sector.[2] It is interesting and, at the time, was fashionable to borrow from business/industrial management to study the state organization, but it is theoretically meaningful to delineate the differences between the two (Rainer 1991; Gortner et al. 1997). It is noteworthy that the generic formulations of organization and management tend to remain blurred on the distinctions between the state and markets.

To begin with, the state differs from the markets in that the former relies heavily on the exercise of command rather than market transactions to achieve coordination among multitude of organizational members. As a form of territorial organization exercising mandatory power for the implementation of a mix of policy purposes, the state is normally funded by tax revenue, and is staffed by appointed officials. In the field of policy studies, authors have borrowed concepts and theories relating to decision-making from business/industrial management and applied these to the state while highlighting its distinctive characteristics centering on mandatory power. To examine the policymaking role of the state in descriptive terms (i.e. what it is), one needs to account for several salient characteristics as follows: policy actors acting on behalf of public authorities and wielding mandatory policy tools; multiple policy actors who are institutionally positioned in the state hierarchy; multiple goals of diverse nature (e.g. economically oriented and non-economically oriented); and policymaking process with limited information, capacity and resources.

Some authors endeavor to use the generic formulation of pure rationality model (or taken as one singular rational actor model) as a starting point to identify the main characteristics of policymaking in the realm of the state organization (Allison 1971; Allison and Zelikow 1999:13–75; Dror 2013: 132–42). The pure rationality model entails a task environment where one singular rational actor strives to attain one chosen goal. Such a goal is often taken as "stake," material interest of some kind. It is often assumed that in the public sector, a singular policy actor only acts upon "material interest" just like the way a businessman pursues profit in commercial circle. The said model is merited for allowing analysts to take an empathetic understanding of the real decision-making situation where policy actors perceive, operate, and grasp key elements of decision-making process (Allison 1971; 10–38; Allison and Zolikow 1999: 19). But empathy is no substitute for what happens in reality.

In the studies of health care policy in China, some authors have applied versions of the pure rationality model in order to reconstruct patterns of policymaking activities, leaving some important theoretical issue untreated (Lampton 1977; Duckett 2013; Huang 2014). First, it is assumed in their analyses that in each policy episode in the public sector, there is only one singular rational actor involved. They implicitly take either the state, government unit, ministry, bureau, or society (or sectors of the people) among others as a policy actor (s), but they leave it unspecified and undefined in operational terms. Second, they take it as given that a policy actor (s) is dictated only by material interest in policymaking, without any genuine policy concern. Policy actors are motivated by only extrinsic values such as power, prestige and status, but never by intrinsic values (for instance, merits in policy itself, principle, or a sense of justice). That is to say, the government unit adopts a tangible goal of material interest (something like profit) and a calculating scheme, acting "rationally" by choosing the best means to attain the goal as if the "stakeholder" is not different from the corporate entity in market transactions. Neither is a policy actor(s) able to differentiate political interest from commercial interest, nor can he/she draw a distinction between power and policy. As the policy actors only pursue material interest in theoretical term, no room is left to considerations of such meta-policy issues such as "social utility," distributive justice, public policy concerns, and ideologies in policymaking—issues raised by Hebert Simon and further spelled out by Yehezkel

Dror (Simon 1957: 45–60; Dror 2013: 161–96). In the existing literature of China studies, for example, Lieberthal and Oksenberg represent one of the earliest attempts to draw an analytical boundary between "policy approach" (taken as "rationality model") and "power approach," suggesting that policy actors might act upon concern of power as much as the merits of policy (Lieberthal and Oksenberg 1988).

Not only are plurality of policy actors (e.g. various government units) involved, but also a mix of policy goals needs to be attained, making policy-making in the public sector distinctively different from that in the private sector. According to Graham T. Allison and Philip Zelikow, the state represents a "vast conglomerate of loosely allied organizations" with multiple policy actors who are institutionally positioned in the hierarchy of government (Allison and Zelikow 1999: 141–96). Although their empirical study is based upon one singular policy issue of war and peace pertaining to the Cuban missile crisis that concerned one singular goal of national security, they are fully aware of great complexity where multiple policy actors often acted with different preferences (and/or interests), perceptions and interpretations given a broad policy goal (Allison and Zelikow 1999: 141–96). One can visualize the complexity and challenges involved regarding domestic social policy where multiple policy actors who represent the concerns of their home departments and work with different goals, and they cannot readily reach an agreement among themselves, given a sense of duty derived from their affiliation to home department, and divergent understandings and interpretations on each policy goal, if so chosen. As being illustrated in the study on energy policy in China, Lieberthal and Oksenberg, in their pioneering effort, try to identify key characteristics of policymaking process in the public sector, highlighting the scenario of multiple policy goals that are held by plural policy actors who are institutionally positioned in a "fragmented structure of authority" (Lieberthal and Oksenberg 1988: 22–3). In conceptual term, "fragmented structure of authority" represents one step forward to address behavioral attributes that might deviate from what a researcher can find in a formal organizational chart. It also highlights considerable difficulty in achieving coordination among many departments which are assigned different functions and duties on the basis of division of labor. This theme of plural policy actors working with multiple policy goals (or sub-goals) is echoed in Yanzhong Huang's volume on health care policy during reform China, illuminating complexity in delivery of public health services in some chosen policy episodes (Huang 2014: 21).

With multiple policy goals that are different in nature, how are policy actors motivated and guided in the policymaking process? In the analysis of three analytical dimensions of policymaking on the basis of the case study of Cuban missile crisis, Allison and Zelikow maintain that pure policy concerns, organizational ethos and politics are relevant albeit they do not assign relative weight to each. Accordingly, two questions arise on the nature and characteristics of relationship among policy actors. First, are policy actors purely policy oriented? In other words, is it true that all officials are only committed to pure policy goals regardless of political interest and organizational ethos? In fact, Allison and Zelikow argue that all three variables are pertinent in the study of policymaking as they review three "cuts" of the Cuban missile crisis, which are taken as "rational actor paradigm," "organizational behavior paradigm," and "government politics paradigm" (Allison and Zelikow 1999). Lieberthal and Oksenberg have made a pioneering adventure by bringing Allison's earlier analytical scheme (Allison 1971) into their study of energy policy in China, and they lend greater weight to analysis of bureaucracy/organization against the intellectual background of "politics taking command" in China studies for past several decades, given available research material during the economic reform (Lieberthal and Oksenberg 1988). In essence, they argue that it is not only theoretically meaningful but also feasible to tackle both the issue of bureaucracy/organization and of politics in policymaking in China. It is noteworthy that Allison and Zelikow in their work (in 1999) have made some revision of Allison's early formulation of the "government process model" (in 1971). Nonetheless they do not intend to assert that the policy approach (or taken as "rationality model") is irrelevant.

Given the scenario of multiple institutional actors in the state organization, how to forge a set of shared goals and thus to achieve some measure of consensus and coordination in policymaking process and subsequent implementation in the public sector? First of all, the principle of unity of command often remains an ultimate solution with which rival actors can always appeal for a final decision from their common superior within the state hierarchy. In an administrative way, moreover, some disagreements can be minimized, if not eliminated entirely, through division of labor among departments, specialization, assignment of duty to subordinates by the superior, and delegation of power from higher echelon to lower echelon. Theoretically speaking, nonetheless, division of labor entails a paradox: on the one hand, in a formal organizational chart, the division of labor is intended to ensure that each department performs its assigned function/duty, and therefore to facilitate coordination; on the other hand, it tends to create some measure of difficulty for coordination in tackling new issues in policymaking which is often controversial and lacking consensus, because each official is expected to represent the position of his or her home department acting upon its assigned function.

Borrowing from Avery Goldstein, Yanzhong Huang's study of public health provides an illustration of dynamic process through which unity of command allies to a continuum from the behavior of compliance, e.g., "bandwagon," to that of non-compliance, e.g., "passing the buck" (Huang 2014). Both authors appear to highlight behavioral features associated with the exercise of command in the context of a flat hierarchy of a relatively large scale territorial organization: a superordinate unit marshals a large number of subordinate units in a Chinese case, for example, one central government versus 34 provincial jurisdictions, and further down, 34 provincial governments versus 334 prefectural/municipal jurisdictions, and further down more than 2,000 counties in addition to numerous urban districts. Directly relevant to health care policy during the reform era, for instance, a focal point pertains to decentralization of power and finance from the central authorities to provincial/local governments within the Party-state hierarchy during the economic reform. In a way, rather than using simple exercise of command, the central government needs to exercise some degree of leadership through persuasion and consensus-building, since considerable power and financial resources have been "transferred downward" to the provincial level or below. Without "influential resources" in Goldstein's term, the central government often makes use of demonstration effects of pilot programs; and this does not necessarily follow a rigid structure of central command that is reinforced by its "influential resources" from time to time.

There is no lack of analysis of the process and mechanisms of coordination in the business sector, for instance, the observation regarding coalition formation and side payments advanced by R. M. Cyert and J. G. March (Cyert & March 1963). How does the state organization differ from the business firm? With reference to mechanisms of coordination achieved through a policymaking process in the public sector, Allison and Zelikow tend to stretch the conception of market-oriented behavior overly to that of command-oriented activities by suggesting that "bargaining" is normally employed as a mechanism to resolve the conflicting preferences among organizational units within the government. As they put it, "political in the sense that the activity from which decisions and actions emerge is best characterized as bargaining along regularized channels among individual members of the government" (Allison and Zelikow 1999: 295). In other words, they assume that government officials act like businessmen. By the same token, Lieberthal and Oksenberg offer a theoretical alternative about conflict resolution among multiple institutional actors by borrowing the notion of "bargaining" from a market economy to account for conflict resolution in the public sector (Leiberthal and Oksenberg 1988). In their words, "the fragmentation is overcome through negotiations, bargains, and exchanges that are struck among the parts of the system ... The way these bargains are struck and the purposes behind them go to the heart of the practice." (Leiberthal and Oksenberg 1988: 32)

Is the market paradigm appropriate to characterize the process of coordination in the public sector? It does not seem that under normal circumstances government officials really "bargain" with each other strictly in term of quid pro quo exchanges in commercial transactions. Professor David Lampton appropriately takes bargaining as just one of several forms of authority relationship in policymaking in the health care sector in China (Lampton 1992: 34). In fact, there is an analytical category of non-transactional interactions, such as persuasion, consultation, exchange of opinions, and all other possible means that could be equally effective to forge consensus among institutional actors for building a foundation for inter-departmental coordination, as will be demonstrated in many cases of policymaking and enforcement in the subsequent chapters.

To study the policymaking role of the state from a descriptive perspective, furthermore, it is necessary to work with multiple policy goals often resulting in a clash of divergent value premises in the realm of the state apparatus rather than to deal with one simple, clearly defined goal such as a concern for profit as in the case of a business or a production target. To address many policy goals in the public sector, first of all, one needs to deal with meta-policymaking issues, namely, how to evaluate a policy goal according to value premises (Dror 2013: 160–1). In fact, one cannot rule out entirely that policymakers might act in an altruistic way, e.g., "stake" as broadly defined in terms of pure merits of policy: for instance, the quest for more resources on behalf of a home department, and defense for interest of their clients, the provision of services to patients, and maintenance of good health of labor forces to ensure productivity of the whole economy, etc. In a way, concern of meta-policymaking makes Lieberthal and Oksenberg's policy approach (or rationality model) relevant as a theoretical alternative to be examined empirically in this study of public policy in China. Moreover, Leiberthal and Oksenberg's "power model" is applicable here in this study too, so long as policy actors often act upon their "political interest," a loosely defined category yet to be defined operationally. It is also realistic and likely for policymakers to be motivated by a mix of formal policy commitment and personal concerns.

How are pure values, ideology, or political belief fused with material interests? It is apparent that policy actors need to address a mixture of non-economic values with economic concerns in the public sector. To go beyond pure economic concerns, some ideologies are pertinent to defining and mandating medical care entitlements in China. For example, sovereign planners uphold the principle of corporatism by legally recognizing the occupational benefits/entitlements, including basic medical care insurance for staff and workers, commensurate with their sacrifices and contributions under the low-wage policy during the early years of CPE (Lee 1987; Lee 1991). Moreover, the state upholds the ideal of universalism by making basic medical care available and accessible to all and by ensuring a safety net of minimal and essential protection extended to citizens regardless of their trades and economic status.

Another descriptive dimension of a policymaking model has to do with the cost of information from a post-Simonian vantage point. This concerns not only the choices of policymaking models, organizational designs, and managerial tools but also the ways to deal with unintended consequences in the process of implementation at both the macro and micro level. In some authors' discussions, cost of information (either equivalent to zero or larger than zero) is key to designs of policymaking models. In his formulation of the "synoptic model," for example, Lindblom implicitly assumes, in a normative sense, that policymakers are assigned by themselves an omniscient and omnipotent role with all information and capacity required in a policymaking episode (Lindblom 1977: 247–60). It is evident that the "synoptic model" does not address cost of information in policymaking process. To put it in another way, the cost of information is taken as "zero" in the "synoptic model." In contrast, the "strategic model" assumes theoretically that the cost of information is larger than zero. Since policy actors do not have access to all the information required in reality, the "strategic model," coupled with incrementalism that it represents makes better sense of policymaking in a political system (Lindblom 1977: 247–60).

At the empirical level, not many authors have extended the use of a generic formulation of "bounded rationality" to research regarding the policymaking role of the state where the cost of information is an issue, as an element of the unknown is constantly present. With reference to China, Peter NS Lee makes an attempt to propose to examine the transformation of policymaking models from Maoist period to reform era, hinging on considerations of cost of information. Lee argues that in the Chinese case, sovereign planners were confronted with uncertainty and the unknown (i.e., cost of information), when they first built the centrally planned economy (CPE). They started with an image of an exceedingly, but unrealistically, large policymaking role of the state in a normative sense during the early years of CPE. Through a learning process as testified by Mao Zedong, top policymakers adjusted to reality by accepting their being limited by an irreducible element of uncertainty and the unknown in the policymaking arena (Lee 1987). Theoretically speaking, once sovereign planners became aware of the cost of information, they started to curtail this cost by adopting uncertainty avoidance measures, e.g., not only by scaling down the scope of direct interventions in the economy, but also by adopting market/transaction-oriented management. For examples, Hu Qiaomu's celebrated paper on policymaking diagnosed the weaknesses of the model of macro-rationality of CPE. To reduce the cost of information and minimize uncertainty, Hu not only advocated the retreat of the state but also proposed the introduction of market-oriented measures, e.g., including a plan of narrower scope, decentralization to lower echelons of government, fewer bureaucratic methods, more financial restructuring, fresh revenue retention schemes adopted in industry, tax reform, and a new monetary policy (Lee 1987: 172–5). And Hu recommended the extensive use of "economic leverages," that is, a market-oriented approach to alleviate the burden to the state, as Naughton has documented and analyzed brilliantly at considerable length (Naughton 1996). To be discussed further in subsequent chapters, one will find that in order to learn from the results of policy implementation, a rational actor often engages in collecting information pertinent to making a right decision not only by conducting search and investigation but also by introducing pilot programs and policy experiments as reflecting on many policy episodes cited in this study. In a more systematic way, policymakers may adopt a "sequential decision model" by learning from the outcomes of a series of policy programs previously implemented (Dror 2013: 142–3).

The path toward marketization

During economic reform, the discussion surrounding market options has gained currency in medical care policy, as markets have become increasingly assertive in the allocation of health care resources in China. This study uses transactions as the core definition of "market," emphasizing quid pro quo exchanges of values as central to economic activity. In China, the market-ization of health care resources embraces two forms: one pertaining to ser-vices and products, e.g., introducing user charges, while the other concerns property rights, e.g., corporatization, privatization, divesture and sales of assets. Moreover, it appears that the market is always embedded in the state structure to varying degrees, from the legal protection of contractual and property rights, licensing of market entry, regulatory and pricing controls, and subsidies for users to direct participation as an institutional actor in buying and selling in the market, just to name a few (Hughes 1998: 81–108).

Is marketization a solution to affordable care in China? One needs to work on the issues of operational definition and classification first, and then deal with substance. Conceptually speaking, one is warranted proposing a classifi-cation scheme comprehending all modes of market restructuring/building in health care reforms in China with all possible combinations of services/pro-ducts and property rights (Chapter 2). In such a classification, partial mar-ketization may include either transactions in the case of services and products (e.g., drugs and medical devices) or the transfer of property rights based on corporatization and asset privatization. And full-fledged marketization may include both. While sovereign planners have placed considerable emphasis on partial marketization in form of "commercialization" by introducing user charges to a variety of services beginning in the early 1980s, they started to undertake property right reforms in the health care sector and to construct a legal and institutional framework for non-public hospitals from the mid-1990s, thereby allowing the entry of services and investments of for-profit providers into the medical care markets (see Chapter 2).

Since the economic reform starting in 1979, sovereign planners have been using three main types of market as policy tools in the allocation of health resources: free markets, regulated markets, and quasi-markets. Free markets mean the kind of transaction basically free from government intervention, for example, private practitioners, the drug market, and the market for medical devices, especially during early stages of economic reform prior to the 1990s. Regulated markets pertain to the type of transaction with observable and sometimes strong regulatory control over market entry, pricing, quality, and safety standards. Examples include basic curative care services with user charges, paid immunization services, and the regulated provision of pre-scription drugs. Quasi-markets refer to transactions within a well-defined administrative boundary where all actors are institutionally positioned in the Party-state hierarchy and governed by administrative laws. The notion of quasi-market owes its origin to the NHS in United Kingdom where tax revenue constitutes the main funding source, and the Chinese brand of quasi-market operates mainly with public insurances in addition to tax exemptions. Moreover, funding sources from public insurances with risk-pooling mechanisms and tax exemptions are mandated; and services/products are legally stipulated as entitlements, a manifestation of the exercise of mandatory power of the state.

Referring to empirical investigation of health care reform in the UK, Ewan Ferlie et al. warn of the danger of applying a "misleading analogy" to internal markets and/or quasi-markets phenomena (Ferlie 1996: 57). For China, it is equally challenging to establish operational definitions and empirical tests when such notions as "internal markets" or "quasi-markets" are used as in the case of UK. Here, this study will refer the "quasi-markets" to transactions encapsulated within a common set of accounting and budgetary rules binding to a group of actors, such as purchasers, providers, and users, within a defined administrative boundary where not only is a measure of choice and competition entertained but also exchanges of equal values take place. In this study, transaction is taken as a requisite in a quasi-markets/internal markets, albeit it varies from one case to another in given jurisdictions. By the same token, one may treat the German health care system analytically as a brand of "internal markets and/or quasi-markets," similar to the Chinese case as both are funded by public insurances.

The introduction and expansion of the markets to the health care sector has created various types of services provided by either the state or markets or both. During economic reform, policy analysts started to work out a conceptual scheme involving four types of service: (1) purely public health care, (2) quasi-public health care, (3) basic medical care, and (4) non-basic medical care (Chapters 2, 7 and 8). By and large, it appears that the state demonstrates strengths in the management of public health care services which involve extensive externality and where costs are neither attributable to, nor retrievable from, the users. Conversely, the markets work more effectively in the delivery of curative care services, which involve limited externality, and as a rule, costs are attributable to and retrievable from users. This study will mainly focus on curative care services, prescription drugs and medical devices, the most controversial issues of which concerns "commercialization." For example, while user charges apply to basic medical care that is partially funded by the government's indirect subsidies, the providing unit is given greater discretion in the pricing of non-basic curative care, for instance, "special care" such as appointments with specialists, upgraded wards, treatment of serious illness, use of imported drugs and drugs not listed as basic catalog drugs, as well as the application of advanced medical devices. Such special care often goes beyond the coverage of basic medical care insurance.

Command-oriented management and transaction-oriented management

From the vantage point of public management, state and market represent different designs of organization and management as mechanisms for coordination of activities in the public sector. For analytical purposes, this study proposes to characterize the state as command-oriented management, and the markets as transaction-oriented management. As illustrated in Table 1.1, command-oriented management is a model, based on a traditional public administration, for coordinating resource allocation.[3] It is applicable to the public sector where policymakers and officials have to implement public policy goals (Pollitt & Geert Bouchaert 2004: 8–15; Massey 1993: 12–16; Rainey 1991: 22–4). As a rule, it adopts a bureau form of organization relying on the exercise of command, tax revenue, and appointed officials to carry out public policy goals. It normally employs an input-centered design: officials organize, control, and operate by making the best use of managerial and organizational input characteristic of means-to-an-end consistency, impersonality beyond face-to-face relations, and procedurally centered tools of management.

Transaction-oriented management is a model of coordination anchored in market transactions, falling into the broad conceptual terrain of either public management or generic management, and sometimes thought of as New Public Management (NPM hereafter) (Hughes 1998: 52–80; Rainey 1991: 15–36; Graham & Hays 1991: 10–27: Pollitt & Bouchart 2004: 6–18). As such, it is an output-centered design to the extent that managerial tasks are organized and carried out on the basis of measurable task performance and financial and economic results. That is to say, it works better to fulfill economic and financial

Table 1.1 Command-oriented management vs. transaction-oriented management

Models dimensions	Command-oriented management	Transaction-oriented management
Value orientation	Public purposes Multiple & vague objectives Non-measurable results	Private concerns Simple & well-defined objectives Measurable results
System characteristics	Public administration Input-centered design Command Public finance (e.g., tax revenue)	Business management Output-centered design Market transactions Profit as resources
Environment	Politics Compulsory interaction Citizens, voters or clients	Market Price-driven transactions Consumers
Organizational form	Bureaus Functions authorized by laws & directives Appointed officials answerable to superiors	Corporations Jobs authorized by contract & property Hired managers accountable to the board of trustees

Sources: Hughes, O. E. 1998. *Public Management and Administration: An Introduction*, 20–88. Houndmills: Palgrave; Gortner, H. F. et al. 1997. *Organization Theory: A Public Perspective*: 16–50. Fort Worth: Harcourt Brace; Rainey, H. G.1991. *Understanding and Managing Public Organizations*: 15–36. San Francisco: Jossey-Bass, 1991; Lindblom, C. E. 1977. *Politics and Market: The World's Political Economic System*: 17–51. New York: Basic Books.

goals which are relatively simple, well defined, and measurable (Carter, Klein, & Day 1992: 5–51).

In endeavors to re-engineer health care, policymakers often adopt ESM and apply market approaches in China. In broad outline, these restructuring endeavors run parallel to NPM and the privatization policy adopted in the West since the early 1980s. The Chinese version of ESM differs from purely transaction-oriented management representing the tenets of NPM. In the context of CPE in China, a significant sector of enterprises is public-owned (i.e. state-owned or collective-owned) and is thus not involved in issues of property rights and corporate governance. By the same token, also public-owned are most providing units (including public hospitals) to which transaction-oriented management can be extended, but not without some limitations. Transaction-oriented management tends to demonstrate its strengths as a public policy tool in the realm of resource management, such as public finance, revenue and funding programs, budgetary reform, compensation schemes, and performance appraisal. And it normally represents an output-centered design for management. To the extent that an output-centered design is able to work effectively, there is much less need for an input-centered design consisting of rules and regulations, direct command and close supervision, extensive hierarchy and centralization, and heavy use of written communication and instructions, just to name a few. As the workload of the supervisory task at the bureau level is simplified and lessened accordingly, managerial autonomy at the providing unit is warranted (Rainey 1991; Carter, Klein & Day 1992; Massey 1993; Gortner, Mahler & Nicholson 1997). As this study intends to show, conversely, diminishing effects are likely to be registered when the output-centered design goes beyond resource management, entering into other types of public policy issues that are non-economic and non-financial concerns. In addition, this study argues that command-oriented (often input-centered) management is applicable more to those policy arenas where goals pertain to the provision of collective goods or quasi-collective goods, often funded by tax revenues. These policy goals are often multiple, less definable and less measurable (Chapters 2, 7 and 8).

By and large, learning from ESM represents an effort to transform a procedurally oriented organization into a result-oriented organization in light of James Wilson's classification scheme for organizations in terms of compliance. That is to say, measurable results/products can be used as tools for performance appraisal in the latter, but with relative difficulty in the former (Wilson 1989: 154–75). By the same token, ESM can be successfully introduced into the health care sector only when the types of service are quantifiable and measurable, most likely in connection with revenue targets and resource management.

Unanticipated policy outcomes

As the study has already tackled the theoretical issues of policymaking, implementation, and day-to-day management, it is germane here to focus on policy outcomes, anticipated or unanticipated, at the final end of a given policy cycle.[4] To implement an affordable care policy in China, unanticipated policy outcomes, including over-provision, issues of pricing and charges, revenue seeking (or maximizing) behavior and other irregularities take place constantly at the providing unit level. From a broad theoretical perspective, the study endeavors to deal with two categories of unanticipated policy outcomes: one treating the public providing unit as a policy enforcing unit at the lowest reach of the Party-state hierarchy, and the other analyzing it as an actor subject to regulatory control in the market transactions. The study argues that medical care personnel, in collaboration with the providing unit, often enjoy upper-hands in a kind of revenue maximizing game often involving in both categories of unanticapted policy outcomes. To begin with, several pioneering scholars have focused on the behavior of knowledgeable and technical competent subordinate in the power game arising from uncertainty in the classic studies on bureaucratic behavior, for example, Gouldner's study of miners (Gouldner 1954), Blau's case of consultants in social services (Blau 1963) and Crozier's case of technical engineers in industrial monopoly (Crozier 1967). These case studies are illuminating with reference to the behavioral pattern of medical doctors who enjoy overwhelming advantage in an asymmetric power game pertaining to the decision-making process in the health care services in China.

Post-Weberian analysis works with the assumption that policy goals are only partly attainable, as policy implementation is partly controllable. Falling in line with post-Weberian analysis, there are four approaches meriting further examination. The first approach is concerned with the basic control cycle within bureaucracy, namely, the cycle from purposive control, unintended outcomes, feedback, and renewed or remedial actions (Crozier, 1964: 175–208; Mouzelis 1967: 59–62; Downs 1968: 144–66). The second pertains to various formulations of bureaucratic pathology and deviant behavior (Lapalombara 1973: 278–309). The third approach, termed uncertainty approach, holds that uncontrollable results are caused by uncertainty embedded in the task environment, coupled with the adaptations made at the decision-making, managerial and institutional level (Thompson 1967; Hall 1980: 32–43; Mintzberg 1983). Last but not least, the fourth is the decision-making approach which is represented by the formulations concerning the issues of unintended consequences and adaptive behaviors regarding the cost of information at the decision-making level. As policymaking process is "satisficing," policy outcomes are sub-optimal in most cases (Perrow 1972: 145–72; Simon 1957).

Among four approaches, the close kinship between the decision-making approach and the uncertainty approach is evident, as both address the cost of information in connection with the emerging behavioral adaptations, managerial designs, and organizational forms. How do they differ from each other in term of emphasis in formulation? The former focues on the actor's behavioral characteristics in facing cost of information. And the latter deals with the behavioral attributes of two actors involved in a set of authority relations in the context of asymmetric information. So far, authors have endeavored to examine the informal relations of the superior to subordinate when the latter is more knowledgeable and better informed than the former—for example, the expansion of subordinate's autonomy (Gouldner 1954; Blau 1963; Crozier 1964).

Both consider, moreover, that unintended consequences are derived from the issue of control rooted in the interaction between the organizational unit and task environment. However, they still work with a premise that policy actors are normally confronted with a fixed structure where policymaking process remains a controllable situation, rather than an open and fluid situation that is ever changing and uncontrollable. In Thompson's view, for instance, policy actors still have hold of "core technology" to protect the organizational integrity from overwhelming contingencies and uncertainties (Thompson 1967: 144–58). Therefore, they do not deal with dynamic and future-oriented issues in the sense that policy actors need to forge consensus on an entirely new set of policies and to create and design new programs without the benefit of policy precedents. Neither Weberian authors nor post-Weberian analysts are theoretically prepared to handle "organized anarchies," where "policy entrepreneurs" need to create something out of nothing, and where no established standard and fixed regulation have ever been in existence to determine, in the first place, what is deviant and undesirable behaviors in implementation (Kingdon 1984: 75–94).

Furthermore, supposed that decisionmakers need to cope with the cost of information, what kinds of remedial measures they would adopt? And how do they proceed to re-invent organization? According to Richard M. Cyert and James G. March, for example, decision-makers tend to engage in four ways of adaptive behavior when wanting to save the cost of information: quasi-resolution of a conflict, uncertainty avoidance, problematic search, and organizational learning (Cyert and March 1963: 116–27). It is assumed that policymakers may choose to develop better organizational designs and managerial measures and to make good use of limited but available information, existing resources, and talents and competence in order to enhance their ability to face uncertainty. For example, James Thompson provides a pertinent analysis of decision-makers' adaptations to uncertainty at the organizational and managerial level through specialization, division of labor, and decentralization (Thompson 1967).

Moving from generic formulations largely rooted in the data base of private firms to policy analysis in a territorial organization, one is confronted with the scenario of multiple policy actors. They represent different departments' concerns, and they hold divergent preferences, varying sets of priorities, and conflicting value premises in order to forge consensus among themselves. The study tries to address the issue of unanticipated policy outcomes, non-compliance, and irregularities that are derived from not only the bureau level but also higher levels mainly because the cases of non-compliance at the providing unit level are often compounded by the dissonance created by interdepartmental tensions on the proper mix of policy goals at the bureau or even higher levels, e.g. municipal, provincial, and ministerial levels. Moreover, a political issue tends to set in whenever regulators themselves are fused with the role of policymakers, or vice versa in the midst of decentralization of power from the central level to provincial/local level during the era of economic reform. As a consequence, divergent policy views are further dictated by vested interests held by various departments at ministerial level and territorial level. In other words, various bureaus are not able to forge a consensus and introduce consistent and effective regulatory controls to deal with the same issue. Not infrequently, regulators encounter conflicts between two established policies (or programs), making it difficult to exercise any form of mandatory power in the first place.

The issue of regulatory control of public hospitals has to do with two dimensions: one pertaining to a vertical dimension involving the exercise of command of supervising bureaus over hospital management together with medical personnel, and the other regarding horizontal dimension concerning two sides in a transaction, for example, between hospital management (often represented by medical doctors) and the patient.

Focusing on the vertical dimension, Post-Weberian analysis deals with the authority relationship of the superior to the subordinate to account for unanticipated policy outcomes, for example, non-compliance of the providing units and medical personnel.

On a horizontal dimension, some theoretical formulations explicitly address the issues of irregularities arising from marketization (e.g., commercialization) at the public hospital level, including, for example, the theory of asymmetric information, the principal-agent theory and rent-seeking theory. First, the theory of asymmetric information, deals with the relations of asymmetric information between the two sides of a given transaction: the doctor and patient, highlighting the former's advantage in choices involving curative care services often inseparable from user charges and pricing (Folland, Goodman & Staton 2004: 187–224). Second, the theory regarding principal-agent relationship, borrowed from the corporate setting, finds illuminating in explaining the doctor's influence not only on curative decisions, but also on actual charges (Folland, Goodman & Staton 2004: 195–6). Third, the rent-seeking theory deals with the issue of franchise: one-sided advantages of choices by the one party in a given area of transactions because of rights of market entry, while the other party's choices are limited because of denial or restriction of the participation in the markets (Tullock 1967; Krueger 1974).

In the Chinese case, one may find that franchising is responsible for aggravating non-compliances of medical personnel and the providing unit. In essence, it is the state that introduces the franchise funding policy, but elements of the said policy are in conflict with the state's low-price policy of medical care services. Through franchising, the providing unit, in collaboration with medical doctors, gains a market share in health care services, making use of user charges to ensure revenue flow to maintain budgetary balance at the providing unit level. Not only does franchising shield doctor's discretion over the purely medical side of curative care services, coupled with drug prescriptions and the use of medical devices, from regulatory control imposed from the above but also protects doctors' say over pricing pertaining to the same discretion from their supervisors outside.

Professor Zhu Hengpeng points to a paradox created by franchising of medical care services including prescription drugs that are associated with regulatory control. On the one hand, it is intended for the providing unit to generating revenue to finance delivery of basic curative care and thus reduce costs for the patient. On the other hand, it inadvertently produces opposite results by charging the patient even more. As he puts it, all regulatory policies, including price control, intended to alleviate the burden of medical expenses, are not likely to succeed unless the government abolishes the monopoly status of public hospitals in curative care services and retail markets in drugs all together. He adds that this monopoly status tends to bring about some undesirable consequences such as over-prescription, abuses of prescription drugs, commercial bribery as well as waste of social resources (Zhu 2011: 64–90). How true is Zhu's observation? This will be further discussed in the remainder of the book.

According to a popular metaphor, in public hospitals in China, doctors are often treated by the government as if they were dogs fed with regular food in fixed amounts in a rigid routine determined by their masters; and yet in theory, doctors ought to be best compensated as if they were free-range chickens: they are their own masters who are choosy when coming to the issue of taste and preference, and always able to find their own ways to feed themselves in free-range environment as such. Therefore, it is not always effective to treat medical personnel as civil servants who are procedurally oriented. While, presumably, the work of civil servants can be better standardized and routinized, leading to reducing the cost of information and minimizing uncertainty, the job of medical personnel often requires considerable discretion facing complexity and the unknown in diagnosis, tests and examination, treatment and drug prescription, all entailing high stakes in terms of health and human life. In fact, the metaphor of feeding free-range chicken raises a big question on what ought to be right policy design, regulatory control, management, and organization pertaining to affordable care programs in China today.

Conclusion

It has been suggested in the foregoing analysis that the state and markets represent alternative policy tools in the allocation of health care resources and provision of health care services. Instead of asking whether the market-oriented approach is most applicable in the public sector categorically, the study proposes to investigate in which functional arena where the market-oriented approach is found effective, for example, revenue targets versus social utility, resource management versus affordable care, and revenue-maximizing and property value. To a considerable extent, the state is found indispensable and in public health care.

Theoretically, the study underscores the differences between the public and non-public sector in examining policymaking, management and policy outcomes. Focusing on policymaking, the study highlights the scenario of multiple policy actors who need to work with several policy goals and face the issue of cost of information. Moreover, it is proposed to draw the distinction between command-oriented management and transaction-oriented management in order to delineate the extent to which the market paradigm applies in the health care sector. While placing an emphasis on organizational behavior in discussion of government process as suggested by Allison and Zelikow, the study has proposed to examine alternative formulations of post-Weberian analysis, in dealing with not only the behavior of the superordinate but also that of the subordinate. To go beyond the analytical concern of sub-optimal policy results and remedial responses, the study suggests to look into the behavior of subordinate who has accumulated substantial discretionary power in case of uncertainty, meaning the unknown and high risks such as the role of medical personnel. In addition, focusing on the issues of non-compliance and regulatory control arising from marketization, medical personnel's discretion is further fortified by the state's franchise funding policy, part of which is found incompatible with the affordable care policy. In subsequent chapters, this study will highlight the challenges to formulating policy, organization and management pertaining to doctors, a thorny issue in the implementation of affordable care policy during China's economic reform.

Notes

1 This study proposes to use transaction rather than "interaction" as a defining feature of the markets. Lindblom's original formulation of "interaction based upon volition" is too broad and too diffuse to be operational. See (Lindblom 1977: 237–60).

2 In conceptual terms, Lindblom takes the two systems as the "preceptoral model" (or Model I) and "strategic model" (or Model II), respectively: the former is characterized as a root (or comprehensive) method, problem diagnosis, theory-guided approach and produces once-for-all answers, while the latter features the branch method (or successively limited comparison), problem-solving, preference and incremental approximation. To lend a descriptive account of the policymaking process, Lindblom adopts a generic approach to decision-making without distinguishing between the state and markets. Nor does he separate normative/prescriptive from descriptive dimension. For example, in Lindblom's Model I (namely a normative, pure rationality model), it is assumed that policy actors have all information and capacity required to make comprehensive and exhaustive review of all options and then choose the right one. That is to say, Model I is too idealistic to differentiate "what ought to be" from "what it is" regarding availability of pertinent information and capacity. And in his formulation of Model II, he too readily and uncritically borrows a "satisficing model" from Simon and James G. March, but he does not address the difference between Models I and II with regard to the cost of information.

3 It is often represented in the Weberian legal-bureaucratic ideal type, Administrative Management, among others (Hughes 1998: 22–51; Gortner et al. 1997:16–50; Downs 1967: 49–74).

4 Some authors, from post-Weberian analysis, take one step forward by treating the decision-making process in term of interaction between a decision maker and task environment with regard to the cycle from decision making, implementation and management, unanticipated policy results and remedial measures, and often a feedback loop connecting the task environment with an organizational unit. This is a reconstruct based upon Anthony Downs' conceptualization of basic control cycle in bureaucracy (Downs 1967: 144–66).

References

Allison, G. T. 1971. *Essence of Decision: Explaining the Cuban Missile Crisis.* Boston: Little, Brown and Company.

Allison, G., & Zelikow, P. 1999. *Essence of Decision: Explaining the Cuban Missile Crisis* (2nd ed.). New York: Longman.

Blau, P., M. 1963. *The Dynamics of Bureaucracy.* Chicago: University of Chicago Press.

Bloom, G., & Gu, X. 1997. Health sector reform: Lessons from China. *Social Science and Medicine,* 45(3): 351–360.

Carter, N., Klein, R., & Day, P. 1992. *How Organizations Measure Success: The Use of Performance Indicators in Government* London: Routledge.

Crozier, M. 1964. *The Bureaucratic Phenomenon.* Chicago: University of Chicago Press.

Cyert, R. M., & March, J. G. 1963. *Behavioral Theory of the Firm.* Englewood, NJ: Prentice-Hall.

Dror, Y. 2013. *Public Policymaking Reexamined.* New Brunswick and London: Transaction Publishers.

Du, L., & Zhang, W. (Ed.). 2009. *Zhongguo yiliao weisheng fazhan baogao, No. 5* (The Report of the Development of Medical and Health Care in China, No. 5). Beijing: Shehui Kexue wenxian chubanshe.

Duckett, J. 2013. *The Chinese State's Retreat from Health.* London and New York: Routledge.

Folland, S., Goodman, A.C., & Stano. 2004. *The Economics of Health and Health Care* (4th ed.). Upperside River, NJ: Pearson Education.

Gortner, H. F., Mahler, J. & Nicholson, J. B. 1997. *Organization Theory: A Public Perspective* (2nd ed.). New York: Harcourt Brace.

Gouldner, A. 1954. *Patterns of Industrial Bureaucracy.* Glencoe, IL: The Free Press.

Gu, X., Bloom, G., & Tang, S. *et al.* 1993. Financing health care in rural China: Preliminary report of a national study *Social Science and Medicine,* 36(4): 385–403.

Ho, L. S. 1995. Market reforms and China's health care system. *Social Science and Medicine,* 41(8): 1065–1072.

Hsiao, W. C. L. 1995. The Chinese health care system: Lessons for other nations. *Social Science and Medicine,* 41(8): 1147–1155.

Huang, Y. 2014. *Governing Health in Contemporary China.* London and New York: Routledge.

Hughes, O. E. 1998. *Public Management and Administration: An Introduction* (2nd ed.). Houndmills: Palgrave.

Krueger, A. 1974. The political economy of the rent seeking society. *The American Economic Review,* 64(3): 291–303.

Lee, P. 1991. The Chinese Industrial State in Historical Perspective: From Totalitarianism to Corporatism. In B. Womack (Ed.), *Contemporary Chinese Politics in Historical Perspective.* Cambridge: Cambridge University Press.

Lieberthal, K. & Oksenberg, M. 1988. *Policy Making in China: Leaders, Structures, and Process* Princeton, NJ: Princeton University Press.

Liu, Y., William C. L., Hsiao, W. C. L., Li Q., *et al.*1995. Transformation of China's rural health care financing. *Social Science and Medicine*, 41(8): 1085–93.

Ma, J., Lu, M., & Quan, H. 2008. From a national, centrally planned health system to a system based on the market: Lessons from China. *Health Affairs*, 27(4): 937–948.

Massey, A. 1993. *Managing the Public Sector: A Comparative Analysis of the United Kingdom and the United States.* Aldershot and Brookfield, VT: Ashgate.

Ng, Y. C. 2008. The productive efficiency of the health sector of China. *The Review of Regional Studies*, 38(3): 381–393.

Pollitt, C. & Bouchaert, G. 2004. *Public Management Reform: A Comparative Analysis* (2 ed.). Oxford, New York: Oxford University Press.

Rainey, H. G. 1991. *Understanding and Managing Public Organizations.* San Francisco: Jossey-Bass.

Simon, H. A. 1957. *Administrative Behavior: A Study of Decision-Making Process in Administrative* New York: The Free Press.

Tam, W. 2010. Privatising health care in China: Problems and reforms. *Journal of Contemporary Asia*, 40(1): 63–81.

Tullock, G. 1967. The welfare costs of tariffs, monopolies and thefts. *Western Economic Journal*, 5 (June): 224–232.

World Bank. 1987. *Financing Health Care: Issues and Options for China.* Washington, DC: World Bank.

Yip, W., & Hsiao, W. C. 2008. The Chinese health system at a crossroads. *Health Affairs*, 27(2): 460–468.

Yip, W., & Mahal, A. 2008. The health care systems of China and India: Performance and future challenges. *Health Affairs*, 27(4): 921–932.

Zhonggongzhongyang & Guowuyuan. 2009. Guanyu shenhua yiyao weisheng tizhi gaige de yijian (The opinion of further reform of medicine and health care system). Retrieved from www.moh.gov.cn//publicfiles/business/htmfiles/mohzcfgs/s7846.

Zhu, H. P. 2010. Guanzhi de neishengxing jiqi houguo: yiyao jiage guanzhi weili (Endogenous causes as well as consequences of regulatory control: The case of price control of medicine). *Tizhi gaige* (System Reform), 10: 64–81.

2 Repackaging health care service and paths to reform

China's health care reform represents a change with considerable magnitude, covering a very broad front and lasting a long period during the economic reform. The change was incremental and path-dependent. It is not a revolution, but a step by step change with limited scope when it is compared with its baseline—the pre-reform construct. The study will start here to examine how sovereign planners deal with two major sets of choice: the choices of the types of health care services to render either by the government or by the markets, and the choices among institutional and managerial means to carry out the reform. In fact, the two sets of issues, regarding what and how, are often intertwined in the re-engineering endeavors of affordable care in last three decades. A brief discussion on the two issues suffices to illuminate the focus, contents and theoretical orientations of the study.

First, the study of health care policy in China, with a focus on affordable medical care, will begin here to address the choices of which types of health care services and entitlements to be made available to the user. And such choices involve re-defining and repackaging of health care services. From the user's point of view, the issue about affordability will not be raised unless the question of availability, e.g., what types health care services and in what quality and quantity, has already been answered. Under the circumstances of economic reform, moreover, the delivery of affordable, often essential, care is not necessarily in contradiction with the provision of a wider variety and upgraded categories of services. They might, in fact, be congruent with each other. Accordingly, questions arise on what a proper mix of health care services is, and how to define affordable care within the mix. In addition, the repackaging of health care services has been associated with the role of the state and markets, as well as the changing balance between the two in the health care sector.

Second, one needs to address the issue of which means are chosen for allocating health care resources in order to answer the question how each type of service is provided. It is evident that marketization carries considerable currency throughout health care reforms in view of plenty of policy proposals and experiments on the subject matter in China. How far can marketization go in tackling the issue of affordable care for all in China? The study argues that sovereign planners were cautious about the adoption of the markets as a policy tool in the realm of public policy at the onset of economic reform. In theoretical terms, can the state perform more effectively than the markets in the provision of various types of health care services? Or vice versa? In organizational and managerial terms, is the state preferable to the markets or a combination of the two in the restructuring of the health care sector? Above all, the state or the markets? Which one is more likely to consolidate in what types of health care services? Let us examine these questions one by one in the remaining passages of the chapter.

Repackaging of health care services

Repackaging of health care services is inseparable from changing health care demands that were dictated by overall policy trends of the transformation from the CPE built during the pre-reform era to the mixed economy starting in 1979. It appears that user charges represent a solution for two different kinds of problem, one concerning revenue aroused first and then the other regarding the quest for health care consumerism that began to assert itself gradually later on. For instance, the government first found it practical and feasible to adopt user charges as a revenue tool to finance various types of health care services, when it was facing financial strains in the midst of a craze for revenue growth and investment fevers among provincial and local jurisdictions in building new industries during the early phase of economic reform. In later phases, user charges to new types of service became an answer to health care consumerism, which was shaped and reinforced by the quest for improvement of living standards and compensation packages among the working population in the early 1990s. With a steady rise of wages and bonuses, meanwhile, the accumulated purchasing power could not be long suppressed, eventually finding expressions in all directions, including the demands for a better and greater variety of health care services.

It is germane to examine classification schemes for policy actors/participants and analysts in order to identify various health care demands for different kinds of user, and to determine the role of the government and markets. And these classification schemes need to make sense to policymakers, enforcing bureaus/ agencies, providers, insurers, and users. For analytical purposes, therefore, the study needs to deal with interpretative schemes that carry subjective meaning of all those interacting with one another in the health care sector.

Overall, this study focuses on medical care services, the scope of which is narrower than that of health care services in the sense that the former deals only with curative care services while the latter embraces all that enhances the health and well-being of people and minimizes and controls illness. Contrary to the optimism of the pro-market analysts, one finds that the markets merely penetrated a part and not the entirety of the health care sector as soon as health care reform began in 1979. While the markets represent a useful managerial tool in the provision of health care services in selected types of non-basic curative care, the government's role is actually essential in other types, such as basic curative care as well as public and preventive health care. It appears that the markets have gained much ground with the rise of new medical care demands and the availability of novel services (e.g., special need and "extravagant" types of curative services) during the last several decades.

Theoretically speaking, policy analysts and policymakers treat health care services as those which promises in part or as a whole, to become "collective goods (or public goods)" on the basis of an assumption that the government plays a significant role in dealing with the externality spilling over from the arena of market transactions between the provider and recipient in terms of costs/benefits analysis; meanwhile, they still hold a view that the markets can also be given a role in the allocation of health care resources and provision of health care services to those patients who enjoy divisible, private services (Downs 1967: 32–3; Savas 1978: 35–57; Hughes 1998: 81–108). To move from theorizing to policymaking, the case of health care reforms in China sheds light on how one can best apply the idea of "collective goods" to health care policy, and how to define the role of the state versus markets from a public policy vantage.

By and large, policy analysts in China have reached a consensual view on the four categories of health care services in the classification scheme of health care services as given in Figure 2.1 (Li 2002; Guan, Dong and Chui 2006; Xia 2006; Ge 2007: 223–9; Wang 2008; Shen, Liang & Yan 2010; Liu 2012: 9–12). For analytical purposes, the classification scheme includes two dimensions: public health care and medical care (or curative care). In general terms, the former deals with enhancing health and preventing illness, while the latter addresses cures for disease and patient recovery. Here public health care is further divided into two categories: Category I, pure-public health care, stands for those services with extensive externality and indivisible costs, while Category II, quasi-public health care, is of limited externality and partially divisible costs.

With reference to policy implications, Category I, the pure-public health care, represents indivisible benefits that are normally shared by multitudes of people, for instances, clean and unpolluted water that prevent spread of germs and effectively control contagious diseases. In managerial and operational terms, it is not feasible to identify who enjoys indivisible benefits, and therefore it is next to impossible for the provider to retrieve the costs. In case of Category I, therefore, the government can play a more effective role than the markets. Category II, quasi-public health care, pertains to the kind of services from which one can theoretically identify individuals who receive it, and thus to attribute to and retrieve costs from it; meanwhile it produces external costs and/or benefits to others to some limited extent. For example, the HIV immunization program that benefits the patient himself/herself while it curtails opportunity of contagion and protect many other residents in the same community.

Medical care services (or curative care services) are targeted at individuals who are sick, producing benefits that are available to individuals who seek a cure only. As given in Figure 2.1, further division of medical care services creates two categories: Category III, basic medical care services, and Category IV, non-basic medical care services. Category III covers barely minimal but essential curative care in order to cure a patient at what would normally be expected to be at relatively low costs, including surgery and hospital services, emergency services, examination and treatment for common and frequent illnesses, and drugs listed in the basic drugs catalog. In terms of managerial and operational feasibility, this is taken as divisible: the user who directly benefits from it can readily be identified, and its costs are therefore attributable and retrievable. From the viewpoint of public policy, however, this is often taken as "merit goods" or "worthy goods," meaning an equivalent to collective goods that produce positive externality in that the maintenance of good health in each individual. Meanwhile, it is considered a benefit to the undifferentiated masses of people, producing positive externality—maintenance of better health and well-being of entire population, supply of needed labor forces, and productivity of the national economy (Savas 1987:52–7; Hughes 1998:97–8). Category IV is often considered as an upgrade of Category III, generating value mostly to the individual patient who can financially afford, for example, "special care" such as appointments with specialists, upgraded wards, serious illness not covered by basic insurance, imported drugs, and special drugs not listed in the basic drug catalog (Ge and Gong 2007: 233–5). In most cases, it goes beyond the essential level that an individual can enjoy. And, it is considered fully marketable, and the users are expected to pay extra for what they get.

Further to the foregoing analysis of the classification of health care, it is worthwhile mentioning that the interpretative scheme of public health care demands has not stayed static, but it has experienced dynamic change in the sense that its scope has broadened, and its contents have enriched, reflecting changing states of the public health care services at various stages of economic development. In an operational sense, the conceptual change of public health care has considerable policy implications in the following several aspects. First, there have been major shifts concerning operational definition

Table 2.1 Classification of benefits and entitlements of health care service in China

Nature of health care \ Types of health care	Public health care	Medical care (Curative care)
Basic (essential)	Category I, Pure-public health care	Category III, Basic medical care
Non-basic	Category II, Quasi-public health care	Category IV, Non-basic medical care

of public health care from the period of the CPE to mixed economy during the reform period. During the CPE period, it was first taken narrowly as the prevention of contagious deceases and improvement of environmental hygiene, while during the economic reform, it embraces a broad scope, including preventive care of both contagious deceases and non-contagious deceases, societal incidents affecting health (such as car accidents and food poisoning), regulatory policy of health care (legislation, monitoring and control), food hygiene and nutrition, environmental pollution, professional illness and labor protection, health care programs for women, infants and youth, protection from radiation, and health care knowledge and education (Ge & Gong 2007: 72). Second, the policy priority of public health care services changed to control of contagious deceases, immunization programs, and five major health care programs (food hygiene, labor health, radiation control, environmental control and youth health). One needs to put some specific policy episodes of public health care in perspective. It is noteworthy, for example, that the emergency mechanisms in public health care which was installed in order to answer a specific incident after SARS event in 2003 only represents one of policy priorities among the broad scope of public health care policy (Ge & Gong 2007: 84–5). Third, from the vantage of implementation and management, public health care is further divided in terms of mass orientation and individual orientation. According to a report filed by the Development Research Center in 2005 (hereafter, 2005 DRC report), purely public health care is mass-oriented type, and quasi-public health care is individual-oriented (Ge & Gong 2007: 230–8; 329–32).

From the perspective of public management and health care economics, the benefits of public health care are treated as "collective goods" as just noted. The separation of quasi-public health care from purely public health took place in the midst of the financial stringency and breakdown of public health care institutes after the Cultural Revolution. Under the circumstance, the government needed to address policy priority with regard not only to funding the existing programs immediately, but also to financing new programs to answer the changing demands in the long term. This appears true also for curative care services to be tackled later.

User charges and revenue retention schemes were parts of a larger policy package, addressing resource management in general and financial stringency in particular. To compensate for the financial shortfall at the providing unit level, the relevant ministerial units inaugurated budgetary reform in 1979, with subsequent amendments in 1985 and 1988, respectively, transforming the total-quota budgetary system into a "budgetary undertaking system" (yusuan baoganzhi; abbreviated as BUS) together with retained revenue schemes (Liu 2008: 5–6). At the end of the day, the inauguration of BUS corresponded with the application of franchise to what is provided under Category II, quasi-public health services, at certain charges/fees, and the creation of new revenue sources through partially paid services.

According to the 1985 Report, for example, user charges were attached to planned immunization, maternity care, and childcare benefits. In addition, the providing units collected user charges (called "cost fees," chengbenfei and/or "services charges," fuwufei) through public hygiene programs, hygiene inspection, physical examinations, and testing and approval of new drugs (Weishengbu, PRC 1992). Emphasis was also placed on the prevention of locally relevant common diseases as first put forth at the 1984 National Conference of Office/Bureau Chiefs and was subsequently incorporated into the 1985 Report (Weishengbu, PRC 1990).

In accordance with a new series of policy papers, some systematic schedules of user charges for preventive care services were formulated and adopted later on (Wu, Ma & Xie 1990). An estimate made in 1990 indicates that around 90 percent of preventive care services units had introduced user charges (Weishengbu, PRC 1990). In an operational sense, all the above changes were based upon the demarcation between Category I and Category II services (Weishengbu 1988). Accompanying user charges with the latter, many preventive care stations adopted the "undertaking responsibility system" (chengbaozhi, abbreviated as URS) to manage revenue retention schemes and to improve remuneration to medical staff (Gao and Wang 1990). Subsequently, in 1992, the State Pricing Bureau and the Ministry of Finance promulgated another set of regulations to make a series of rulings regarding the items and schemes for fee collection at immunization stations throughout the country. And this completed the task of introducing user charges to Category II services in China.

Associated with the budgetary reform, user charges and revenue retention schemes were only piecemeal solutions to problems emerged randomly at the early phase of economic reform. In retrospect, there has remained a conspicuous gap between the claimed importance of public health care and actual performance throughout China's health care reform (Geng and Legge 2009; Li et al. 2002). In the records, for example, China was in 2000 put in a very bad light as it received a near-bottom ranking among 199 membership countries of WHO on the basis of an equality index and funding for public health care.[1]

Basic and non-basic types of medical care services

As the state and markets found their respective roles in the realm of public health care, it is germane to examine how each was able to find entry into the territory of curative care services that were undergoing repackaging process during the economic reform. First of all, it became apparent in the early stage of commercialization that the markets were able to establish a foothold only in selected types of curative care services. Beginning in 1985, curative care had become differentiated into two types, the essential and non-essential types, in conjunction with the commercialization of medical care services. The former is termed "basic medical care," which remains heavily subsidized by the state and public funding/insurance programs like public financed medical care (or PFMC) and labor insurance medical care (or LIMC), and the latter is described as "non-basic medical care" including "special care," upgraded services, whose provision depends mainly on transactions and choices in the market place. Furthermore, as the restructuring of public funding/insurance programs into basic medical care insurance programs picked up momentum in the mid-1990s, the operational definition of essential curative care services assumed importance as attempts were made to broaden insurance coverage to a larger number of residents in each municipal jurisdiction.

In theoretical terms, overall, the state has to assume a heavier financial burden when medical care services are deemed to fall under the basic (i.e., essential) type, while the markets find their place once services are defined as the non-basic type. However, it is a slippery exercise to demarcate a boundary between basic and non-basic types of medical care services, as stakeholders tried to argue on where the boundary ought to be drawn. In order to continue medical care reforms, it became important to install an operational definition of basic medical care services and to curtail public spending as various jurisdictions are confronted with the unintended and undesirable tendency of excessive provision driven by franchise funding, inadequate state subsidy and deficient remunerative designs, excessive use of prescription drugs, excessive dependency upon medical devices, and excessive health care insurance (Liang, Zhu & Zhao 2005: 10). In operational and managerial terms, moreover, the several key actors who were stakeholders in the provision of basic medical care services, and each actor was inclined to work with his or her own version of the operational definition in the fight for a share of revenue, and this was often done with considerable deviation from the medical-technical standards.

As a matter of operational and managerial concerns, each case or disease would have to fall into either the basic or non-basic category, given that different operational definitions of basic medical care entail varying extents of financial liability for different stakeholders. While the former was normally subsidized by public finance, the latter was funded through user charges in market transactions (Xue 2006: 13). According to Xue, the non-basic type of medical care often included expensive options of special care or extravagant services that were covered by out-of-pocket payment (hereafter, OPP) (Xue 2006:13).

In practice, public hospitals are given a franchise to provide an undefined mix of services of medical care, including both basic and non-basic types, to patients, and, given slippery of operational definition, it is often optional to treat a given case either as basic or non-basic type. According to Wang Bingyi, the health care providers, especially public hospitals, are entrusted with an undifferentiated mix of jobs, embracing not only private goods but also public services. And it has never been clearly defined which kinds of jobs are to be provided through the markets and which by the government through public means. When coming to the public hospitals' responsibility for providing affordable care, Wang points out that the root of the issue has to do with the lack of a clear conception on the boundary between different types of services (Wang 2008: 299).

Because of medical/professional strengths, meanwhile, medical doctors are in a position to have a say on whether a medical care case ought to fall into the basic or non-basic types of curative services, entailing considerable difficulties of spending control as basic medical care can easily be treated as non-basic category. In order to fulfill revenue targets, it is in hospital management's advantage to increase non-basic medical care services proportionally and fetch a bigger income from user charges. In Liang et al.'s view, there was considerable blurring of the boundary between basic and non-basic medical care services, titling towards over-stretching the definition of the latter, which was often driven by financial concerns (Liang, Zhu & Zhao 2005: 9). First, some patients themselves might take advantage of a loose operational definition of basic type in laying claim for an expanded government subsidy for some better but expensive services (e.g., treatment, prescription drugs, and advanced medical devices) which were often beyond their means, but often were absorbed willingly by the insurer, a third-party payer. Second, medical personnel tended to yield to the pressure for excessive medical care demands from patients and insurers, even for those services that were under tight price control. And third, the providing unit and medical personnel who were driven by revenue maximizing motives were inclined to narrow financial shortfalls and opted for over-provision (Liang, Zhu & Zhang 2005).

The study argues that medical personnel, in collaboration with hospital management and often with the drug industry, were able to gain considerable discretionary room to choose options for diagnosis, tests, medical devices, and drugs at the higher end of the price range in light of the unknown area of modern medicine, namely, the personal nature of illness, the great variety of illnesses, and the multiple alternatives for diagnosis and treatment (Chapter 1, 8 & 9). As it turned out, implementing an operational definition of basic medical care services often came down to a case-by-case exercise, due to substantial difficulties where policy lacks clarity and accuracy, concreteness, and uniformity (Liang, Zhu & Zhao 2005: 9). Besides, the outsider's (e.g., government's) monitoring and supervision often encountered limitation in view of asymmetry of information. Nor was it easy to establish a standard curative procedure in order to control provision, since medical care practices could not be fully standardized and routinized. This meant that with discretion, medical personnel tended to recommend/induce patients to move from basic to non-basic type of medical care, entailing higher payments for treatment, medical devices, and drugs.

Taken together, the basic and non-basic types of medical care services can be treated as a variety of demands at different levels, but they often overlap. Thus, in operational and managerial terms, it remains a challenge to separate basic from non-basic medical demands. In a general sense, basic medical care services ought to satisfy the essential demands of medical care for common and frequently seen illnesses, meaning low tiers in the hierarchy of needs at lower costs. From the perspective of public policy, Xue finds a great complexity involving several criteria relevant to drawing the boundary between

basic and non-basic medical care services.[2] For the sake of policy implementation, various policy analysts tended to be more selective by recom-
mending a shorter list of criteria for basic curative care. According to Xue,
for instance, the definition for a basic type of medical care services needed
to meet the following requirements: the medical-technical standards as
suitable as possible, the curative procedure as simple and convenient as
possible, the kinds of curative services as inexpensive as possible, and the
results as reliable as possible (Xue 2006: 13). In a different version, Liang
et al. argued that the basic type of medical care services had to meet three
requirements: medical-technical rationality, necessity of curative care, and
economic acceptability to the patient.[3]

Regardless of various attempts, policymakers had yet to settle on an
operational definition of basic curative care services and to contain the pressure of increasing costs in the midst of reform. For the purpose of cost containment, accordingly, the relevant authorities resort to certain administrative
approaches in conjunction with health care reform at different stages. First,
they applied the mechanisms of "basic list/catalog of prescription drugs,"
"basic list/catalog of diagnoses," and "basic rules/procedures of treatment,"
often in connection with introducing basic medical care insurance across jurisdictions (Hu 2007). The second approach concerned defining basic medical
care services through the list/catalog of common and frequently seen diseases,
coupled with re-establishing a referral system with the hospitals of higher tiers
(Jin, Yao & Chen 2007). Third, the operational definition of basic medical
care services pertained to the kind of curative services rendered at the basic
level, e.g., urban community health care centers and health care institutes at
the village/town level being linked to hospitals at higher tiers through a
referral system (Chen 2007; Jin, Yao & Chen 2007; Yao 2008). Fourth, the
implementation of basic curative care services was accompanied by a variety
of funding arrangements, for instance, Basic Medical Care Insurance (BMCI)
for staff and workers in cities and towns, Urban Resident Medical Care
Insurance(URMCI) in cities and towns, and the New Rural Cooperative
Medical Care Insurance (or NRCMCI) (Du 2007). In parallel fashion, non-
basic care services were funded by supplementary insurance programs, such
as supplementary medical care subsidy schemes for civil servants, major illness subsidy schemes, and mutual medical care funds. Once the kinds of
medical care services are taken as non-basic, the markets quickly take them
over, and users had to foot the bills. This entails a shifting balance between
the markets and the state, which emerged as a constant theme throughout
health care reforms—an issue to be discussed further (Chapter 4).

Alternative paths to health care reform

In examining alternative paths to health care reform which have emerged
since 1979, one may identify a variety of modes of coordinating, organizing,
managing, and funding that have been explored and experimented with. And

these modes can be taken as either market-oriented or non-market-oriented or a combination of both. In a broad sense, the journey of the health care reform has followed four developmental paths, including purely administrative reorganization, property rights-centered reforms, commercialization of services, and full-fledged marketization reform. With their diversity and complexity, curative care services, either basic or non-basic, have been in the limelight, being most controversial throughout the health care reform for more than three decades.

From a theoretical perspective, there has been considerable debate over the issue of "marketization" (shichanghua) and "commercialization" (shanyehua) of the health care sector among policy analysts and policymakers in China. Commercialization refers to expanding transactions for health care services often measured in terms of volume of user charges and/or revenue from market transactions. As a concept, "marketization" pertains to the full extent of economic exchanges of health care resources broadly embracing property rights, organized services, equipment and devices, fixed assets, and so forth. Commercialization is narrower than marketization, for the former is concerned with transactions of services and products but does not normally include considerations of fixed assets and other property rights.[4] By and large, non-transactional activities such as "managed competition," "contractualism" (e.g., undertakings by subordinates for some sort of superordinate entity), and "clientelism" (e.g., service orientation toward clients) that often involve the exercise of power are not treated as market activities.

To sharpen operational definition of market, this study suggests that a requisite for market activities is an irreducible ingredient of economic exchange of equal values, namely, quid pro quo transactions. The non-market realm might include command-centered activities of the modern state, voluntary activities relying upon charity, welfare, and reciprocity among others. According to Lindblom, non-command-centered form of coordination is taken as "interaction" which is actually broader than market activities, and, in this study, therefore, ought not to be taken as market activities as such (Lindblom 1977: 247–60).

By design, market behavior features the pursuit of a narrow set of goals, such as revenue/profit targets, which are definable, measurable, and amenable to performance appraisal. Property rights lay a solid institutional ground in order to enhance the value of assets, often derived and accumulated from profits. By budgetary and accounting rules, revenue/profit-oriented endeavors tend to externalize costs and thus ensure its maximization. The study argues that theoretically speaking, the markets, as a public policy tool, are most effective for the purpose of resource management, but its utility tends to become diminished once it moves to deal with multiple and less measurable policy goals.

It has become apparent that in health care reforms, commercialization is closely associated with the revenue-generating activities relating to providing health care services, a main part of which pertains to curative care services. With reference to curative care services, one may find several groupings relevant as objects of transactions: (1) the essential core of the diagnosis, examination, and treatment; (2) hospital care, nursing, and therapy by medical personnel; (3) the use of medical devices in laboratory tests, treatments, and examinations for diagnosis and treatment; (4) prescription and dispensing of drugs; (5) medical materials, utilities, and facilities; and (6) logistic and administrative services. In fact, these groupings are often overlapping and difficult to separate from one another. For instance, the input and services of doctors, nurses, and technicians (e.g., medical skill, judgment, and knowledge) are medically inseparable from the drug prescriptions, use of medical devices, hospital care, and logistic and administrative services.[5]

To study the developmental paths from the command-centered mode of coordination to market-centered mode, it is proposed here to adopt a classification scheme that is based upon two analytical dimensions: de-regulation and property rights restructuring as given in Figure 2.1. The former refers to the mode of coordination where not only is entry into transactions of certain types of services allowed, but also all other legal restrictions are lifted. For instance, it is often taken as "commercialization" when providing units are given space in the markets for the provision of curative care services.[6] The latter pertains to a property-rights-centered dimension, namely a change normally converting all health care resources into property rights and thus potentially making them objects of market transactions. Examples include denationalization of ownership, corporatization, asset privatization, divestiture, etc. It entails development from bureaucratic governance to corporate governance, promising full autonomy to the providing unit in decisions over assets and facilities, services and products, medical device sales and marketing, finance, and personnel in the market context. As a result, sovereign planners stand as equal to, but not above

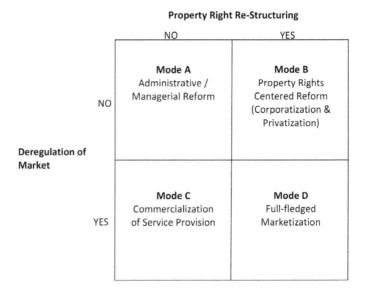

Figure 2.1 Paths to the reform: De-regulation of market and property rights restructuring

other actors in the market places in accordance with civic code (Ma & Wu 2006; Miao 2005). The scheme produces four types which will be briefly treated here. Furthermore, Mode A, Administrative/managerial reform, will be extensively examined in Chapters 3, 4, 5 and 6, and Mode C, commercialization of services, will be further elaborated because of the relatively large scale of implementation during the era of economic reform (See Chapters 7, 8, 9 and 10).

To begin with, the administrative mode, Mode A, represents one type of ongoing non-market-oriented reform focusing on restructuring within the conventional bureaucratic framework in the context of CPE. Examples include both the conventional type of rectification, "reorganization" (chongzu) and novel designs of public management reform (to be elaborated in Chapter 3). Rectification represents an effort of streamlining in order to put the work unit back to operational and effective shape. Reorganization pertains to optimizing deployment and allocation of health care resources through institutional rebuilding and adjustments in order to make better of use of health care resources, especially clinics and hospitals, the workload of which is insufficient and where beds, equipment, and facilities lie idle (Liang 1988; Li 1989; Xia 1990). Such kinds of restructuring often cut across jurisdictions and echelons of administrative hierarchy, sectors of the economy, and/or ownership systems; for instance, in the case of "jointly managed health care institutes," the jurisdictional line between state-owned health care units and collective-owned units is crossed. And through "horizontal combination" (hengxian lianghe), for instance, providing units make collaborative arrangements with industrial and mining enterprises and/or military establishments to make health care services and facilities available to local residents (Luo 1990).

Moreover, new designs of public management address the issues of the multiplicity of supervising bureaus, the separation of managerial tasks of production and provision from policymaking and regulatory functions, and the establishment of new executive agencies to handle separately asset management, supervisory work, and other routine managerial jobs in the public sector (Hou 2001; Ma 2005; Ma 2006a; Ma 2006b; Ma 2006c; Ma 2006d; Ma 2006e). Since 2005, priority has been given to three tasks. The first pertains to the constructing of community service networks in both urban districts and rural counties and townships coupled with a rebuilt referral system connected with public hospitals, promising to alleviate the workload of large, over-crowded modern hospitals (Du 2007; Chen 2008; Wang 2008). In the name of optimizing use of health care resources, the second task aims to reorganize and transfer to local jurisdictions those providing units managed by SOEs, commercial enterprises, transportation systems, and the military (Chen 2008; Wang 2008). The third task, since the early 2000s, has concentrated on a major restructuring effort in building the network of contractual or quasi-contractual arrangements between executive agencies of insurance and designated hospitals and pharmacies in most of county jurisdictions and in a small number of municipal jurisdictions (Laodong he shehui baozhangju & Guojia Yaopin Jiandu Guanliju 2003). (See Chapters 3 and 5).

Theoretically speaking, Mode B represents a pattern of property-rights-centered restructuring including denationalization, corporatization and asset privatization, promising to optimize use of assets and enhance the property value of the providing unit as a whole (Yang 1994). In China, the progress of property-rights-centered reform in the health care sector has been dictated by the overall pace of building a modern property rights system in the public sector, which started in the late 1980s.[7] Generally speaking, the property-rights-centered reform requires two steps to complete: the first step, to initiate the transformation from bureaucratic governance to corporate governance and to delink from the state bureaucracy in both financial and personnel management (Chen 2008). By doing so, it is better equipped to mobilize financial resources for investment projects from multiple sources. For instance, it can encourage more investments by non-public entities to enter into infrastructure, public utilities, industries, and other sectors. And the second, to make it possible to move in the direction of divestiture and other forms of asset privatization through the dilution and sale of publicly owned stocks and shares, as was the case when Britain privatized its public owned assets.[8]

Sovereign planners put the first step of the property-rights-centered reform as an important item on policy agenda of new health care reform that started in 2009, proposing to carry out policy experiments in various jurisdictions (Guowuyuan 2009). The first step of the property-rights-centered reform is likely to present potential advantages in restructuring the health care system in the following ways: first, the organizational status of the providing unit shifts from "service work unit" to that of a corporate unit. Accordingly, providing units can shed their status as appendices to the Party-state entity and acquire legal autonomy, becoming fully accountable for their own decisions on the value of the property in the market place.[9] Second, the providing unit operates in accordance with corporate laws rather than administrative laws, lending the providing unit an option to establish a set of legal mechanisms, and to work efficiently through market transactions rather than coordinate through the costly exercise of administrative command. Meanwhile, both the budgetary system and personnel management are to be separated from the state bureaucracy. Third, as the transformation from administrative governance to corporate governance takes place, the bureau's command yields to decisions by a board of directors. It would facilitate corporatization, shedding the heavy workload of handling both policymaking and micro-management of publicly owned hospitals at the same time, as well as reducing the high administrative costs, complexity, and political liability (Shao 2006; Du 2007a; Du 2007b; Du 2007c; Chen 2008).

Toward full-fledged marketization mode

The fully fledged marketization mode, Mode D, involves both property-rights-centered restructuring and commercialization of service-delivery. Such a development covers two time periods in China. The first period lasted from the 1950s to 2000 with the tendency toward Mode D remaining at an embryonic stage as further development was interrupted by policy excesses during the Great Leap Forward and the Cultural Revolution. When the economy returned to normal after 1979, policymakers allowed some market space to licensed private practitioners in view of their "supplementary role" to publicly owned providing units.[10] In better articulated fashion, the 1985 Report and 1988 Opinion continued to affirm the policy of licensed private practices (Weishengbu 1992). Introducing a new form of governance over the private sector, various ministerial units assumed a regulatory role by applying mainly economic and legal levers, such as issuing provisional measures of management in 1988, promulgating standards for charges in 1992, and introducing an income tax for licensed practitioners in 1997 (Qu & Meng 2004).

As a landmark in history of health care policy, the second period began in February 2000, when fully fledged property rights restructuring accompanying the commercialization of medical care services were formally proposed in a policy paper known as the 2000 Advisory Opinion.[11] Going far beyond the policy of licensed private practices of previous decades, the 2000 Advisory Opinion foretold the rise of privately owned and managed large-scale modern hospitals and medical care service conglomerates. At the providing unit level, sovereign planners proposed a new "classification management" by establishing two new categories of health care providing units, namely, non-profit-oriented and profit-oriented categories, taking into consideration the nature, social function, and mission of the health care providing unit. At the bureau level and above, sovereign planners intended to curtail direct state intervention in the midst of an expanding market economy (Guowuyuan tigaiban et al. 2001).

When installing a new system to govern profit-oriented providing units, it is reasonable and feasible for government to retreat to macro-management when publicly owned, non-profit-oriented units adopt corporate governance (e.g., Mode B). In theoretical terms, this entails a restructuring of the bureaucratic governance under CPE by addressing such issues as the multiplicity of bureaus over the work unit (either the production unit or the service unit). To minimize procedural complexity and reduce administrative costs, some analysts recommend an organizational alternative, which is to designate one sole bureau to be in direct charge of the publicly owned providing unit.

Through the implementation of the 2000 Advisory Opinion, the establishment of the said two categories of hospitals was intended to introduce "mechanisms of competition," including competition among providing units, and between public and non-public hospitals.[12] Deputy Minister of Health Wang elaborated this point further: the health care managerial system that evolved under CPE lacks competition and vitality, and therefore it is not adaptable to a market economy system. In Wang's view, it was necessary to apply mechanisms of competition in order to drive price levels downward and to improve quality of service to the public (Wang 2002). According to State Councilor Li, the creation of two categories of providing units meant breaking the monopoly of publicly owned hospitals and subjecting them to the pressure of competition from non-public hospitals (Li 2001).

Taking the developmental direction toward Mode D, profit-oriented medical units would neither enjoy government subsidies, nor would they be able to claim tax exemption. Yet, they can possess extensive managerial autonomy and full pricing power, coupled with minimal government interference. The development toward Mode D leads to a process of institutionalization by curtailing direct administrative intervention to the providing unit level while installing an entirely new set of macro-managerial and indirect control mechanisms for market transactions. The 2000 Advisory Opinion urges ministries and bureaus concerned to establish a "market entry" system (zhunru zhidu) and to control entry into the market at three points: the medical care providing units, practitioners, and various types of medical devices. First, accompanying registration exercises under classification management, profit-oriented providing units were to be licensed in accordance with the Rules of Management of Medical Care Institutes. Second, the Ministry of Health Care instituted its own procedure to issue a Certificate of Eligibility of Medical Doctors and the Certificate of Practice of Medical Doctors beginning in 2001. Third, control and managerial measures were extended to new clinical technology, new medical services, and the use of key technologies (Wang 2002; Guowuyuan Tigaiban et al., 2001).

Through the 2000 Advisory Opinion, the classification of the two categories of providing unit was established within a short time span of two years. As a further step toward Mode D, profit-oriented providing units became further legitimized in a new policy perspective recognizing variegated and multi-tiered health care needs, diverse financial sources, as well as the advantages of mechanisms of competition among all providing units, and between profit-oriented and non-profit-oriented sectors.

Mode D has been gaining currency as the 2000 Advisory Opinion was put into implementation across provincial and municipal jurisdictions, coupled with a series of supplementary measures, rules and regulations since 2000 (Qu & Meng 2004). It has grown numerically and has consolidated functionally in some areas of expertise as well as in special needs services as noted. By the end of 2003, of the total number of medical care institutes registered, non-profit-oriented units and profit-oriented units consisted of 48.35 percent and 51.65 percent respectively. However, profit-oriented units remained marginal, consisting of 8.04 percent of medical personnel from a total of 493,400 and 3.21 percent of beds from a total of 314,400 (Zhang & Sun 2006). For illustration, Jiangsu Province had a modest beginning for property-rights-centered reform among public-providing units: out of 264 units, 22 units adopting the full-fledged corporate system, 239 working with the corporate-cooperative system, two working with joint ownership with foreign investors, and one falling into the category of joint ownership with investors from Hong Kong and Taiwan. And in the case of Jiangsu Province, it is estimated that public-providing units amounted to 57.46 percent while non-public units to 42.34 percent (Liu 2006).

Most profit-oriented providing units are taken as so-called "privately managed institutes" (minying yiliao jigou), while the remaining are "publicly managed" (likely non-profit-oriented) (Qu & Meng 2004). For the moment, privately managed institutes consist of only 3 percent of the medical care market, about slightly less than one half (or 48 percent) of which are clinics (Qu & Meng 2004). Overall, privately managed units are small-scale and specialty-oriented, and in term of geographical distribution, they tend to concentrate in coastal cities and provinces. After gaining recognition in the early 2000s, nonetheless, privately managed providing units encountered considerable pressure in terms of taxation burden, enlisting as insurance-designated units, problems with recruitment of medical personnel, and other tight and rigid policy measures in various jurisdictions, on top of the risks and competition in the market place (Zhang & Sun 2006; Shao 2006; Shao 2008). However, due to their organizational design, privately managed providing units enjoy advantages which tie the interest of investors to the appreciation in the value of their assets. They have emerged as a potentially attractive sector for interested investors both inside and outside China.

Last, but not least, Mode C refers to the commercialization of goods and services, representing the case of de-regulation, without property-rights-centered restructuring in most cases (Miao 2005). Mode C commercialization represents the predominant form of market-oriented health care reform in China, in which public hospitals are allowed to make use of franchising as a revenue tool in market transactions for medical care services (including drugs and devices) although the allocation of other health care resources remains largely within the realm of administrative command (Lin 2005: Miao 2005). "Deregulation" here pertains to the relaxation of restrictions over the entry of goods and services into market transactions (e.g., pricing, types of commodities and services, technology and equipment, and liquid capital and investment). Often found in CPE, a franchise is built upon a set of rights of market entry that specifies the qualifications of agents, types and pricing of goods and services, and rules and procedures governing access to the market. Some observers characterize this as "industrialization of medical care" (yiliao chanyehua), imitating the reform of state-owned enterprises (Ma & Wu 2006).

Concluding remarks

The foregoing analysis has been considering the question what the state can do better than the markets and vice versa in the health care policy. While the study reaffirms the merits of the state in health care, it endeavors to chart the farthest frontier in health care sector which the markets can reach. First for funding considerations and then for satisfying the rise of medical consumerism, all in all, the study finds that through the repackaging of health care services, the reform has created four categories: Category I, purely public health services; Category II, quasi-public health services; Category III, basic medical care services; and Category IV, non-basic medical care services. As one notes that the market approach of management has expanded its territory in the case of Category II and IV which are funded more and more by user charges, so one finds that the role of government has been strengthened in Category I and III, which still rely heavily on public finance. Sovereign planners make repeated attempts to consolidate the government's role in Category I, pure-public health care and Category III, basic medical care.

It appears in the foregoing discussion, moreover, that China's health care reform has taken place on a very broad front, including all four modes of restructuring in the realm of organization and management. In fact, all four modes represent alternative developmental paths, and each has profound policy implications regarding not only the allocation of health care resources, but also the delivery of affordable care to people throughout China. In order to provide affordable care, sovereign planners intend to stay with the public hospital system and to follow Mode C commercialization, featuring user charges and franchise funding for the time being. This represents one step forward toward marketization, but only half way through, still remaining within the institutional framework and managerial style under legacy of the CPE (Gu 2000; Guowuyuan Tigaiban et al. 2001).

As being put on policy agenda since 2009, the policy experiments concerning Mode B property-rights-centered reform is indicative of policy-makers' concern of the insensitivity of appreciation of asset value of public hospitals. Through both, the policymakers are given options to move away from the CPE.

Notes

1 As often cited in WHO statistics from the year 2000, China is ranked 188th out of a membership of 191 countries with regard to an equality index, meaning that the low-income family tends to shoulder a heavier financial burden than a high-income family (Du and Ding 2008: 56). In WHO's assessment, China is ranked 132nd with reference to the overall improvement of heath care; overall efficiency of China's health care system is ranked 144th (Ge and Gong 2007: 54–6).

2 Examples include a kind of entitlement for the citizen, i.e., a constitutional right and cornerstone of a "harmonious society"; a minimal but essential provision of medical care services in light of optimal use of health care resources; the essential category of medical care service delineated and established in accordance with the standards and assessments of cost-benefit analysis and medical/technical research; a culturally acceptable level of health for the maintenance of normal life and work; and standards of health care compatible with the given stage of economic-social development. See (Xue 2006: 12).

3 Accordingly Liang Hong et al. put forth a policy definition for basic medical care services: "Given a certain level of social-economic development, medical-technical standards, and characteristics of the population, the type [of basic medical care services] which is intended to provide for the whole population has to fulfill the

requirements of medical-technical rationality, economic acceptability of the user, and necessity of curative services" (Liang, Zhu & Zhao 2005: 8–9).

4 In common usage, "markets" is more than a place and is actually taken as activities/behaviors surrounding transactions. According to Yuan et al., "markets" is defined originally as the place where the transactions of commodities occur. See (Yuan, Chang & Chang 1995: 7).

5 To go beyond the provision of services, however, one finds that property rights including equipment and devices, building and facilities, and R&D and patents, which can command monetary value, become objects of marketization but not necessarily commercialization.

6 The term "commercialization" (shangyehua) highlights the kind of transactions involving commodities produced and services rendered solely for the value of exchange, for example, in the case of "special care services" (texu fuwu) in reform China.

7 For instance, the first property transactions market of public enterprises was not established on an experimental basis in Wuhan until 1988. The State Council did not put forth the Provisional Measure of Enterprise Property Rights Management until 1994. The state asset management bureaus were not established at the ministerial and municipal levels until 2002. As a conservative projection, China had not taken the first step in asset privatization in the industrial sector until November 2003 when the construction of a modern property rights system was formally put on the policy agenda for the first time in the 3rd Plenum of the 16th Party Congress. For the purpose of implementation, the State Council, the State Asset Committee, and the Ministry of Finance jointly promulgated the Provisional Measures of Transactions of State Assets among Enterprises on December 30, 2003. See (Sun & Du 2006; Ma & Wu 2006).

8 Thatcher's government was able to privatize these public corporations through sales of shares and stocks for about one decade from 1979 to 1990. See (Gormley 1991; Massey 1993; Savas 1987; Starr 1989).

9 According to Ma and Wu, the property-rights-centered reform will lead to a real separation of health care institutes from the bondage and protection of the government and to their becoming genuine entities in the marketplace. See (Ma & Wu 2006).

10 For example, the Ministry of Health issued the Circular Regarding the Report on the Issues of Permission of Medical Care Practice by Individuals on September 2, 1980 (hereafter, the 1980 Circular) with regard to licensed private medical care practices, granting licenses to unemployed doctors, maternity nurses, nurse assistants, dental technicians, and retired doctors, some of whom had been licensed prior to the reform era. See (Weishengbu 1992).

11 The full title of the policy paper reads as follows: The Advisory Opinion on Institutional Reform of Medical and Health Care in Cities and Towns. It was first circulated by eight ministerial units led by the Institutional Reform Commission of the State Council in February 2000 (Guowuyuan Tigaiban et al., 2001).

12 For the details of implementation, see the Opinion on Implementation of Management by Classification of Various Categories of Medical Care Institutes in Cities and Towns (abbreviated as the 2000 Opinion). See (Weishengbu, Guojiazhongyiyaoguanliju, Caizhengbu, & Guojiajiwei 2000)

References

Bo, X. 1996. Gufenzhi banyi—xiangzheng weisheng yuan ziwo fazhan de chenggong xuanze (The system of stocks and shares in running hospitals—a successful option of self-propelling development of health care institute in township and town). *Gaige neican* (Internal Reference for Reform), 2: 32–34.

Cai, J. 2007. Shehui shichang hezuo moshi: Zhongguo yiliao weisheng tizhi gaige de xinsilu (Cooperative model of socialist market: New ideas of health care reform in China). *Shehui baozhang zhidu* (Social Security System), 8: 27–33.

Cai, R., & Li, W. 1999. Zhongguo yiliao jigou changquan zhidu gaige xianchuang jiqi fazhan qushi (The current reform situation of property system as well as its developmental tendency in china's medical care institutes). *Shehui baozhang caiwu guanli* (Financial Management of Social Insurance), 3: 14–17.

Chen, C., & Zhou, J. 2009. Woguo caizheng gonggong weisheng zhichu zhengfujian fudang fenxi (An analysis of the structure of burdens among governments in the expenditure of public health care in China's public finance). *Zhongguo weisheng jingji* (China's Health Care Economics), 28(8): 15–17.

Chen, S. 2007. Xinshiqi woguo xiangzhen weishengyuan de fazhan yu biange (The development and change of health care institutes of administrative village and towns in China). In L. Du, W. Zhang & Zhongguo Weisheng Chanye Zazhishe (Eds.), *Zhongguo yiliao weisheng fazhan baogao, No. 3* (The Report of Development of Medical and Health Care in China, no 3), 241–262. Beijing: Shehui kexue wenxian chubanshe.

Chen, S. 2008. Woguo gongli yiyuan ruhe yingjie xin de yigai (How to face the new medical care reform in China). In L. Du (Ed.), *Zhongguo yiliao weisheng fazhan baogao No. 4* (The Report of the Development of Medical and Health Care in China No. 4), 197–266. Beijing: Shehui kexue wenxian chubanshe.

Downs, A. 1967. *Inside Bureaucracy*. Boston: Little, Brown and Company.

Du, L. 2005. Yilia feiyong biaosheng de linglei guandian (A different view on the soaring expenditure of meidcal care). *Zhongguo Weisheng* (China's Health Care), 7: 29–31.

Du, L. 2007a. Hongguan jingji he weisheng fazhan de liangxing xunhuan ho exing xunhuan—ershihnian weisheng zhengce yanjiu huigu (Positive and vicious cycles of macro economy and health care development). In L. Du, W. Zhang, & Zhongguo Weisheng Chanye Zazhishe (Eds.), *Zhongguo wesheng yiliao fazhan baogao, No. 3* (The Report of Health Care Development in China, No. 3): 25–40. Beijing: Shehui kexue wenxian chubanshe.

Du, L. 2007b. Jianli jiben weisheng baojianzhidu, goujian duoyuan banyi xingeju (To establish basic health care system, to construct new framework for a diversified health care management). In L. Du, W. Zhang, & Zhongguo Weisheng Chanye Zazhishe (Eds.), *Zhongguo yiliao weisheng fazhan baogao, No. 3* (The Report of Development of Medical and Health Care, No. 3), 296–307. Beijing: Shehui kexue wenxian chubanshe.

Du, L. 2007c. Zhongguo yiliao jigou chanquan gongsi hezuo moshi he fazhan qianjin zhanwa (The model of public-private partnership through property rights in medical care institutes as well as its prospect for development). In L. Du, W. Zhang, & Zhongguo Weisheng Chanye Zazhishe (Ed.), *Zhongguo yiliao weisheng fazhan baogao, No. 3* (The Report of Development of Medical and Health Care, No. 3), 194–211. Beijing: Shehui kexue wenxian chubanshe.

Du, L. & Ding, Z. 2008. Zhongguo tese jiben weisheng fuwu de linian, zhengce he shijian (The ideal, policy and practice of basic health care services with Chinese characteristics). In L. Du, W. Zhang, & Zhongguo Weisheng Chanye Zazhishe (Eds.), *Zhongguo yiliao weisheng fazhan baogao, No. 3* (The Report of Development of Medical and Health Care, No. 3), 53–71. Beijing: Shehui kexue wenxian chubanshe.

Ferlie, E., Ashburner, L., Fitzgerald, L., & Pettigrew, A. 1997. *The New Public Management in Action*. Oxford and New York: Oxford University Press.

Fu, X. 1993. Yiyuan zhuanhuan jingying jizhi de youyi changshi (A fruitful attempt in the transformation of managerial mechanisms in hospitals). *Zhongguo weisheng jingji(China's Health Care Economics)* 4: 19–21.

Fu, X. 1995. Shenhua weisheng gaige de jidian silu (Some considerations on further reform in health care). *Zhongguo weisheng jingji* (China's Health Care Economics), 5: 5–6.

Gan, B., Duan, L., & Hou J., et al. 1999. Yiyuan zhijishi shixing gufenzhi gaizao de shexiang (Considerations on the introduction of stock sharing system to the pharmacy office in hospitals). *Zhongguo weisheng jingji* (China's Health Care Economics), 3: 133–136.

Gao, S., & Wang, M. 1990. Fangyizhan shixing chenbbaozhi de tantao (Discussion on the implementation of chengbao system in the immunization station). *Zhongguo weisheng jingji* (China's Health Care Economics), 7: 39–40.

Ge, Y., & Gong, S. 2007. *Zhongguo yiliao gaige: Wenti, genyuan, chulu* (China's Health Care Reform: Problems, Roots and Solutions). Beijing: Zhongguo fazhen chubanshe.

Geng, Y., Pei, L., & Legge, D. 2009. Zengjia zhengfu touru tigao yiyao weisheng fuwu de gongpingxing he kejixing (Improve equality and accessibility of healh care services through the increase of governmental input). *Zhongguo weisheng jingji* (China's Health Care Economics), 28(3): 12–18.

Gormley, W. T. J. 1991. The privatization controversy. In W. T. J. Gormley (Ed.), *Privatization and its Alternatives*: 3–16. Madison, Wisconsin and London: The University of Wisconsin Press.

Gu, W. 2000. Yiliao jigou gaige yunliang xinyilun tupo (A new round of breakthroughs fomented in the hospital organizational reform). *Liaowan* (Lookout), (March 13): 53–54.

Guan, Z., Dong, C., and Chui, S., 2006. Zhongguo yiliao weisheng tiaozhan yu chulu (China's medical and health care: Challenges and solutions). *Zhongguo weisheng jingji* (China's Health Care Economics), 10: 5–9.

Guowuyuan 2009. Yiliao weisheng tizhi gaige jinqi zhongdian shishi fangan 2009–2010 (The plan of implementation priority for medical and health care reform for the near future). In L. Du, W. Zhang, & Zhongguo Weisheng Chanye Zazhishe (Eds.), *Zhongguo yiliao weisheng fazhan baogao No. 5*. (The Report of Development of Medical and Health Care in China No 5. 2009) Beijing: Shehui kexue wenxian chubanshe.

Guowuyuan Tigaiban et al. 2001. Guanyu chengzheng yiyao weisheng tizhi gaige de zhito yijian (The advisory opinion concerning the institutional reform of medical care and pharmacy in cities and towns). In Weishengbu Fazhi Yu Jiandusi Ed., 15–19. Beijing: Beijing falu chubanshe.

Heilongjiang Sheng Weishengting Zhengcefaguichu. 1994. Heilongjiang sheng weisheng gaige zongshu (A summary of health care reform in Heilongjiang). *Zhongguo weisheng jingji* (China's Health Care Economics), 6: 19–22.

Hou, Y. 2001. Ershiyi shijichu goujian zhongguo weisheng guali xintizhe de tantao (Discussion on the reconstruction of china's health care management of the early 21th century). *Zhongguo weisheng jingji* (China's Health Care Economics), 1: 26–27.

Hu, S. 2007. Jianli guojia jiben yaobing zhidu de zhengce (To establish the national policy of basic medicine system). In L. Du, W. Zhang, & Zhongguo Weisheng Chanye Zazhishe (Ed.), *Zhongguo yiliao weisheng fazhan baogao, No. 3* (The

Report of Development of Medical and Health Care in China, No. 3), 340–352. Beijing: Shehui kexue wenxian chubanshe.

Hu, S. 2005. Jiankang yu fazhan: Zhongguo yiliao weisheng zhidu de lilun fenxi (Health and development: Analysis on the theory of medical and health care system in China). *Shehui baozhang zhidu* (Social Security System), 10: 39–45.

Hu, S. 2010. Touzi yuren de jiankang, goujian youxiao de weisheng tixi (Investing in health of man; building up an effective health care system). In H. Lu (Ed.), *Shanghai shehui fazhan baogao 2010* (The Report of Social Development in Shanghai 2010), 266–292. Beijing: Shehui kexue wenxian chubanshe.

Huang, C., Pang L., & Zhang, L. 2011. Yiliao weisheng fuwu xuqiu de xianguan gainian tantao (Discussion on relevant concepts of the demand of medical and health care services). *Zhongguo weisheng jingji* (China's Health Care Economics), 30(11): 5–7.

Hughes, O. E. 1998. *Public Management and Administration: An Introduction* (2nd ed.). Houndmills andNew York: Palgrave.

Jin, S., Yao, N., & Chen, Q. 2007. Shequ weisheng fuwu de fazhan (The development of community services). L. Du, W. Zhang, & Zhongguo Weisheng Chanye Zazhishe (Ed.), *Zhongguo yiliao weisheng fazhan baogao, No. 3* (The Report of Development of Medical and Health Care, No. 3), 212–240. Beijing: Shehui kexue wenxian chubanshe.

Laodong he Shehui Baozhangbu, & Guojia Yaopin Jiandu Guanliju. 2003. Chengzhen zhigong jiben yiliao baoxian dingtian lingshou yaodian guanli zanxing banfa (The provisional measures of management of designated retail stores for the basic medical care insurance of staff and workers in cities and towns). In Guowuyuan Jiuzheng Hangye Buzhengzhifeng Bangongshi (Ed.), *Jiuzhen yiyao gouxiao zhong buzheng zhi feng gongzuo zhinan* (Guidelines for the Eradiction of Irregular Work Style in the Procurement and Sale of Drugs), 78–79. Beijing: Zhongguo fangzheng chubanshe.

Lee, P. N. 1987. *Industrial Management and Economic Reform in China, 1949–1984*. Hong Kong, Oxford and New York: Oxford University Press.

Lee, P. N., & Wing-Hung Lo, C. W. (Eds.). 2001. *Remaking China's Public Management*. Westport, Connecticut, and London: Quorum Books.

Li, F. 1989. Jundui yiyuan dui shehui kaifeng de xiaoyi he xingxhi yanjiu (Research on the form and results of the opening up of military hospitals to the public). *Zhongguo weisheng jingji* (China's Health Care Economics), 8: 21–25.

Li, N. (2001). Li nanqing fuzhongli zai quanguo chengzhen zhigong jiben yiliao baoxian zhitu he yiyao weisheng tizhi gaige gongzuo huiyi shan de jianghua (Vice-premier Li Nanqing's speech at the national conference on the institutional reform of basic insurance system and medical and health care in cities and towns). In Zhongguo Weisheng Nianjian Bianji Weiyuanhui (Ed.), *Zhongguo weisheng nianjian 2001* (China's Health Care Yearbook 2001), 3–7. Beijing: Renmin weisheng chubanshe.

Li, S., Ma, W., & Li, S. 2002. Woguo yiliao weisheng zhichu de gonggong zhengce yanjiu (A study of public policy on the expenditure of medical and health care in China), *Zhongguo weisheng jingji* (China's Health Care Economics) 21(7): 17–18.

Liang, H., ZhuY., & Zhao D. 2005. Woguo xianxing jiben yiliao fuwu jieding de biduan jiqi chongxin jieding de fangfa yu zhengce (The deficiencies of the current definition of basic medical care services as well as the methods and policies of its re-definition). *Zhongguo weisheng jingji* (China's Health Care Economics) 24(12): 7–10.

Liang, Z. 1988. Shenhua weisheng tizhi gaige de sikao (consider in depth the reform of health care system). *Zhongguo weisheng jingji* (China's Health Care Economics), 12: 13–15.

Lin, F. 2005. Yiliao weisheng tizhi gaige bu yinggai zou huitoulu (No return for medical and health care reform), *Shehui baozhang zhidu* (Social Security System), 11: 45–47, 59.

Lindblom, C. E. 1977. *Politcs and Markets, the World's Political-economic Systems.* New York: Basic Books.

Liu, J. 2008. Gaige kaifan sanshi nianlai woguo zhengfu weisheng touru ji zhengce huigu (The health care input and policy review of the Chinese government for the last 30 years of reform and openning up). *Weisheng jingji yanjiu* (Research on Health Care Economics), 12: 3–9.

Liu, J. 2012. *Zhongguo yigai xiangguan zhengce yanji* (Study on Policies related to China's Medical Care Reform) Beijing: Jingji kexue chubanshe.

Liu, Xian, Yu Runji and Gao Ping. 1999. Ershi shiqi woguo weisheng fazhan qushi guankui (A look at the developmental trend of health care development in 20th century China). *Zhongguo weisheng jingji* (China's Health Care Economics), 3: 21–23.

Liu, X. 2006. Jiangsusheng yiliao jigou chanquan zhidu gaige xianzhuang yu duce yanjiu (Research on the current reform situation and policy proposal of the property rights system in medical care institutions in Jiangsu province). *Zhongguo weisheng jingji* (China's Health Care Economics), 25(1): 54–58.

Luo, Y. 1990. Woguo weisheng gaige ruogan tezheng de yanjiu yu shkao (Study and thoughts on some salient characteristics of health care reform in China). *Zhongguo weisheng jingji* (China's Health Care Economics), 3: 4–8.

Ma, A. 2005. Guanyu dangqian weisheng shiye fazhan wenti de sikao (Some considerations on the issues of development of the current health care enterprises). *Zhongguo weisheng jingji* (China's Health Care Economics), 24(4): 10–11.

Ma, A. 2006a. Guanyu weisheng shiye fazhan yu gaige jige zhangce wenti de sikao (Some thoughts concerning several issues of development and reform of health care enterprise). *Zhongguo weisheng jingji* (China's Health Care Economics), 11: 5–8.

Ma, A. 2006b. Weisheng gaige guilu lun (Theory on the law of health care reform). *Zhongguo weisheng jingj(China's Health Care Economics)*, 9: 13.

Ma, A. 2006c. Weisheng shiye gaige yu fazhan ying chulihao shege guanxi (Handle the ten relations well in reform and development of health care enterprise). *Zhongguo weisheng jingji(China's Health Care Economics)*, 1: 16–17.

Ma, A. 2006d. Weishengtizhi "guanban yiti" yu "guanban fenli" moshi yanjiu (Research on integration between supervision and managment and separation between supervision and management in health care institution). *Zhongguo weisheng jingji (China's Health Care Economics)*, 25(8): 48–52.

Ma, A. 2006e. Xinxingshi xiao de weisheng xingzheng jiguan dingwei yanjiu (Research on the positioning of health care administrative apparatus under the new situation). *Zhnoguo weisheng jingji (China's Health Care Economics)*, 25(12): 10–11.

Ma, L., Wu Qifei. 2006. Gongli yiyuan gaige moshi de huigu yu fansi (Retrospect and reflection on the reform model of public hospitals). *Zhongguo weisheng jingji (China's Health Care Economics)*, 2: 16–19.

Massey, A. 1993. *Managing the Public Sector: A Comparative Analysis of the United Kingdom and the United States.* Aldershot and Brookfield, VT: Ashgate.

Miao, S. 2005. Yiliao weisheng tizhi gaige: Pinggu yu zhanwang (The assessment and prospect of medical and health care reform). *Shehui baozhang zhidu* (Social Security System), 11: 36–40.

Peng, R., Cai, R., & Zhou, C. (Ed.). 1992. *Zhongguo gaige quanshu, yiliao weisheng tizhi gaige juan 1978–1991* (Encyclopedia of China's Reform). Dalian: Dalian chubanshe.

Qiao, J. 2009. Gonggong weisheng fuwu jundenhua yu zhengfu zeren: Jiyu woguo fenquanhua gaige de sikao (The equalization of public health care services and responsibility of the government: Some thoughts on the basis of China's reform of decentralization). *Zhongguo weisheng jingji (China's Health Care Economics)*, 28 (7): 5–7.

Qu, J., & Meng, Q., 2004. Shichang jingji zhuangui shiqi de zhengce yu minying yiliao jigou fazhan (The policy during the transformation towards market economy and development of private hospital institutes). *Zhongguo weisheng jingji (China's Health Care Economics)*, 23(9): 8–10.

Savas, E. S. 1987. *Privatization, the Key to Better Government*. Chatham, NJ: Chatham House Publishers.

Shao, G. 2006. Zhongguo minying yiyuan jiannan qianxing (China's privately managed hospitals moving forward in hardship). In L. Du (Ed.), *Zhongguo yiliao weisheng fazhan baogao No. 2* (The Report of Development of Medical and Health Care in China No. 2), 318–350. Beijing: Shehui kexue wenxian chubanshe.

Shao, G. 2008. Zhongguo minying yiyuan de huigu he zhanwang (China's privately managed hospitals in retrospect and prospect). In L. Du (Ed.), *Zhongguo weisheng fazhan baogao, No. 4* (The Report of Development of China's Medical and Health Care, No. 4), 508–539. Beijing: Shehui Kexue Wenxian Chubanshe.

Shen, X. 2006. Shilun gongli yiliao jigou de gongyixing (A tentative discussion of the public utility characteristics of public medical institutes). *Weisheng jingji yanjiu* (Research on Health Care Economics), 1: 10–12.

Shen, X. 2009. Gongli yiliao jigou 'guanban fenli' zhi wojian (A view on the 'separation between managing and running' of public medical care institutes). *Weisheng jingji yanjiu* (Research on Health Care Economics), 11: 5–7.

Shen, X., Liang, Q., & Yan, Y. 2010. Jianchi gonggong yiliao weisheng gongyixing de ruogan wuqu (Some erroneous issues on the insistence of pubilic welfare characteristics of public medical and health care). *Zhongguo weisheng jingji (China's Health Care Economics)*, 29(9): 7–9.

Starr, P. 1989. The Meaning of Privatization. In S. B. Kamerman, & A. J. Kahn (Eds.), *Privatization and the Welfare*, 15–48. Princeton andLondon: Princeton University Press.

Sun, N., & Du, L. 2006. Gongli yiyuan gaizhi gaizao (The reform and reconstruction of public hospitals). In L. Du (Ed.), *Zhongguo yiliao weisheng fazhan baogao No. 2* (The Report of Development of Medical and Health Care in China), 86–118. Beijing: Shehui kexue wenxian chubanshe.

Wang, B. 2008. *Zhengfu yiliao guamzhi moshi ghonggou yanjiu* (Research on the Restructuring of Modes of Governmental Control). Beijing: Renmin chubanshe.

Wang, F. 2008. Qiye yiyuan gaizhi sikao (Some considerations on reform of enterprise hospitals). In L. Du, (Ed.), *Zhongguo yiliao weisheng fazhan baogao No. 4* (The Report of Development of China's Health Care, No. 4), 171–174. Beijing: Shehui kexue wenxian chubanshe.

Wang, L. 2002. Weishengbu fubuchang wang longde zai 2001 nian quanguo weisheng gongzuo huiyi shan de zongjie jianghua, zhaiyao (Deputy Minister of Health Care Wang Longde's concluding speech at the national conference on health care work, a summary). In Zhongguo Weisheng Nianjian Bianji Weiyuanhui (Ed.), *Zhongguo weisheng nianjian 2002* (China's Health Care Yearbook 2002), 41–48. Beijing: Renmin weisheng chubanshe.

Weishengbu. 1988. Weishengbu guanyu weisheng gongzuo gaige ruogan zhengce wenti de baogao (The report of the Ministry of Health care concerning several policy problems in the reform of health care tasks). In Z. Y. Weishengbu Bangongting (Ed.), *Zhonghua renmin gongheguo weisheng fagui huibian, 1984–1885* (The Collection of Laws and Regulations of Health Care of the PRC, 1984–1985). Beijing: Falu chubanshe, Xinhua shudian.

Weishengbu. 1992. Guanyu yinfa 'guanyu yongxu geti xinyi wenti de qingshe baogao' de tongzhi (The general circular regarding the report to seek advice on the problems of permission of practicing medicine by individuals). In R. Peng, R. Cai, & C. Zhou (Ed.), *Zhongguo gaige quanshu* (Encyclopedia of China's Reform), 112–114. Dalian: Dalian chubanshe.

Weishengbu, PRC. 1990. Yufang baojian sihixing youshang fuwu de huigu yu sikao (Review and observation on the implementation of paid services in preventive care). *Zhongguo weisheng jingji(China's Health Care Economics)*, 6: 26–28.

Weishengbu, PRC. 1992. Guanyu weisheng gongzuo gaige ruogan zhengce wenti baogao (The report concerning the policy problems of reform of health tasks). In R. Peng, R. Cai, & C. Zhou (Ed.), *Zhongguo gaige quanshu* (Encyclopedia of China's Reform), 139–142. Dalian: Dalian chubanshe.

Weishengbu, Guojiazhongyiyaoguanliju, Caizhengbu, & Guojiajiwei. 2000. Guanyu chengzheng yiliao jiguo fenlei guanli de shishi yijian (The opinion of implementation of the classification system of medical care institutes in towns and cities). nhfpc.gov.cn.

Wu, W., Ma, X., & Xie, Y. 1990. Yao chang fuwu shoufei biaozhun xianzhuang fenxi (An analysis of the state of the schedules of charges to paid services). *Zhongguo weisheng jingji(China's Health Care Economics)*, 5: 46–47.

Xi, W. 1994. Heilongjiang sheng weisheng gaige de zongti guoxiang (Overall considerations on health care reform in helongjiang province). *Zhongguo weisheng jingji (China's Health Care Economics)*, 6: 15–18.

Xia, Q. 1990. Ying jiaqiang weisheng bumen yu guomin jingji ge bumen de lianhe (Strengthen collaboration among various health care sectors and among different economic sectors). *Zhnoguo weisheng jingji (China's Health Care Economics)*, 7: 41–44.

Xiao, Z., & Li, H. 1994. Gufenzhi shi wanshan yiyuan jingying jizhi de haozhidu (The system of stocks and shares is a good managerial mechanism for a perfect hospital). *Zhongguo weisheng jingji(China's Health Care Economics)*, 3: 27–28.

Xue, Y. 2006. Lun fazhan jiban yiliao (On the development of basic medical care). *Zhongguo weisheng jingji(China's Health Care Economics)*, 12: 12–15.

Yang, Z., & Liang Z. 1994. Shenhua weisheng tizhi gaige de sikao (Some considerations on further institutional reform in heatlh care). *Zhongguo weisheng jingji (China's Health Care Economics)*, 11: 12–14.

Yao, N. 2008. Shequ weisheng fuwu de fazhan yu jiben yilao weisheng zhidu de goujian (The development of community health care services and construction of basic medical and health care system). In L. Du *et al.* (Eds.), *Zhongguo yiliao weisheng fazhan baogao, No 4* (The Report of Development of Medical and Health Care in China, No. 4), 452–465. Beijing: Shehui kexue wenxian chubanshe.

Yu, R. 2006. Yuanchang fuzezhi xian faren zhili jiegou guodu yingtisu (Accelerate the transformation from the hospital director system to legal person' governance). *Zhongguo weisheng jingji (China's Health Care Economics)*, 25(2): 23–25.

Yuan, D., Chang, T., & Chang, Y. 1995. Yiliao weisheng fuwu shichang tanxi (Analysis on the market of medical care services). *Zhongguo weisheng shiye guanli* (Management of Health Care Enterprises), 1: 7–9, 19.

Yuan, G. 1989. Qianlun yiyuan gugen shehuihua, gerenhui (A preliminary discussion on socialization and privatization of the system of stocks and shares). *Zhongguo weisheng jingji(China's Health Care Economics)*, 3: 33–35.

Zhang, W., & Sun, N. 2006. Yiliao jiguo fenlei guanli (Classification managment of medical care). In L. Du (Ed.), *Zhongguo yiliao weisheng fazhan baogao, No. 2* (The Report of Development of Medical and Health Care in China, No. 2), 195–219. Beijing: Shehui kexue wenxian chubanshe.

Zhang, Y., & Wei, G. 1989. Dui yiyuan shixing gufenzhi de tantao (Discussion on the adoption of the system of stocks and shares). *Zhongguo weisheng jingji(China's Health Care Economics)*, 11: 35–37.

Part II

Rebuilding the state in the health care sector

3 Institutional framework and managerial mechanisms

Overall, the study endeavors to examine on how policy actors employed institutional and managerial tools for the purpose of allocation of health care resources, and provision of health care services. On the basis of the policy actors' interpretive scheme, the study here will be first devoted to the issues of restoration of organization and management in the aftermath of Mao. And the second step will focus, in a broad outline, on those reform attempts that have been most active and visible in regard to three policy arenas: care delivery and revenue-generating activities at the providing unit level that commenced in 1985 and 1988, the installation of basic medical care insurance at the municipal level that was initiated in 1994 and formally launched in 2001, and planning and deployment of health care resources at the municipal level and above that was first advocated in 1997 and reaffirmed in 2000. With these highlights, let's proceed to address some key issues concerning what are their novel institutional and managerial designs dealing with resource management at both the micro and macro level.

Rebuilding command-oriented management

As a standard operational procedure, sovereign planners undertook the tasks of organizational "rectification" and streamlining in the health care sector, that were followed by rebuilding institutional structure and reinventing managerial mechanisms during the early phase of reform from 1979 to the early 1990s. In these reform attempts, they tried to look backward first in tackling the problems created in the past, before they started to look forward. Like many programs and functions of social services elsewhere in the public sector, the delivery of health care throughout China was adversely affected during the Cultural Revolution. As the "old scores" of radical politics were settled, from the mid-1990s onward, the rebuilding of the institutional framework and the introduction of new managerial mechanisms were inseparable from the increasing market orientation in the reform policy. In the meantime, strengthening command-oriented management accompanied with improving transaction-oriented management took China's health care one more step forward to the market paradigm.

With a close look at the policy design, one may characterize China's health care reform at the providing unit level beginning in 1979 as "partial marketization": it neither intended to provide all categories of health care services through market transactions in a comprehensive fashion, nor did it touch the issues of property rights involving either corporatization or asset privatization. Trying not to move away from the existing institutional framework, this commercialization in Mode C took place within the Party-state hierarchy while command-oriented management remained intact, and it was even strengthened and rebuilt further throughout the reform.

As the very first step of the health care reform, this endeavor of "rectification" was made a prerequisite to admission to a pilot program of "economic management" (jingji guanli; EM hereafter) in a given jurisdiction.[1] While "rectification" endeavors placed an emphasis on rebuilding command-oriented management (often taken as general management), EM strengthened resource management (broadly treated as part of transaction-oriented management). The design of pilot programs of EM required all the participant providing units to go through a brand of organizational auditing exercise.[2] For instance, the Ministry of Health and other ministerial units issued the 1979 Supplementary Circular, requiring the providing units to fulfill five criteria before they could be admitted to the pilot programs of EM in various jurisdictions.[3] These five criteria are of input-centered design for building the institutional structure of what is often taken as Weberian "legal-bureaucratic ideal type" in the field of Public Administration (Henderson & Parsons 1964: 324–40; Bendix 162: 385–457). They are as follows: first, a relatively strong and competent leadership team; second, a set of rules and regulations centering on the work post responsibility systems as well as standard operating procedure of hospital management; third, the reform of prescription drugs management; fourth, the trial implementation of quota management at the department and office level; and fifth, an inventory check (Weishengbu & Guojialaodongzongju 1980).

It appears in the process of implementation that the fulfillment of five criteria of "rectification" was provided a strong incentive that came with joining the pilot programs of EM. With the prospect of a revenue-retention system and other bonus and incentive packages, the pilot programs of EM did generate considerable enthusiasm among the providing units. Some kinds of "bandwagon" phenomenon took place in the case of EM similar to Huang's observation of a health policy episode during the economic reform period (Huang 2014). For example, 676 hospital units in 25 provincial jurisdictions had succeeded in earning admission to take part in the pilot programs of EM within the two months from April to June 1979, after the promulgation of the 1979 Supplementary Circular (Weishengbu & Guojialongdongzongju 1980).

As the second step, the directors' responsibility system (DRS) was installed, and it was taken as pivotal to the rebuilding of general management. As the pilot programs of EM picked up momentum in the early 1980s, the ministerial ranking policymakers tried to install the DRS in order to curtail unnecessary interferences from the bureau officials and from the Party organization at the providing unit level (Cui 1992b: 129). According to Xie Honggang and Li Xinmin, this would help merge "two governments" into "one government" by combining two parallel hierarchies (i.e., the administration and the Party organization) into one (i.e., the hospital director system) and improve performance in terms of lower costs with higher efficiency; moreover, this would simplify the complex and clumsy hospital organization by transferring a considerable number of Party cadres and filling administrative posts (Xie & Li 1988).

As a conceptual term, the DRS is understood to be a "unity of command" or monocracy in the existing literature (Fayol 1996: 55–6). In the Chinese context, it represents the so-called "one-man management" (yichangzhi) that was borrowed from the USSR during the early phases of forced industrialization (Lee 1987: 26–31; Shurmann 1968: 253–84). It was then employed as a remedy to excessive interferences by the Party Committee (headed by the Party Secretary) with the managerial and operational works in the production units (Lee 1987:138–40). It also meant delegation of full power to one person in the managerial and technological realm, ensuring the best use of autonomy that was central to all aspects of the health care reform, especially regarding a variety of "responsibility [accountability] systems" (zerenzhe) (Cui 1992b: 131–2). Through the introduction of the DRS, for example, enhanced managerial autonomy tended to strengthen the attribution of responsibility, facilitate the application of performance appraisal, and sharpen the use of incentive tools. Similarly, according to Minister Chen Minzhang, the DRS could help build a hospital director's "unified leadership" over not only general administrative tasks but also resource management (e.g., financial accountability, performance appraisal, revenue retention, incentive schemes, and other economic tasks) (Chen 1992: 136). Additionally, the director could also act on behalf of the state entity administratively with regard to public policy concerns of the work unit (be it service unit or enterprise unit).

During the 1980s, the restoration of the DRS was an integral part of an ongoing, nation-wide policy concern of building a young, knowledgeable, and professional generation of leadership teams in each echelon of the Party-state hierarchy in the midst of the rectification campaign. The campaign was under the auspices of Premier Zhao Ziyang and Yuan Baohua, Director of the State Planning Commission and concurrently Head of the Enterprise Rectification Leadership Team for state-owned enterprises starting in 1982.[4] Three years later, in 1984, a parallel endeavor was made in order to install the DRS in the health care sector, according to ministerial ranking official Cui Yueli (Cui 1992b:129). To lend needed policy support, Chen Minzhang, another ministerial ranking official, made mention of Hu Yaobang's statement to restore the DRS to all enterprise units, service units, schools, and research institutes immediately in 1984 (Chen 1992: 136). In the midst of inaugurating the DRS in the health care sector in 1984 and 1985, Hu stated: "It [the restoration of the director's responsibility system] should go faster with no need for further pilot experimentation" (Chen 1992: 136). Upon a suggestion made by Secretary General Zhao Ziyang early on at the 13th Party Congress, the hospital director assumed an increasingly important responsibility in charge of all administrative, managerial, and financial matters from 1985 to 1990, while the role of the Party Committee shrank and was only confined to supervisory, supportive, and ideological functions (Xie & Li 1988: 15).

Beginning in 1984, the installation of the DRS took place not only in state-owned hospital units above the county level, but also in collective-owned units below the county level (Cui 1992b: 131–2). Some forms of democratic management were introduced in order to create room for participation of staff and workers, and more importantly, to impose checks and supervision of possible abuses of administrative power at each hierarchical level. For example, the Congress of Representatives of Staff and Workers (CRSW) was often restored to state-owned hospital units to serve as a counterweight to the growing power of the director, similar to the case of industrial management (Lee 1987: 138–43). In the collective-owned units, moreover, their directors enjoyed even greater latitude than that of their state-owned counterparts in personnel, finance, and management as they practiced the system of "independent accounting, full accountability for earning and loss, remuneration according to labor contribution, and democratic management." (Cui 1992a: 156; Cui 1992b: 129). In those collective-owned providing units, democratic management was even more important than CRSW in the state-owned unit to maintain checks and balances in relation to the director, who acted on behalf of the collective unit exercising collective property rights as well as discretion over retained revenue, compensation issues, and financial matters, e.g., allocation of wages, bonus, collective accumulation funds, and charity funds in accordance with relevant rules and regulations (Weishengbu 1988).

As articulated in a policy paper issued in 1981, the improvement of EM ought to be integrated with that of administrative management, coupled with the upgrading of the levels of technical, scientific, and professional management.[5] Overall, the installation and strengthening of the DRS were put on the top of the policy agenda of health care reform starting in the early 1980s and remained as a policy emphasis consistently into the late 1990s and beyond. In accordance with the policy paper, the 1997 Decision, for example, all health care institutes are required to install and improve a DRS in conjunction with the expansion of autonomy in business and management and further improvement of personnel management and the compensation system.[6]

Management by multiple bureaus

There are three types of work unit in China (i.e. enterprise work unit, service work unit, and government/quasi-government work unit), all of which are given a role in policy implementation, and they work together with the bureau in translating policy into action (Sil 1997; Straus 1997; Warner 2000; Duckett 2004). In the health care sector, most work units play the roles as the employers who are mainly responsible for funding and in some cases, as the health care providers in organizing and managing clinics/hospitals for delivery of health care services. The providing unit (e.g., the public hospital) is taken as the service work unit, acting as an institutional vehicle through which health care services are rendered, while the bureau level assumes main supervisory and regulatory responsibility over a host of major functions (Yang, Gao & Ai 2006; Wang 2008: 253–4). Within the framework of the CPE, the providing unit operates under bureau management, even though it is understood to be self-contained in operational and functional terms.[7]

To study the implementation of public policy in China, the providing unit needs to work with multiple counterpart bureaus operationally and managerially at the next higher level (Yang July 1989; Yang et al. 2006; Wang 2008: 253–4). The scenario of multiple bureaus differs from that of one singular rational actor in the pure rationality model in the sense that the former entails several perspectives and evaluating criteria in policymaking and policy implementation. And these perspectives and evaluating criteria are often in conflict, and coordination is a constant job in the process of implementation. In the health care sector in China, each providing unit is subject to so-called "dual command."[8] On the one hand, as a general principle, each providing unit is under direct and overall command of a government unit mainly at the territorial level, e.g., county, municipal/prefectural, and provincial level in a horizontal fashion (Wang 2008: 251–2). Representing an exception, however, the Ministry of Health (MOH) often plays a dual role: on the one hand, it is considered as "staff organization" according to the logic of generic management, lending technical and professional advices on policymaking on health care to the Premier, head of the State Council. On the other hand, it assumes the role of "line organization" by taking direct charge of a small group of public hospitals at the central level, often being placed, along with several relevant functional areas (health care, financing, pricing, personnel, etc.), under the regulatory control, management, and supervision of several bureaus in a vertical fashion from the central/ministerial level down to the provincial, municipal/prefect, and county level (Wang 2008: 253–4).

Within the framework of the CPE, a government within territorial jurisdiction takes major managerial responsibility over the delivery of health care services (Wang 2008: 252). The workload of health and medical care service is determined roughly by the number of clients and often grouped by the size of a territorial jurisdiction. As a rule, the delivery of health care services is defined in terms of missions, contents, and the qualitative and quantitative standards and is governed by various financial and pricing policies. It is coordinated, organized, and managed through the chain of command of health care departments running from the central echelon to provincial and local echelons within the administrative hierarchy of the Party-state (Wang 2008: 252). And as regards residential management, each jurisdiction is given sufficient power to deal with the matters of policy implementation of health care as well as most, if not all, of their impacts (namely, policy outcome and feedback so to speak) within its defined area of authority in order to be held accountable (Yang et al. 2006).

As the task of health care services is exceedingly complex, accompanying considerable workload and the thorny issue of accountability to policy outcomes, it is rational and more effective to group the providing units in terms of classes and categories. In accordance with the Measures of Management of Hospitals by Echelons as updated and reintroduced in 1989, public hospitals are classified into three tiers according to their functions and missions. As given in Figure 3.1 below, the county government (or urban district administration) with all its relevant bureaus are in charge of either county-affiliated hospitals (or urban district administered hospitals), most of which fall into Tier 1; the prefectural/municipal government with its relevant bureaus has jurisdiction over the prefectural/municipal affiliated hospitals, most of which are in Tier 2 and a few of which belong to Tier 3; provincial governments and ministerial units, coupled with their relevant bureaus, are in charge of provincial/ministerial affiliated hospitals, a majority of which are Tier 3 hospitals. Tier 3 hospitals represent the highest quality and professional standards of services, catering of specialized medical and health care services, and teaching and scientific research at the advanced level. In each tier, hospitals are divided further into three grades: A, B, and C. With an additional, special grade created on top of Tier 3, there are three tiers and ten grades in total. As it is

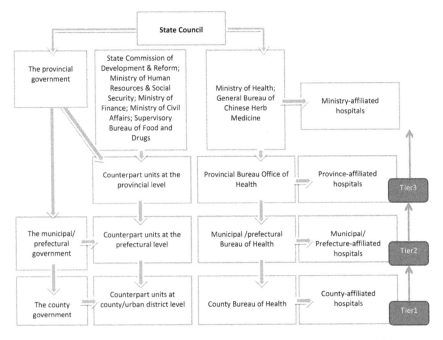

Figure 3.1 The supervisory and managerial system of public hospitals in China

implemented, the managerial power is allocated vertically to various echelons within the administrative hierarchy (Wang 2008: 251–2).

In fact, there is considerable overlap among the health care bureau, the committee of development and reform, the finance bureau, the price bureau, the bureau of personnel and human resources, and social insurance over a series of policy issues such as the investment, planning, and allocation of medical care resources, pricing of medical care services, quality and quantity of medical care services, and entry into and regulatory control of medical care markets (Wang 2008: 253–4). Such a design of multiplicity of bureaus entails irrationality as well as inherent problems of coordination, meaning that each providing unit is faced with complexity, difficulties, and a heavy workload with its counterpart bureaus in the next higher echelon. Such problems call for solutions in terms of restructuring at both institutional and administrative levels, a topic to be tackled further in the remaining passages.

Re-engineering administrative structure

The administrative restructuring and rebuilding represent an attempt in the search and adoption of institutional and managerial tools to attain chosen policy objectives in the health care sector, often placing an emphasis on resource management in the exercise of "reorganization" similar to the industrial sector (Lee 1987: 149–69; Solinger 1991: 194–220). Through Mode A administrative reform mode, sovereign planners have endeavored to allocate health care resources by following two distinct approaches: the first approach focusing on restructuring of work units and institutions in order to make better use of existing stock of health care resources, and the second approach concerning the creation of entirely new organizational units and functions, often involving fresh investments (Fu 1989; Si 1990).

Representing the first approach, one of the largest scales of restructuring effort in the health care sector was devoted to the task of reorganizing underused medical care facilities which had been controlled and managed by the SOEs, and this was carried out in conjunction with the establishment of a modern enterprise system.[9] The issue is rooted in the developmental strategy of the CPE and also closely tied to the consideration of optimal use of health care resources.[10] In accordance with a policy paper put forth by the State Planning Commission (SPC) in collaboration with the Ministry of Health (MOH) and Ministry of Finance (MOF) in 1997, for example, some jurisdictions started to take action to stop establishing providing units within the SOEs; some others began to adjust and restructure their existing providing units through closure, merging, transfer, joint management, and contracting-out arrangements (Chen 1999: 219). Two years later, furthermore, the Party Center of the CCP and the State Council put forth the policy paper entitled the 1999 Decision, urging various jurisdictions across the country to separate social functions (including medical care services) and alleviate the social burden of the SOEs in the perspective of regional health care resources planning.[11]

In fact, the policy of separation of hospitals from industrial enterprises was implemented with visible results in some local jurisdictions. For example, the number of enterprise-managed hospitals was recorded as 7,348 or 44.1 percent and the number of hospital beds was counted as 600,000 or 27.4 percent of the national total in 1999; they were brought down within a period of seven years to 4,382 or 22.8 percent and 355,000 or 13.9 percent of the national total in 2006 (Fang & Wang 2010). This policy represents an attempt to set a brake on the expansion of "work unit collectivism" which was considerably reinforced during the early phase of economic reform when public enterprises had diverted retained revenue to building "collective welfare," communal amenities and facilities, including clinics and hospitals, in order to counter the government's tight wage control.

The second approach is future-oriented in the sense that it attempts to channel new investments and resources according to some chosen targets and plans. For example, the adoption of a "unified planning system" (abbreviated as UPS) represents one of the most salient reform attempts at rebuilding medical care providing units amid the economic reform. On March 17, 1994, the State Council, for the first time, promulgated a set of regulations, namely, the 1994 Regulations, requiring each government at the county level or above to adopt a UPS for the establishment of new health care institutes at the community level with regard to the size of the population, medical care resources and needs, and the deployment of the existing medical care institutes within a given jurisdiction.[12] Accordingly, the providing units (or "medical care institutes") of all tiers and categories, various affiliations, and ownership systems were required to be placed under one unified planning system (Guowuyuan 1994). The UPS worked as a set of managerial mechanisms aiming at making the best use of health care resources and providing public and preventive health care as well as basic medical care services in a convenient, accessible, quality, and equitable way for each community (Guowuyuan 1994).

Not only was the set of 1994 Regulations community-centered but it was also market oriented in the sense that it was procedurally tied to the licensing and franchising of medical care practices with explicit reference to market situation. It specified the standards and requirements of the market entry of medical care providing units and medical personnel into medical care services. It was also trade-wide oriented to the extent that it ensured that only professionally qualified personnel were allowed to practice medicine and permitted to diagnose cases of illness, treat the patients, and issue documents and certification of medical care conditions and results of treatments of the patients (Guowuyuan 1994; Li 1996; Li & Lu 2008). In the same year, the MOH issued a set of guidelines to specify in concrete terms the principles, contents, standards, and procedures regarding the planning for the medical care institutes, placing emphasis on the lower level. The guidelines proposed to establish a system of health care services with three echelons and to divide the planning tasks among county, municipal/prefecture, and provincial levels (Li & Lu 2008).

Moreover, in 1997 the Party Center of the CCP and State Council put forth the 1997 Decision, proposing to build the network of community health care services as an additional tier at the community level in each city throughout China: while the existing public hospitals (with all three tiers) continue to perform their conventional role in the provision of curative care (such as emergent, serious, and difficult cases), training, and research, a newly added tier of community medical care facilities will focus on primary and family health care services as well as the cases of common and frequent diseases.[13] The building of community health care services was formally put on the policy agenda in 1999 when the MOH and other ministerial units promulgated the policy paper known as the 1999 Several Opinions.[14] In 2000 and 2006 respectively, a new set of policy papers provided further details concerning community health care facilities and services that are functionally equivalent to the gatekeeper's role of General Practitioners in the UK and the family doctors system in the USA (Jin, Yao & Chen 2007; Gu 2008: 300–29; Li & Lu 2008).

The proposal of community health care service facilities addressed the issue of the top-heavy pyramid of the health care system where most health care resources were concentrated at the large and modern public hospitals, but the small providing units were left inadequately funded and under-utilized at the bottom. By design, the former is more effective in dealing with emergent, serious, and difficult cases of illness while the latter is more suitable for treating the common and frequent diseases. In an explicit and articulate fashion, Minister of MOH Gao Qiang was among one of the highest ranked health care officials to characterize this problem at the system level as a "reverse pyramid" and described it as suboptimal in the deployment of heath care resources.[15]

Since 1979, large public hospitals of a high class (mostly Tier 3) have registered considerable growth in terms of service capacity, number of beds, medical personnel, and advanced medical devices. They were able to capture a large market share of the patients, many of whom fell into the category of frequent and common illness that could have been suitably treated by those small-sized hospitals (i.e., in Tier 1) or clinics at the community level in a much more accessible, convenient, and inexpensive way. The disparity between the large and small hospitals (and even clinics and community medical care facilities) was further aggravated because of the biased policy of financial appropriation in favor of the former. To narrow down the gap of health care resources between large and small public hospitals, it required a considerable injection of funding into the building of community medical care facilities in both urban and rural settings (Gu 2008: 300–20). This policy trend is registered on the increase of community health care centers/stations from 8,211 in 2002 to 17,128 in 2005 (Gu 2008: 307).

Organizing basic medical care insurance programs

In conjunction with the pilot programs and policy experiments of medical care insurance from 1994, 1996, and 1998 to the early 2000s, sovereign planners were confronted with choices regarding not only the institutional designs for managing basic medical care insurance (BMCI) but also the right scales for the organizational unit and at an appropriate level of the Party-state hierarchy (Guojia Tigaiwei et al. 1999a; Guojia Tiegaiwei et al. 1999b). Among several policy alternatives, sovereign planners have finally chosen the municipal government as the principal locus for establishing an entirely new set of institutions to handle policymaking, regulatory control, and management and supervision of BMCI in respective jurisdictions. At the end of the day, however, most of the BMCIs were built at the county level.

Theoretically speaking, the program of basic medical insurance has a larger scope than that of both public-financed medical care (PFMC) and labor insurance medical care (LIMC) programs combined in light of an expanding sector of mixed economy, and therefore, a managing body needs to be established to supersede the previous government departments in charge of the new insurance related functions. Emerging from the pilot programs including Jiujiang and Zhenjiang, two organizing principles were put forth: the first is residential management principle requiring the BMCI to be organized and managed in the community where the insured can have easy access to the medical care services; the second proffers that the municipal level (equivalent to prefectural level) or as an alternative, the county level, should assume principal responsibility in policymaking, funding, operation, and management (Guowuyuan 1995).

In order to perform the role of financial risk pooling (called "unified funding," tongchou), it was originally proposed that the municipal/prefectural level or above is to be designated as the unified funding unit in accordance with the 1998 Decision as promulgated by the State Council in 1998.[16] As an alternative, however, the county could be chosen when a given prefectural-status municipality enjoys too great a geographical size and too much in economic variations to render managerial task of health care effective. In addition, Beijing, Tianjin, and Shanghai, three directly administered metropolitan areas are each authorized to be a unified funding region. Accordingly, a unified policy of medical care insurance is to be followed in any region where the collection, use, and management of the program of BMCI are to be handled at municipal level (Guowuyuan 1998). According to Wu Mutu and Chen Jinpu, officials of the Ministry of Labor and Social Security, the choice of the level of hierarchy for the BMCI should hinge on two considerations: the capacity of risk absorption, mutual help, and levels of managerial services, and the balancing between the variations of consumption and economic development across each region (e.g. municipality/prefecture). They argue that in general the provincial level is too high a level to accommodate regional differences and too administratively taxing because of excessively large-scale and organizational complexity, while the county level entails a smaller revenue basis, coupled with lesser capacity to cope with financial risks (Wu & Chen 1999).

In the process of implementation, however, provincial policymakers have built majority of jurisdictions over public insurances at the county level rather than municipal/prefecture level as originally intended. According to Ma &

Gui, public insurance programs were managed by the municipal level and at the county level—2,620 jurisdictions of unified social funding (USF) during the 2010s, and the average size of each amounting to an average of 500,000 enrollees. Given the total of municipal units (with prefectural status) are numbered 330 or so, it appears that county level was undoubtedly favorite choice for the BMCI and other public insurance programs, meaning that the scale of risk pooling is too small to address the issues of labor mobility, and market economy beyond the local confine.[17]

In accordance with the residential management principle, the 1998 Decision proposes that all qualified employing work units as well as staff and workers are required to join the program of BMCI of the unified funding region, together with special arrangements for those trades whose employees are scattered in wide and remote locations (Guowuyuan 1998; Wu & Chen 1999: 365). Examples include railways, electricity, and oceanic shipping whose employees can be better served as the provision of medical care insurance is organized in a "relatively concentrated fashion" in a designated unified funding region (Wu & Chen 1999: 365).

Evolving from the pilot programs in 1994, a non-departmental public body called "executive agency" (jingban jiguo) is chosen to be responsible for managing a given medical care insurance program (Guowuyuan 1995). It acts as the sole agent of the BMCI fund in charge of collection, management, and payments in a given jurisdiction. By design, the government is therefore able to keep "one arm length" with the executive agency that takes over the workload created by the BMCI programs in each municipality/county by adhering to the principle of separation of policymaking and regulatory control from day to day management in medical care insurance.[18] The executive agency was then treated independently of the government, and its staff members were not taken as government officials (Guojia Tigaiwei et al. 1999a). These staff members were paid by the government, however, in order to avoid the issue of conflict of interests, as they were in a better position to handle the financial matters of the BMCI independently (Guojia Tigaiwei et al. 1999a).

To strengthen management and supervision and ensure rational use of funds, the government drew a clear demarcation between the "administrative departments in charge" (xingzheng zhuguan bumen) and executive agency. The former was responsible for making policies, rules and regulations, and schemes and standards, including the scope of medical care services, the standards and accounting measures of medical expenses, the catalogs of basic drugs, the measures of management, and the standards of medical devices, among others (Guowuyuan 1998). And the latter acted as a "relatively independent body," taking charge of the collection, payment, and operation of the funds of medical care insurance (Guojia Tigaiwei et al. 1999a).

While the Ministry of Labor and Social Security (MLSS) and other relevant ministries were responsible for making the standards and procedures of eligibility for designated providing units and designated pharmacies, the executive agency acquired considerable powers, becoming a controlling core of a managerial network of a cluster of "designated" (dingdian) providing units and designated pharmacies on the basis of contractual arrangements (Guojia Tigaiwei et al. 1999a; Guojia Tigaiwei et al. 1999b; Guowuyuan 2001). With reference to the provision of prescription drugs, the designated hospital still managed its own pharmacy department for inpatients, while the designated pharmacy provided dispensary services to outpatients. The designated pharmacy was intended to give the insurer and outpatient an option and to enhance its competition with the hospital pharmacy for inpatients (Guowuyuan 1988). As a result, the designated pharmacy, that enjoyed exclusive right to serve inpatients, was only given a share of the drug market for outpatients, and often a smaller share relative to what was given to the providing unit that serves inpatients.

This managerial network over designated providing units and designated pharmacies was quasi-governmental to the extent that it was created by relevant policies and regulations, playing an important role not only in upholding the standards of quality and safety but also enforcing spending control measures. It was taken as "quasi-market" oriented in the sense that its operation hinged on a cluster of contracts for medical care services that were signed by the executive agency with designated hospitals and designated pharmacies, and thus curative care and prescription drugs were to be provided through transactions paid by the insurer and insured. These designated providing units and designated pharmacies were screened and chosen by relevant bureaus in accordance with the measures and regulations promulgated by ministerial authorities. Meanwhile the executive agency enforced the policies and directives, regulations and rules, and standards and other requirements of the government, for example, the list of basic medical care services and the catalog of basic drugs (Laodong he Shehui Baozhangbu et al. 2003; Laodong he Shehuibaozhangbu, Weishengbu & Guojia Zhongyiyao Guanliju 2003).

According to Gu Xin, the executive agency performed three functions: first, as the purchaser, it determines the content of services, e.g., clinical services, hospitalization, and dispensary services; second, as negotiator, it worked with designated hospitals and designated pharmacies on the pricing of various items of services; and third, as payers, it decided how to pay for relevant services, for example, schemes of payments (e.g. global pre-payment, individual user, or type of illness) to be adopted (Gu 2010:127–33). Moreover, the executive agency acted on behalf of the insurer according to their needs, conveniences, and accessibility of the insured. The executive agency also signed contracts with the designated providing units and designated pharmacies with reference to their responsibility, rights, and obligations, normally for a term of one year (Guojia Tigaiwei et al. 1999b). The contract specified the scope and contents, quality of services, measures of accounting, schemes of payments, and procedures of auditing and control (ibid.). As the executive agency was installed, China's medical care system could choose to phase out the office of the PFMC program and the union organization/enterprise administration that managed the LIMC program.

Managing health care resources

The issue of managing health care resources gained considerable currency beginning in the second decade of health care reform, which started in the late 1980s. This was then marked by the introduction of mechanisms of management and planning of health care resources from the central, provincial to municipal/prefectural level, including so-called comprehensive trade-wide oriented residential management (abbreviated as CTORM hereafter) and the regional health care planning (abbreviated as RHCP hereafter).

The earliest idea of CTORM was proposed in 1991–2000 Outline after a process of fermentation from the early 1990s.[19] And it was formally put on the policy agenda on March 15, 1999, as the State Planning Commission (SPC) and other ministerial units put forth the 1999 Advisory Opinion. The CTROM is concerned with a macro-managerial system where all health care resources are subject to planning, management and supervision, regulatory control, licensing, and enforcement of quality and safety standards at the municipal level. In exceptional cases, a directly administered municipality, separate/single-listed municipality, or provincial capital takes charge over the same function, depending upon the planning and managerial considerations (Ren 2007; Ma 2007: 4–5).

In theoretical terms, the CTORM deals with the practical issues of suboptimal deployment and allocation of health care resources evolving in various organizational contexts and being created during different eras in the past, for example, including the under-utilized facilities of enterprise-managed providing units and the redundancy of providing units affiliated with different administrative establishments within the same territorial jurisdictions (Zhongguo Weisheng 2006; Ma 2007: 4–5). As illustrated by Ma Anning et al., for instance, one would normally find several clusters of medical care providing units that operated at the same municipal level but were affiliated with and managed by ministerial and provincial authorities at the next higher hierarchical level; there were also providing units that worked in a municipal jurisdiction but were affiliated with and managed by county governments at the next lower level (Ma 2007: 4–5). And each rendered the same kinds of services to the residents but each ran into the issue of redundancy and under-utilized health care resources such as personnel, facilities, and equipment within a given jurisdiction (Ren 2007: 168–9; Ma 2007: 5). As previously noted, moreover, there were the cases of the so-called "reverse pyramid" regarding medical care facilities sitting idle at the community level, while big, modern hospitals, which were supposed to work on rare and difficult cases, were overly packed with the patients ailing with common and frequent cases of illness (Ren 2007: 167–8).

The CTROM is a managerial design intended to ensure the proper match between the health care demands of residents and the deployment/allocation of health care resources within a given municipal jurisdiction. It consists of two components, namely, "residential management principle" (shudi zhuyi) and "trade-wide oriented management" (hangye guanli) (Ma 2007: 4–6). The former pertains to the matters of structure of command, mainly dealing with the decentralization of managerial power of personnel, quality and safety standards, licensing of market entry and investment, and property rights to the municipal/prefectural level in order to satisfy the demands of the users. The latter focuses on the issues of optimal use, deployment, and macro-management of health care resources such as personnel, technology, equipment, and facilities from the vantage and relevant considerations of the medical profession on a trade-wide basis (Ma 2007: 4–6).

What are new roles that a municipality can assume in CTROM? So far it has been proposed that the municipal level should be expected to undertake several new responsibilities. At the municipal level, the design of the managerial and supervisory system should follow the residential management principle, namely, those units which authorize market entry (i.e., "granting franchise," called zhuenru in Chinese) should be those units which exercise supervisory authority (Ma 2007: 5). In principle, the municipality (normally with prefectural status) should be in charge of market entry, application and approval, and supervision and management on a routine basis (Ma 2007: 6–7). The municipal government is also expected to play the role of gatekeeper in the market entry of new providing units, fresh investments, admission of medical interns and trainees, certified use of advanced devices, and advertisements and commercials for medical care services (Wang 2008: 244–7).

Furthermore, the municipal government will be in charge of setting up the professional standards of the medical care services and ensuring consistency and uniformity in management, policy enforcement, and supervision within a given municipal jurisdiction (Ma 2007: 4–5). It is suggested ideally that the municipal government be given the responsibility to implement the BMCI of workers and staff among the providing units whose affiliation is above the county level (Ma 2007: 4–5). To enforce the residential management principle, the newly built providing units with ministerial and provincial affiliations should be subject to municipal management and regulatory control, and follow the unified planning as prescribed by the municipal government (Ma 2007: 4–5) The CTROM is also intended to provide guidelines and establish priorities not only in the introduction of fresh funding and investments, but also the regrouping, restructuring and management of the existing stock of the fixed assets and facilities at the municipal level (Ren 2007: 168–9; Ma 2007: 5–8).

In a conceptual and functional sense, the CTROM is closely related to the regional health care planning (abbreviated as RHCP hereafter). With the installation of CTROM at the municipal level, the health care reform also propelled a salient trend of building the mechanisms of RHCP at the State Council, provincial, and municipal level respectively commencing in the late 1990s and gaining further momentum in the early 2000s. Accordingly, in two installments, the central authorities first introduced the 1999 Advisory Opinions concerning the concrete tasks of planning for regional health care resources in 1999 as just noted (Ren 2007: 163). And then they adopted the 2000 Advisory Opinions regarding the dismantlement of barriers of jurisdictions and ownership systems in 2000 (Ma 2007: 3; Ding 2009: 6). Subsequently in 2001, 2006, and 2007, a series of policy papers made recommendations specifically to incorporate into RHCP the following: the licensing of market entry of hospital units, medical professionals, advanced medical technology, large and expensive medical care devices, and social insurance programs (Ma 2007: 3–5).

Representing an entirely new set of planning mechanisms and procedures, the RHCP is an exercise following a five-year cycle, but it differs from the conventional central planning regarding purposes and methods (Ren 2007). In Ren's observation, it is organized, coordinated, and conducted by a work team/leadership team on an ad hoc basis at three levels: The State Council, provincial, and municipal levels. At the State Council level, the work team is responsible for coordinating and advising in terms of general policy direction. The provincial leadership team is mainly in charge of creating the deployment standards of health care resources. Municipal leadership takes command of drafting and enforcing the regional health care plan (Ren 2007: 169–70). As Ren further suggests, the 1999 Advisory Opinion advised various provincial governments to adopt RHCP within the municipal jurisdiction and other cities in order to take geographical advantage of a nuclear city incorporating the adjacent rural area within its radiating perimeter. In Ren's view, accordingly, RHCP dealt with the allocation of health care resources and defined the scope and activities of health care services, but the existing administrative affiliations and investment channels remained intact. It also provided guidelines for the eligibility and admission of medical personnel, evaluation and certification of providing units, unified technical standards of health care services, and the criteria of quality management, among other things. In addition, it put forth the principle for setting priority for those investing units to enjoy health care services (Ren 2007: 169–70).

As reported, various provincial jurisdictions started the task of drafting the deployment standards in the late 1990s, and they were completed and put into implementation in twenty-nine provinces, directly administered cities, and autonomous regions up to 2001 (Ren 2007: 177). These deployment standards served as the foundation for drafting and enforcing RHCP at the municipal level. As a rule, the contents of RHCP included analyses of social and economic situations, health conditions and available health care resources of the residents, main health care problems, targets of the plan, the deployment standards, measures, implementation and methods of review, and the requirements of inter-departmental coordination (Ren 2007: 165–6). At the provincial level, the deployment standards of health care resources would normally embrace quantitative indicators and requirements of health care resources (such as the number of personnel and hospital beds) with reference to the establishment of the providing units (Ren 2007: 174–9). Retrospectively in a way, RHCP tended to reinforce the State Council's initiatives to streamline the installation and management of medical care institutes at the community level beginning in 1994 (Li 1996; Li & Lu 2008).

Concluding remarks

The foregoing analysis suggests that, overall, the entire health care system has gradually moved away from the conventional structure of the CPE amid the creation of new institutions and evolution of novel managerial tools throughout the reform era, which began in 1979. In stark contrast to various market options, these reform attempts follow Mode A—largely administrative in nature, performing tasks and functions in the health care provision. From the low echelons to high echelons, there witnessed considerable efforts not only to restore and streamline the conventional institutions and managerial mechanisms but also to rebuild and reinvent new organizational and managerial designs. At the providing unit level, for instance, much attention was drawn to installing director's responsibility system to beef up a competent leadership team, armed with rules and regulations, and financial and budgetary system, and all effective SOP for care services and dispensary services. At the municipal level, the three tier hospitals system has been rebuilt, and strengthened by community health institutes together with referral procedures, intending to absorb a large number of common and frequent cases of illness and to alleviate the excessive workload of large, modern hospitals. Moreover, the government endeavored to optimize use of health care resources by opening up the facilities of enterprise-managed hospitals and clinics and making them available to the patients in the same community. With the advent of BMCI programs came a novel institutional framework in which the executive agency, a non-governmental public entity, serves as the organizational vehicle in charge of collection and allocation of insurance funds, and build contractual ties with the providing units. Such a framework bears a resemblance to a brand of quasi-market through which public funding is channeled to users by market mechanisms. However, the Chinese version of quasi-market differs from its UK counterpart in the sense that the former is encapsulated into an administrative system of basic medical insurance, operating with insurance funding rather than tax revenue as it is in United Kingdom.

The reformers are confronted with new issues of optimal use of health care resources, e.g., the gap between small hospitals and overly congested large hospitals. In addition, they need to build up community health care centers/ stations in order to render primary care services in both urban districts and neighborhood organizations and rural counties and townships. In the place of the work unit and local bureaus under the CPE, furthermore, there has been the effort to promote the municipal jurisdiction as the organizing core, not only in care delivery but also in medical care insurance. In principle, the designs of BMCI is intended to create entirely new institutional forms such as the executive agency, a non-departmental public entity that replaces the work unit and supervising bureaus that ran conventional programs of PFMC and LIMC prior to the reform. Additionally, in retreat from the CPE, new ideas and designs of planning mechanisms (e.g., CTROM and RHCP) have been put forward in the arenas of planning, deployment, and use of health care resources at the municipal level, representing a rising trend in China's health care system.

Notes

1 The Ministry of Health, and Ministry of Finance and the State General Bureau of Labor accordingly authorized pilot experiments in various jurisdictions by issuing the Opinion Concerning the Pilot Work of Strengthening Hospital Economic Management (abbreviated as the 1979 Opinion hereafter) on April 28, 1979 (Weishengbu Guojialaodongzhongchu 1979); Qian Xinzhong, Ministry of Health Care, outlined the policy priority of "rectification" as well (Qian 1983).
2 This is reminiscent of Lord Derek Rayner's scrutiny exercises adopted during Margaret Thatcher's government in the United Kingdom (Massey 1993: 40–5).
3 In 1979, the Ministry of Health, the Ministry of Finance, and the State General Bureau of Labor issued the Supplementary Circular Concerning the Pilot Task of Hospital Management (abbreviated as the 1979 Supplementary Circular hereafter) (Weishengbu & Guojialaodongzongju 1980).
4 It is noteworthy that the rebuilding of leadership teams and directors' responsibility system in the health care sector did not start until 1984, about three years behind the industrial sector. The industrial sector began its rectification campaign in 1982 and was basically concluded in 1984 under the auspices of Premier Zhao Ziyang and Yuan Baohua, Director of the State Planning Commission and concurrently Head of the Enterprise Rectification Leadership Team (Lee 1987: 141–2).
5 The policy paper is taken as the Provisional Measures of Hospital Economic Management (draft) 1981 (abbreviated as the 1981 Provisional Measures) (Weishangbu 1985: 458).
6 The policy paper is entitled: The Decision of the Central Committee, Chinese Communist Party (CCP), and State Council on Health Care Reform and Development (promulgated on January 15, 1997, abbreviated as the 1997 Decision hereafter). See (Zhonggong Zhongyang & Guowuyuan 1999: 46).
7 Henderson and Cohen did an early piece of study focusing on the public hospital at Wuhan, but their focus was not placed on the larger bureaucratic hierarchy in which their chosen unit was situated (Henderson 1984).
8 In a broad conceptual scheme of "line and staff," "line" represents a chain of command of chief executives positioned from the highest level to the lowest level in an administrative hierarchy. Staff refers to those personnel who serve the chief executive in advisory, logistical and secretarial jobs at each hierarchical level from the central level running downward to the provincial level, municipal, and county level. Under the command of the Premier, the chief executive at the central level, for example, the ministerial units act as "staff" And the governors directly under the command are taken as line officers. See (Schurmann 1968: 105–308; Mintzberg 1983: 1–23; Yang et al. 2006; Wang 2008; Ding 2009).
9 In Du Lexun's view, the establishment of the modern enterprise system created the imperative of shedding the LIMC programs as well as enterprise-managed medical care facilities from SOEs and other establishments in order to improve efficiency and productivity of the industrial sector. See Du, 2007: 34–6)

10 China adopted the CPE as the main thrust of its developmental strategy, meaning that it built industry well ahead of urbanization, and health care facilities were organized as part of the organizational infrastructure of enterprise units. That is to say, the SOEs undertook the provision of welfare programs, a large part of which consists of the medical care services to staff and workers in a form of "welfare functions" of work units (Qiye Weisheng Ziyuan Youxiao liyong youhua peizhi (ASEM) ketizu 2001).

11 The policy paper is entitled the Decision on Several Problems of the Reform and Development of SOEs (abbreviated as the 1999 Decision) (Ma, 2007: 3).

12 The full title of the policy paper is the Regulations of Management of Medical Care Institutes (abbreviated as the 1994 Regulations hereafter). See (Guowuyuan, 1994; Li, 1996).

13 The full title of the 1997 Decision is: The Decision of Health Care Reform and Development (abbreviated as the 1997 Decision) (Li & Lu, 2008).

14 The title of the policy paper reads as follows: The Several Opinions Regarding the Development of Community Health Care Services in Towns and Cities (abbreviated as the 1999 Several Opinions hereafter) (Gu, 2008: 305).

15 Minister Gao Qiang also points to the problem that the best-trained medical personnel and advanced medical devices were overly concentrated at large and modern hospitals in urban centers while the shortage of medical personnel could not be alleviated at the level of rural areas and communities in cities. See Gao, 2006: 50.

16 The full title of the policy paper is as follows: The Establishment of the Basic Medical Care Insurance System in Towns and Cities (abbreviated as the 1998 Decision) (Guowuyuan 1998).

17 Ma & Gui (2012), 5: 78.

18 See the Opinion of the Expansion of Pilot Programs of Medical Care Insurance System of Staff and Workers (abbreviated as the 1996 Opinion hereafter) as promulgated by the State Institutional Reform Commission, Ministry of Finance, Ministry of Labor, and Ministry of Health Care on April 22, 1996 (Guojia Tigaiwei et al. 1999a)

19 The earliest idea of CTORM was first proposed in The Outline of China's Health Care Development and Reform, 1991–2000, draft for soliciting opinions (abbreviated as the1991–2000 Outline hereafter). See Article 17, (Weishengbu et al. 1992: 44). Subsequently the State Planning Commission took the lead on collaboration with the Ministry of Health Care and Ministry of Finance, in drafting another policy paper in 1997, titled Several Opinions on the Tasks of Regional Health Care Planning (abbreviated as the 1997 Several Opinions), highlighting the issues of deployment, allocation and restructuring of health care resources (Chen 1999: 219).

References

Chen, M. 1992. Chen Mingzhang tongzhi zai yijiu bawu nian quanguo weisheng tingjuchang huiyi shang de zongjie jianghua (Comrade Chen Mingzhang's concluding speech at the 1985 national conference of chiefs of bureaus/offices of health care). In R. Peng, R. Cai, & C. Zhou (Eds.), *Zhongguo gaige quanshu (Encyclopedia of China's Reform)*, 135–138. Dalian: Dalian chubanshe.

Chen, M. 1999. Chen Minzhang buzhang zai 1998 nian quanguo weisheng tingjuzhang huiyi shang de baogao (The report of Minister Chen Minzhang at the 1998 national conference of office/bureau chiefs of health care). In Zhongguo weisheng nianjian bianji weiyuanhui (Ed.), *Zhongguo weisheng nianjian 1999 (China's Yearbook of Health Care 1999)*, 7–10. Beijing: Renmin weisheng chubanshe.

Cui, Y. 1992a. Cui Yueli tongchi zai yijiu baqi nian guanguo weisheng tingjuchang huiyi shang de zongjie jianghua (Comrade Cui Yueli's concluding speech at the

1987 national conference of chiefs of /bureaus/offices of health care). In R. Peng, R. Cai, & C. Zhou (Eds.), *Zhongguo gaige quanshu (Encyclopedia of China's Reform)*, 155–156. Dalian: Dalian chubanshe.

Cui, Y. 1992b. Cui Yueli tongchi zai yijiu bawu nian quanguo weisheng tingjuchang huiyi shang de jianghua (Comrade Cui Yueli's speech at the national conference of chiefs of bureaus/offices of health care). In R. Peng, R. Cai, & C. Zhou (Eds.), *Zhongguo gaige quanshu (Encyclopedia of China's Reform)*, 129–134. Dalian: Dalian chubanshe.

Ding, Z. 2009. Woguo yiliao weisheng tizhi gaige ying zhengque chuli de jige wenti (Correctly handle several issues in medical and health care reform in China) *Zhongguo weisheng jingji (China's Health Care Economics)*, 11: 5–8.

Du, L. 2007. Hongguan jingji he weisheng fazhan de liangxing xunhuan ho exing xunhuan—ershihnian weisheng zhengce yanjiu huigu (Positive and vicious cycles of macro economy and health care development). In L. Du, W. Zhang, & Zhongguo Weisheng Chanye Zazhishe (Eds.), *Zhongguo yiliao weisheng fazhan baogao, No. 3 (The Report of Development of Health and Medical Care in China, no. 3)*, 25–40. Beijing: Shehui kexue wenxian chubanshe.

Duckett, J. 2004. State, collectivism and worker privilege: A study of urban health insurance reform. *China Quarterly*, 177: 155–173.

Fang, P., & Wang, X. 2010. Woguo qiye yiyuan zhuangzhi jizhong moshi de bijiao (Comparison among alternative models of transformation of enterprise hospitals in China). *Zhongguo weisheng jingji (China's Health Care Economics)*, 1: 74–76.

Fayol, H. 1996. General Principles of Management. In J. M. Shafristz, & J. S. Ott (Eds.), *Classics of Organization Theory* (4th ed.), 54–65. San Diego: Harcourt Brace.

Fu, X. 1989. Danqian weisheng gaige de jige xintedian (New characteristics of current health care reform). *Zhongguo weisheng jingji(China's Health Care Economics)*, 6: 15–17.

Gao, Q. 2006. Fazhan yiliao weisheng shiye, weigoujian shehui zhuyi hexie shehui zuogongxian (Develop further the enterprises of medical and health care, contribute to building a harmonious socialist society). In Zhongguo weisheng nianjian bianji weiyuanhui (Ed.), *Zhongguo weisheng nianjian 2006 (China's Yearbook of Health 2006)*, 48–56. Beijing: Renmin weisheng chubanshe.

Gu, X. 2008. *Zouxiang quanmin yibao: Zhongguo xingyigai de zhanlue yu zhanshu (Toward Comprehensive Medical Insurance: Strategy and Tactic of China's New Medical Care Reform)*. Beijing: Zhongguo laodong chubanshe.

Gu, X. 2010. *Quanmin yibao de xintansuo (The New Exploration of National Health Insurance)*. Beijing: Shehui kexue wenxian chubanshe.

Guojia Tigaiwei *et al.*1999a. Guanyu zhigong yiliao baozhang zhidu gaige kuoda shidian de yijian (Opinions concerning the expansion of pilot experiment of the reform of medical care insurance system). In D. Zheng, D. Liu, & B. Zhang (Eds.), *Shehui baozhang zhidu gaige zhinan* (Guidelines for the Reform of Social Insurance System), 104–108. Beijing: Gaige chubanshe.

Guojia Tigaiwei *et al.*1999b. Guanyu zhigong yiliao zhidu gaige de shidian yijian (Opinions concerning the reform of medical care system of staff and workers). In D. Zheng, D. Liu, & B. Zhang (Eds.), *Shehui baozhang zhidu gaige zhinan* (Guidelines for the Reform of Social Insurance System), 100–103. Beijing: Gaige chubanshe.

Guowuyuan. 1994. Yiliao jigou guanli tiaoli (The regulations of management of medical care institutes). *Guowuyuan gongbao* (Bulletin of State Council), 3: 84–89.

Guowuyuan. 1995. Guowuyuan guanyu jiangsu sheng zhenjiangshi, jiangxi sheng jiu-jiangshi zhigong yiliao baozhang zhidu gaige shidian fangan de pifu (The reply of the State Council to the proposal of the pilot reform of medical care insurance system of staff and workers in Zhenjiang municipality, province of Jiangsu and jiu-jiang municipality, Jiangxi province). *Renshi zhengce fagui zhuankan* (Journal of Personnel Policy and Laws), 6: 4–12.

Guowuyuan. 1998. Guowuyuan guanyu jianli chengzhen zhigong jiben yiliao baoxian zhidu de jueding (The decision of State Council concerning the establishment of basic medical care insurance system of staff and workers in urban area). *Guowuyuan gongbao* (Bulletin of State Council), 33: 1250–1254.

Guowuyuan. 2001. Guowuyuan guanyu jianli chengzheng zhigong jiben yiliao baox-ian zhidu de jueding (The decision of the State Council concerning the establish-ment of basic medical care insurance of staff and workers in cities and towns). In Weishengbu Weisheng Fazhi Yu Jiandusi *(Ed.), Zhonghua renmin gongheguo weisheng fagui huibian* (The Collection of Laws and Regulations of Health Care of the PRC), 10–14. Beijing: Falu chubanshe.

Guowuyuan Tigaiban, Guojia Jiwei, Guogji Jingmaowei *et al.* 2000. Guanyu chengz-heng yiyao weisheng tizhi gaige zhidao yijian (The advisory opinion concerning the reform of medical and health care system in cities and towns). *Guowuyuan gongbao* (The Bulletin of State Council), 11: 10–13.

Henderson, G. & Myron, S. 1984. *The Chinese Hospital: A Socialist Work Unit.* New Haven: Yale University Press.

Jin, S., Yao, N., & Chen, Q. 2007. Shequ weisheng fuwu de fazhan (The development of community services). In L. Du, W. Zhang, & Zhongguo Weisheng Chanye Zaz-hishe (Eds.), *Zhongguo yiliao weisheng fazhan baogao, No. 3* (The Report of the Development of Medical and Health Care, No. 3), 212–240. Beijing: Shehui kexue wenxian chubanshe.

Laodong he Shehui Baozhangbu *et al.* 2003. Chengzhen zhigong jiben yiliao baoxian yongyao fanwei guanli zanxing banfa (The provisional measures of management of the scope of drug use for basic medical care insurance of staff and workers in cities and towns). In Guowuyuan Jiuzheng Hangye Buzhengzhifeng Bangongshi (Ed.), *Jiuzheng yiyao guoxiaozhong buzheng zhifeng gongzuo zhinan* (Guidelines for the Tasks of Eradication of Irregular Work Style in Procurement and Sales of Drugs), 74–77. Beijing: Zhongguo fazheng chubanshe.

Laodong he Shehui Baozhangbu, Weishengbu, & Guojia Zhongyiyao Guanliju. 2003. Chengzhen zhjigong jiben yiliao baoxian dingtian yiliao jigou guanli zanxing banfa (The provisional measures of designated medical care institutes for basic medical care insurance of staff and workers in cities and towns). In Guowuyuan Jiuzheng Hangye Buzhengzhifeng Bangongshi (Ed.), *Jiuzheng yiyao gouxiao zhong buzheng zhi feng gongzuo zhinan* (Guidelines for the Tasks of Eradication of Irregular Work Style in Procurement and Sale of Drugs), 68–72. Beijing: Zhongguo fazheng chubanshe.

Lee, P. N. 1987. *Industrial Management and Economic Reform in China, 1949–1984.* Hong Kong, Oxford, and New York: Oxford University Press.

Li, W., & Lu, Z. 2008. Guanyu jiaqiang yiliao jigou shezhe guihua de tantao (Dis-cussion on strengthening the establishment and planning of medical care institutes). *Zhonguo weisheng jingji (China's Health Care Economics)*, 27(6): 26–27.

Li, Y. 1996. Guanyu yiliao jigou guanli tiaoli de jidian yijian (Several opinions on the regulations concerning the management of medical care institutes). *Zhongguo weisheng zhengce (China's Policy on Health Care)*, 2: 30–31.

Ma, A. 2007. Tujin yiliao jigou quanhangye shudi guanli de zhangai yu zhengce cuoshi yanjiu (The obstacles to the promotion of the territory-based management of medical care profession and study of policy measures). *Weisheng jingji yanjiu* (Research on Health Care Economics), 6: 3–8.

Massey, A. 1993. *Managing the Public Sector: A Comparative Analysis of the United Kingdom and the United States.* Aldershot, and Brookfield, VT: Ashgate.

Mintzberg, H. 1983. *Structure of Fives: Designing Effective Organizations.* London, and Englewood Cliffs, NJ: Prentice-Hall International.

Qian, X. 1983. Zai quanguo weisheng tngjuchang huiyi shang de jianghui (Speech at the national conference of office/bureau chiefs). In Zhongguo weisheng nianjian bianji weiyuanhui (Ed.), *Zhongguo weisheng nianjian 1983* (China's Yearbook of Health Care 1983), 41–46. Beijing: Zhongguo weisheng chubanshe.

Qiye Weisheng Ziyuan Youxiao liyong youhua peizhi (ASEM) ketizu. 2001. Fenli guoyou qiye yiyuan de shizhi yu xianshi tantao (The discussion on the substance and forms of separated enterprise hospitals). *Zhongguo weisheng jingji (China's Health Care Economics)*, 20(1): 54–55.

Ren, R. 2007. Chuyu weisheng guihua (The regional health care planning). In L. Du (Ed.), *Zhongguo yiliao weisheng fazhan baogao, No. 3* (China's report of health care development, No. 3), 161–179. Beijing: Shehui kexue wenxian chubanshe.

Schurmann, F. 1968. *Ideology and Organization in Communist China.* Berkeley and Los Angles: University of California Press.

Si, G. 1990. Guanyu weisheng bumen zhili zhengdun shenhua gaige de sikao (Considerations on the further reform and rectification in health care sector). *Zhongguo weisheng jingji (China's Health Care Economics)*, 9: 4–7, 34.

Sil, R. 1997. The Russian 'village in the city' and Stalinist System of Enterprise Management: The Origins of Worker Alienation in Soviet State Socialism. In X. Lu, & E. J. Perry (Eds.), *Danwei: The Changing Workplace in Historical and Comparative Perspective*, 114–144. Armonk, NY: M. E. Sharpe.

Solinger, D. J. 1991. *From Lathes to Looms, China's Industrial Policy in Comparative Perspective, 1979–1982.* Stanford: Stanford University Press.

Straus, K. M. 1997. The Soviet factory as community organizer. In X. Lu, & E. J. Perry (Eds.), *Danwei: The Changing Chinese Workplace in Historical and Comparative Perspective*, 142–168. Armonk, NY: M. E. Sharpe.

Wang, B. 2008. *Zhengfu yiliao guamzhi moshi ghonggou yanjiu* (Research on the Restructuring of Mode of Governmental Control). Beijing: Renmin chubanshe.

Warner, M. (Ed.). 2000. *Changing Workplace Relations in the Chinese Economy.* Houndmills: Palgrave Macmillan.

Weishangbu. 1985. Yiyuan jingji guanli zanxing banfa, xiugaigao (The provisional measure of hospital economic management, revised draft). In Weishengbu Bangongting (Ed.), *Zhonghua Renmin Gongheguo weisheng fagui huibian, 1981–1983 (The Collection of Laws and Regulations of Health Care 1981–1983)*, 485–492. Beijing: Falu chubanshe.

Weishengbu. 1988. Weishengbu guanyu weisheng gongzuo gaige ruogan zhengce wenti de baogao (The report of the Ministry of Health concerning several policy problems in the reform of health care tasks). In Z. Y. Weishengbu Bangongting (Ed.), *Zhonghua Renmin Gongheguo weisheng fagui huibian, 1984–1885* (The Collection of Laws and Regulations of Health Care of the PRC, 1984–1985), 1–6. Beijing: Falu chubanshe, Xinhua shudian.

Weishengbu, PRC. 1992. Caizhengbu, Renshibu, Guojiawujiaju and Guojiaxeiwuju. Guanyu kuoda yiliao weisheng fuwu youguan wenti de yijian (Opinions on the problems regarding the expansion of medical care and health services). In R. Peng, R. Cai, & C. Zhou (Eds.), *Zhongguo gaige quanshe* (Encyclopedia of China's Reform), 177–179. Dalian: Dalian chubanshe.

Weishengbu *et al.*1992. Zhongguo weisheng fazhan yu gaige gongyao, zhengqiu yijiangao (The outline for China's health care development and reform, draft for soliciting opinions). In R. Peng, R. Cai, & C. Zhou (Eds.), *Zhongguo gaige quanshu* (Encyclopedia of China's Reform), 211–220. Dalian: Dalian chubanshe.

Weishengbu & Guojialaodongzhongchu. 1979. Guanyu jiaqiang yiyuan jingji guanli shihdian gongtso di yijian (Opinions concerning the strengthening of pilot work of hospital economic management). *Laodong zhengce he fagui huibian* (The Collection of Policies and Laws of Labor). Beijing: Falu chubanshe.

Weishengbu & Guojialaodongzongju. 1980. Guanyu yiyuan jingji guanli shidian gongzuo de bucong tongzhi (The general supplementary circular concerning economic management of hospitals). *Laodong zhengce fagui huibian* (The Collection of Policies and Regulations of Labor), 563–566. Beijing: Falu chubanshe.

Wu, R., & Chen, J. 1999. Jianli chengzhen zhigong jiben yiliao baoxian zhidu, quanmian tuijin woguo yiliao baoxian zhidu gaige (Build the basic medical care insurance system of staff and workers, propel the reform of medical care insurance system in China). In D. Zheng, D. Liu, & B. Zhang (Eds.), *Shehui baozhang zhidu gaige zhinan* (Guidelines for the Reform of Social Insurance System), 358–374. Beijing: Gaige chubanshe.

Xie, H., & Li, X. 1988. Zouchu kunjing zhenqiang huoli (Step out of the difficult situation, revive vitality). *Zhongguo weisheng jingji(China's Health Care Economics)*, 7: 14–17.

Yang, J., Gao, J., & Ai, P. 2006. Shilun weisheng gaige yu xingzheng tizhi, gonggong caizheng gaige (Tentative discussion on the reforms in health care, administrative system and public finance). *Weisheng jingji yanjiu* (Research on Health Care Economics), 11: 5–8.

Yang, M. M. 1989. Between state and society: The construction of corporateness in a Chinese socialist factory. *The Australian Journal of Chinese Affairs*, 22 (July): 31–60.

Zhonggong Zhongyang & Guowuyuan. 1999. Guanyu weisheng gaige yu fazhan de jueding (The decision concerning the reform and development of health care). In D. Zheng, D. Liu, & B. Zhang (Eds.), *Shehui baozhang zhidu gaige zhinan* (Guidelines for the Reform of Social Insurance System), 43–51. Beijing: Gaige chubanshe.

Zhongguo Weisheng. 2006. Gongli yiliao jigou gaige—ying tupao tizhi jizhi pingjing (Institutional reform of public hospitals—breakthrough of the bottleneck of institution and mechanisms). *Zhongguo weisheng* (China's Health Care), 11: 19–20.

4 Financing Medical Care Services

The health care reform heralds a new era not only in the fundamental restructuring of the role of the state in financial management in the public sector, but also a major shift of financial strategy of health care in the transition to a mixed economy. Funding modes represent various patterns of the allocation of health care resources, directly affecting how health care services are to be rendered. The study will focus on balancing among three funding modes of health care, namely, the government's subsidies, public insurances and user charges through franchising, in light of financial implications for the provision of health care for the period of economic reform.

To gauge the direction and magnitude of this change, the study will first look at the role of the state in financial management of health care in such arenas as subsidies and pricing, taxation and revenue, budgeting and spending control, pricing and regulatory control, among others. The study will also address the question whether or not the changing balance among the three funding sources was attributable to politics. Some analysts suggest that so far the government did not acted timely to rebuild public insurances, nor did it address the government's subsidies to health care in China, diverting health care resources to the other sectors for the sake of pro-growth policy. This is taken mainly as a political act. As a result, both the providing units and patients were made victims of the reform. Therefore, the case of commercialization cannot taken as the sole cause for the failure of health care reform, and, instead, it is the result of overall financial management.[1]

Financing health care is inseparable from the state's macro-management of the economy, and it is often intertwined with other issues of economic policies. It is appropriate for the study to tackle the broad policy implications of financial management in the health care sector. In this chapter, the study will first try to make sense out of the ups and downs of the government's share of health care expenditure and will then deal with public insurances in next chapter, Chapter 5. The issues concerning franchise funding and user charges, characteristic of commercialization, will be briefly touched on here, but extensively discussed in Chapters 7, 8, 9 and 10.

Public finance in the medical care sector

One of the most salient features of China's medical care reform is concerned with the restructuring of financial management, involving in the transformation from a basically subsidized mode of medical care provision to a franchise-funded mode (Liu 2008a: 6–7). Under the centrally planned economy (CPE) prior to economic reform, health care provision was funded by the government. That is to say, the government absorbed the main portion of costs of infrastructure, facilities and equipment, medical personnel, and operation and management; and accordingly, patients received the medical care services either at nominal costs or even free of charge. While all citizens were universally given access to essential medical care services provided at regulated prices, a privileged sector of people who were employed in the public sector were provided with something additional—insurance benefits through their enrollment in public insurance/funding programs such as the Labor Insurance Medical Care (LIMC) and Public Financed Medical Care (PFMC) program (Chen 1988: 232–7; Liu 2008a: 6–7).

Under the new funding mode, namely franchise funding, that is inaugurated during the period of economic reform, health care services are partially subsidized by the state, and partially paid for by users on the basis of differentiation of basic (or essential) medical care services from non-basic types. In other words, users have to pay for part of the expenses in accordance with the basic categories of curative care, examination, tests with medical devices, and dispensary services, while those who can afford to pay extra for upgraded services are open to the choices of the non-basic category of medical care services, e.g., special care services, upgraded drugs, and advanced medical devices. Franchise funding, together with user charges, have to do with a new revenue strategy to answer not only the relative shortage of state financial appropriation but also the rising demands for upgraded health care services during the reform era. Also, the reduction of the share of government subsidies to the providing unit, as has been the case throughout the reform, is often compensated for by an increase of revenue through market transactions on the basis of franchises of various categories of services, ordinary or upgraded (Liu 2008a: 6–7).

Through re-engineering financial management in the health care sector, the balancing among three financial resources has emerged as a much-debated policy issue during the era of economic reform. Some authors take the three as follows: the government, society, and individuals respectively. In operational terms, first, the government refers to those units in the central, provincial and municipal echelons that are held mainly responsible for financing health care services in the reform era. Second, the so-called "society" pertains to public organizations (e.g., labor unions, work units, insurance institutes, etc.) that are in charge of the provision of basically free service financed by welfare fund of the work unit, and/or public insurances (for instance, the LIMC program, PFMC programs, and RCMC programs). It is noteworthy that several public insurances were introduced in 1998 and 2001, 2003 and 2007 during the reform era (Chapter 5). Third, the individual patients shoulder a substantial portion of expenses through user charges or out of pocket payment (i.e., OPP) prior to the reform and they assume heavier financial burden during the reform period (Wang, Cui & Li 2010). Since 1979 the policymakers have entertained the view that user charges are not only a useful tool in enhancing patients' costs awareness, but also an effective instrument for spending control in order to make better use of health care resources (Wang 2002).

It appears that the government continues to play an important managerial and financial role in the delivery of medical care services through the policy of financial subsidies and, meanwhile, maintains a skeleton of budgetary control over the providing units in the ongoing reform era (Weishengbu 1990). As an interpretive scheme, the government, on the spending side, adopts two kinds of financial appropriation to make funds available to the health care sector: direct subsidies and the indirect subsidies. The former are understood as "open subsidies" (mingbu), referring to those subsidies that are made directly to the users to cover part of their expenditure for medical care services, for instance, reimbursement either to public personnel of the government through the PFMC program or to the staff and workers of SOEs through the LIMC program (Gu 2008: 109–29). The latter are often called "hidden subsidies" (anbu), meaning that the government provides financial appropriation to the providing unit through which the medical benefits are passed onto the users (e.g., insurers and patients) at regulated and low prices. In accounting terms, the hidden subsidies include the "special item subsidy" (zhuanxiang buzu) and "differentiated quota subsidy" (chae buzhu). While the "special item subsidy" absorbs the costs of infrastructure, facilities, equipment, and medical devices, the "differentiated quota subsidy" covers current expenditures such as the costs of personnel, operations, and management. And the "differentiated quota subsidy" is normally calculated on a proportional basis, e.g., relative to the number of hospital beds (Weishengbu & Guojialaodongzongju 1979; Weishengbu 1982; Weishengbu 1990). Conceptually speaking, one may take open subsidies and hidden subsidies as equivalent to the government subsidies to the user and to provider respectively.

There have been two major changes in the government's financial role through the health care reform since 1979. Proven to be a landmark in health care reform, first, the government's funding role has changed in the midst of the repackaging of various categories of health care services. In a new classification scheme of the health care benefits and entitlements given in the foregoing analysis (Chapter 2), the government still assumes a major role in subsidizing Category I pure-public health care and, to a lesser extent, Category II quasi-public health care and Category III basic medical care through the hidden subsidies just noted (Ding 2009). Through user charges, the providing units have been able to earn revenue through franchising in Category IV non-basic medical care and to a lesser extent from Category II and III in order to compensate the shrinking share of the state financial appropriation (i.e., hidden subsidies) from the mid-1980s onward.

Second, public hospitals have been able to fetch revenue from franchise services with user charges amid the rapid growth of the drug industry and the increased use of medical devices, as the government has been able to scale down proportionally its financial appropriation to subsidize medical care services. Starting in 1979, the rise of markets for drugs and medical devices has resulted in the visible decline in the government's funding in conjunction with tightening of pricing control over curative care services at the providing unit level (World Bank 1997: 5) (also see Chapters 8 and 9). Overall, the portion of revenue from prescription drugs has stayed relatively high, especially among small-sized hospitals at the county/urban district level or below. Many large and modern hospitals have found it profitable to make use of advanced medical devices to earn extra revenue and maintain their financial balance sheets (World Bank 1997: 42–3). The funding of health care provision is of a managerial concern at the micro level, but it is not separable from the broad context of allocation of health care resources at the macro level, an issue to be tackled below.

Allocation of health care resources

It is germane here to re-examine some broad consensual views among certain Chinese policy analysts on several salient issues concerning the state versus markets in the allocation of health care resources in China. As financial resources are measured in terms of expenditure, some authors observe that, as a general tendency, the growth of health care expenditure has been in line with the GDP since 1979 (Du 2006: 20–31; Liu 2008a). However, not only is the total expenditure in health care services relatively small compared with other countries but also the government has been slow in addressing the disparity between the urban and rural sector. As shown in Figure 4.1, for example, the total expenditure in health care relative to the GDP climbed upward in a slop shape in four phases: the first phase from 3.02 percent in 1978 to 3.62 percent in 1989; the second phase from 4 percent in 1990 to 4.36 percent in 1998, and the third phase from 4.51 percent in 1999 to 4.63 percent in 2008. And for the fourth phase, it hit the mark of 5.15 percent in 2009 for the first time and even higher at 5.36 in 2012. True, in relative terms, the growth of total expenditure for health care in the total of GDP appears slow during the reform, but one cannot dismiss lightly that its observable increments in Figure 4.1 do reflect steady increase of consumption level and purchasing power on the part of users over years. In absolute terms, the total of three funding sources has grown in the midst of the increase of GDP, albeit the share of each has fluctuated over time.

Some policy analysts claimed, from a comparative perspective, that such an increase in expenditure in the health care sector is not fast enough, given that most countries follow the general pattern of increase corresponding with

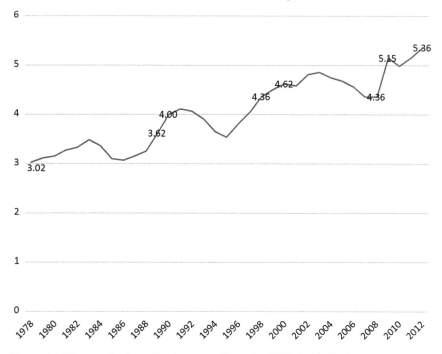

Figure 4.1 The trend of total health expenditure in GDP, 1978–2012

economic growth (Du 2006: 20–31). For instance, China was just comparable with Russia (5.4 percent in 2001) but was obviously behind Brazil (7.6 percent in 2001), both countries being at the same stage of development as China (Ge & Gong 2007: 50–1).

The medical care reform represents a drastic change of funding pattern in terms of balancing of financial contributions among three funding sources as just mentioned. At the starting point of the reform in 1978, contribution to medical care expenditure is divided into three shares among the government, society and individual: 32.13 percent, 47.41 percent, and 20.14 percent respectively as given in Figure 4.2. One of the most striking features concerns the share of individual that reach the historic peak 59.98 percent in 2001, as shown in Figure 4.2. For a whole decade between 1996 and 2005, the percentage of user charges (or OPP) by individuals exceeded the high watermark of 50 percent as indicated also in Figure 4.2. In Ruo Wang's view, the percentage of user charges in per capita health care expenditure goes excessively high at the risk of loss of accessibility as well as equality (Wang 2009: 31).

The salient trends of ups and downs of shares of the government and society deserve further analysis. Referring to Figure 4.2, the shares of two public funding sources, the government and society combined, witnessed drastic shrinkage and then expansion over more than three decades from the late 1970s to the early 2010s. First, as a long-term trend, the government's

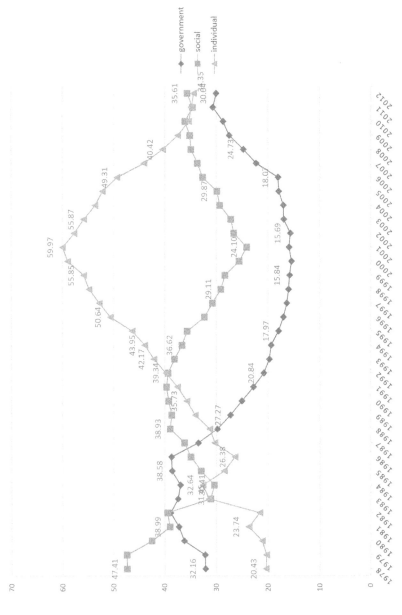

Figure 4.2 Percentages of medical care expenditure in GDP, 1978–2012

share went down for about one half for approximately two decades from 32.16 percent in 1978 to a very low point at 15.84 percent in 2000 and then, moved upward for more than one decade back to 30.04 in 2012, except for some mild fluctuations in between. Similarly, second, the society's share shrank for more than two decades from 47.41 percent in 1978 to the lowest point 24.10 in 2002, and gradually recovered to 34.57 percent in 2012.

With regard to the ups and downs of shares of expenditure in health care among three funding sources as noted in Figure 4.2, Jane Duckett's early study has treated it extensively, raising a number of issues meriting further discussions. Her original focus is on the shrinkage of the shares of two public funding sources of health care until the early 2000s, but she takes note on indications of the state's restoration (i.e. represented by two public funding sources combined) rise from the early 2000s onward (Duckett 2013). Huang also made the same observation on the decline of both the government and society in their shares of expenditure in health care from 1978 to the early 2000s and they surged from the early 2000s (Huang 2014: 64–72).

Duckett's analysis of the relationship between the state and society is in line with some analyses on financing of health care in China cited from various sources. In a broad conception, the role of the "state" is measured in terms of public expenditure, e.g., the total of the public sector (i.e., government's subsidies plus government-sponsored insurances). On the basis of WHO (2004) and UNDP (2004) data sets, China's public expenditure on medical care in proportion to the total of global medical care expenditure is only at 40 percent, one of the lowest points in 2001, considered comparable to 41.6 percent for Brazil but significantly lower than 68.2 percent for Russia, both at a similar stage of development (Ge & Gong 2007: 49–52). According to OECD Health Care Data, one finds overall that in the 1990s the public sector's contribution of health care was weighted higher than 70 percent on average throughout the majority of countries, suggesting a relatively small funding role assumed by the public sector (or the "state") in China (Ge & Gong 2007: 49–52). There were only three countries whose public sector's contribution was less than 50 percent: in Korea's case, 36.6 percent in 1990 and 46.2 percent in 1998; in Mexico's case, 40.8 percent in 1990 and 48.0 percent in 1998; and in America's case, 39.6 percent in 1990 and 44.8 percent in 1998 (Ge & Gong 2007: 49–52).

In an attempt to explain the trend of ups and downs, Duckett appears to work on one brand of the pure rationality model, assuming that the state, an abstract entity, acted upon one well-chosen goal with full knowledge and full capacity available to "cut back" not only budgetary financing, but also engineer retrenchment of public insurance programs. The changing balance among three funding sources is also taken politically as the result of a zero-sum game between the state and society. On the one hand, the state is measured in terms of government's subsidies and public insurances, and on the other, society is represented by share of expenditure by users. As she suggests, other "stakeholders" (meaning users at large) were too weak to assert their interests and resist the state.

In her analysis, Duckett started with the state, seemingly a rational actor in the "pure rationality model" as mentioned, who cuts the budget for health care at will with one stroke. Duckett tries to characterize the decline of public spending in the total of health care expenditure in China with a military metaphor, in which a commander is in the position with his/her full knowledge and control to marshal disciplined troops to take a well-coordinated action—"retreat," for instance. When coming to the concrete policy process, however, she soon shifted from the "pure rationality model" to a version of "government process/organization behavior model," suggesting that the "state" might represent multiple policy actors, and therefore the decline prior to the early 2000s might be attributed to the actions taken by various policy actors in less than coordinated fashion.

Can the trend of ups and downs of funding sources be treated as a zero-sum game in the sense that one sector's gain is made at the expense of the other? In agreement with Duckett, in fact, some analysts from the policy circle in China tend to view the shrinkage of shares of public finance (i.e. government subsidies and public insurances) as something resembling the tension between "have" versus "have not." According to analyst Xu Xiulan, overall, the state's financial appropriation to the health care sector was substantially reduced in order to force the providing unit to earn revenue to sustain itself in a context where doctors, hospitals, pharmacies, and examinations were incorporated into a common body of interests during the reform era. (Xu, 2009: 37). Li Shuxia, Ma Weiwei and Li Shuwen state in 2002 that "A majority of the medical care providing units are not-for-profit institutes built by the governments. However, public hospitals have become commercialized due to inadequate [financial] input and revenue-generating pressure [from the state]." (Li et al., 2002: 18). The 2005 Report also takes a position of dichotomy between the state and markets. The problems affecting the health care sector were mainly created by commercialization, which in turn had been caused by inadequate government subsidies. It underscores that point that the proportion of the government's health care expenditure in the total of national health expenditure dwindled from 36 percent in 1978 to 15 percent in 2000, and correspondingly, the OPP to curative care services had to increase in order to compensate the discrepancy created by the proportional decrease of the total of government's expenditure during the same period (Ge & Gong Sen 2007: 29).

To propose an alternative view to the image of one singular rational actor playing in a zero-sum game, it is appropriate, first of all, to examine the changing balance among the three funding sources in the light of expanding financial pie in the midst of economic growth often measured in terms the increase of GDP. It is noteworthy, for example, that the total expenditure for health care at the national level has been multiplied by 67.87 for 25 years from 11,021 million RMB in 1978 to 759,029 million RMB in 2004 (Wang & Wang 2007: 17–18). Thus, the dwindling of share of public expenditure in health care can only be treated in relative terms. In other words, the shrinkage of share of public expenditure in health care might be read as the slower growth rate of the share of public expenditure relative to accelerated expansion of franchise funding source through user charges. It is evident that in Figure 4.1, percentage of actual health care spending has climbed up steadily as the GNP increases. In absolute terms, one can take that as a whole the government's expenditure on health care has grown as the GDP has been on the increase. Therefore, one cannot take the "state's retreat" in a literary sense.

Furthermore, the study suggests that the government, representing a conglomerate of policy actors in various echelons, adopts a positive interventionist strategy, employing a variety of policy tools, involving a series of policy episodes, and working with shifting priorities at various stages of economic reform in order to lend priority to pro-growth policy and meanwhile, to maintain a measured pace of growth of health care sector. In other words, the government did not act passively to take financial resources away from the health care sector in one stroke, and then put them back into other sectors in order to fulfill a given political agenda. Besides, the government's control over financial input into the health care sector does not mean that it adopts a hand off policy in other closely related policy arenas either. Instead, it has played an active role to address the issues of financing, management, and regulatory control in the health care sector. No less rigorous than the endeavors in promoting pro-growth policy, the government intervened heavily in propelling franchise funding to health care, a policy commonly applied to other spending programs in welfare, educational and cultural arenas (Chapters 7, 8, 9 and 10). Regardless of the changing balance among three funding sources as well as the related financial impacts, one can find such change is more of the issue of managerial and organizational process than the politics dictated by one singular rational actor, and in a zero-sum game. It is represented by an aggregate of statistical results of many accounting items, involving multiple policy episodes rather than one single policy event.

It is noteworthy that among several public insurances, the government was nominally in direct charge of PFMC, but in actual budgetary and accounting terms, PFMC was entrusted to many units positioned in various echelons of the government. Even for PFCM program which was under budgetary and financial control by the government, it was not a simple and easy task to meet challenges to building a set of organizational apparatuses and installing cost containment measures in order to cope with mounting spending pressure. LIMC and RCMC often operated outside the parameter of direct command of the government, and each work unit had considerable say, working with their own budget and account for medical care expenditure, the funding of which depended upon the policy package of compensation, and was often dictated jointly by the work units and supervising authorities at respective levels through a complex set of procedures. Each faced a different set of issues. Neither could a singular organizational unit be held responsible for the decline of public expenditure in health care, nor could a ready-made formula be found for its solution. LIMC needed to be re-structured in view of deficiencies inherent in the work-unit-centered risk pooling design which was funded by welfare fund of each enterprise unit. Moreover, an entirely new risk pooling design to substitute for the breakdowns of RCMC was required to satisfy the health care demands of rural population because of collapse of agricultural collectivization in the early 1980s. Overall, the restoration of the financial role of public insurance funding has to wait until the government could complete its task of re-making of public insurances, including the basic medical care insurance (BMCI) for staff and workers introduced formally in 2001, the New Rural Cooperative Medical Care Insurance(NRCMCI) for the peasants in 2003 and the Urban Resident Basic Medical Care Insurance (URBMCI) for the unemployed, dependents and retirees in cities in 2007 (Chapter 5), in addition to insurance schemes for flexibly employed personnel and agricultural laborers in cities (Gu 2008: 161–72: Wang 2009).

The issue of disparity

The success or failure of China's health care reform has to be assessed with multiple policy goals, among which is equality of allocation of health care resources. The issue of equality is concerned with how to alleviate disparity between various sectors of the economy. As well as being slow to assume its funding responsibility during economic reform, the government was not forthcoming in addressing the two types of disparity of health care provision: one pertaining to the gap between the urban and rural sectors and the other referring to the discrepancy between the large, modern hospitals and the small, inadequately endowed providing units.

According to Geng Ying et al., there has been a serious imbalance in the allocation of health care resources between urban and rural areas: for a long period, the government's financial input tended to pour into the urban areas, which consisted of 30 percent of the total population, while the rural areas, with 70 percent of the population, had been long neglected up to the 2000s (Geng, Pei & Legge 2009: 12–13). As they add, moreover, health care resources (in both quantity and quality) tended to flow towards those geographical areas close to power centers or those institutes that were ranked at a higher status in the administrative hierarchy of the CPE. Conversely, those rural regions that were remote from power centers often gain a share of 20 percent of the health care, while the cities and towns that were close to power centers have a large portion at 80 percent (Geng, Pei & Legge 2009: 12–13).

The government did not act quickly to fill the gap of risking-sharing mechanisms between urban and rural residents until recent two decades, leaving the latter largely unprotected and vulnerable to illness, especially of catastrophic nature. The weakening of government-sponsored insurance schemes was due largely to the collapse of rural cooperative medical care (RCMC) programs inadvertently resulting from agricultural de-collectivization and the introduction of household undertaking (contracting) system. A set of statistics shows that rural residents who are taken as OPP categories and without public insurance totaled 87.3 percent in 1998 and was subsequently reduced to 76 percent in 2003. In contrast, the urban residents who did not subscribe to any public insurances stood at 44.1 percent in 1998 and 44.8 percent in 2003 (Zhonghua renmin gongheguo weishengbu 2012: 175).

Partly due to limited government subsidies and partly because of a low-income level, rural people can't afford to spend as much on medical care services as their urban counterparts. Therefore, the disparity between urban residents and rural peasants persists. The State Statistics Bureau provides a set of data regarding the average expenditure of individuals from 1990 to 2012, indicating considerable disparity between the rural and urban people as follows: per capita health expenditure of each individual in rural areas is only 24.11 percent of that of urban areas (38.8 RMB versus 158.8 RMB) in 1990 and registers considerable improvement to 37.9 percent (214.7 RMB versus 813.7 RMB) in 2000. It returns to a low level again, namely 23.62 percent (358.11 RMB versus 1,516.29 RMB) in 2007, and 28.12 percent (1055.89 RMB versus 2,969.01RMB) in 2012 (State Statistics Bureau, PRC, China Statistics Yearbook 2013, Beijing, Zhongguo Tongji Chubanshe, 2013: 769).[2]

Like other lower income and vulnerable sectors of population, the peasantry would likely be hit hard with a high percentage of OPP. Huang Xiaoping et al. produced a set of statistics indicating the pattern of an excessively high percentage of OPP by individuals. In relative terms, the share among the individual's payment, the government's health care input, and the society's health care input in rural China are: 80.73 percent, 12.54 percent, and 6.73 percent respectively in 1991, and the pattern of excessively high individual payments relative to the government input and the society's input in heatlh care worsen even after more than one decade: 88.72 percent, 6.53 percent, and 4.85 percent respectively in 2005. It appears that rural residents were completely left alone in facing the odds of medical care issues while the government's input was proportionally cut at about one half—from 12.54 percent in 1991 to 6.53 in 2005, well before the NRCMCI had been introduced (Huang & Fang 2008: 20–3).

Moreover, many policy analysts provide evidence to confirm this observation with regards to considerable suboptimal allocation of health care resources among the public hospitals within cities. An estimate by Zhao Yuxin suggests that from 1990 to 2003, the weight of health care expenditure tends to tilt in favor of advanced and higher graded hospitals, for instance, from 32.76 percent in 1990 growing to 51.16 percent in 2003, albeit it slides down slightly below 50 percent in 2006 (Zhao et al. 2008: 358). Covering 2002 and 2005 respectively to demonstrate the over-representation of city hospitals in the allocation of health care resources, Du Lexun's statistics indicate that in the year 2002, the government's appropriation (measured in term of health care expenditure) to public providing units consists of 67.68 percent, the breakdown of which includes 50.52 percent for city hospitals, 8.7 percent for county hospitals, 0.45 percent for urban community health care centers, and 7.26 percent for rural health care clinics; in the year 2005, 65 percent was given to the providing units, including 50.09 percent for city hospitals, 7.36 percent for county hospitals, 0.77 percent for urban community health care centers, and 6.26 percent for rural health care clinics (Du 2008: 370–1). As of 2006, furthermore, urban community health centers and rural health care clinics were only given a negligible percentage. Zhao cites the figures of 2006 indicating that in the total of expenditure of providing units that stands at 64.67 percent, the breakdown of which is 49.26 percent for city hospitals, 7.30 percent for county hospitals, 1.11 percent for urban community health centers, and 6.45 for rural health care clinics (Zhao et al. 2008: 358).

Financial reform and funding of health care services

The foregoing analysis has examined the issue of advantages or disadvantages which various organizational units encountered in re-engineering health care provision. In light of the government politics model, one may treat these organizational actors (e.g., government, units in higher versus lower echelons, big hospitals versus small hospitals, urban residents versus rural peasants) as "winners" or "losers" in the new budgetary and financial game of the reform era. The study will demonstrate in the remaining that the "load shedding" practices—high echelons pushing responsibility of essential curative health care and public health care to lower echelons without lending adequate financial support—is a matter of government process featuring incongruence among policy goals and lack of coordination among government units.

The phenomenon of load shedding did not take place in isolation, and it occurred in in conjunction with the introduction of the revenue raising policy. Yanzhong Huang borrows from Avery Goldstein in the study of policy-making in China, observing the cases of both "bandwagon" and "passing buck" phenomenon covering not only the policy episodes of extraordinary times such as the Cultural Revolution but also ordinary times when social policy was given priority (Huang 2014). It is noteworthy that in the midst of the financial reform during the economic reform, the contagious phenomenon of "passing buck" took place simultaneously with the "bandwagon." The former pertains to "load shedding" in terms of pushing responsibility downward to lower echelons, albeit retaining financial resources in the same echelon as much as possible. The latter refers to endeavors to propel those revenue-generating programs, such as URS among others, and encourage providing units to go commercialized.

As a part of the readjustment policy in the post-Mao era, sovereign planners introduced financial reform in two phases—in 1980 and then in 1994—delegating considerable managerial power to provincial jurisdictions, albeit with dwindling portion of revenue to the provincial/local governments (Ge and Gong 2007: 26–8). In a broad context, the financial reform is pivotal to the restructuring of the CPE, in one way or other, affecting the balance between the public sector and non-public sector, causing the strains of central-provincial relations, and exacerbating the tensions of the role of government in a wide range of health care issues from basic (or essential) curative care services to public and preventive cures among others (Yang, Gao & Ai 2006).

The first phase of financial reform began in 1980 when the central government introduced a "financial undertaking system" (caizheng chengbaozhi, or abbreviated as FUS hereafter) to allow each provincial jurisdiction to retain a share of revenue commensurate with its assigned responsibilities through five schemes on the basis of either a fixed rate or a classification of various categories of revenue and expenditures or both.[3] The second phase commenced with the "revenue-sharing system" (fensuizhi; abbreviated as RSS hereafter) in 1994 (Ge & Gong 2007: 28–31). It is argued that the transformation from the first phase to the second phase was warranted in order to stop further erosion of the financial strength of the central government (Chen 1988: 296–9). The RSS allocated a given amount of revenue to each government in a respective echelon according to the well-defined categories of tax that each enjoys (Yang, Gao & Ai 2006: 6–7). Also, the RRS ensured a greater share of revenue to be returned to the central government through fixing two sets of figures: the percentage of revenue of the central government in overall GDP and the share of central government in the national total of revenue (Ge & Gong 2007: 26–8).

From FUS introduced in 1980 to RSS initiated in 1994, there witnessed a drastic decline of the provincial/local government's share, from a range between the lowest at 59.5 percent (1984) to the highest at 78 (1993) percent during the 1980-1993 period, to that between the lowest at 44.3 percent (1994) and the highest at 50.6 percent (2011) during the 1994–2011 period, as cited in China's Yearbook of Finance (Zhongguo Caizheng Zazhi She 2012: 459–60). On average, there was a shrange of share of the local governments about 20 percent before and after the watershed of 1994, meaning that the provincial/local government had to work with much tighter budget after 1994.

With needed adjustments to FUS, the RSS was able to turn the tide of the continuing decline of financial strength of the central government against the provincial and local governments. As a final result, through financial reform in the name of the FUS and RSS, the central government held respective jurisdictions accountable for their own revenue and loss. Paradoxically speaking, this encouraged better management and entrepreneurship in the public sector by providing incentives to each jurisdiction through the retention of an amount of funds in proportion to saving practiced or revenue generated, forcing each provincial or local jurisdiction to undertake development projects in spite of proportionally smaller share of finance than that before the financial reform starting in 1980 and 1994. (Liu 2008a).

Although the central government was a big winner in financial reform of 1980 and then 1994, it only allowed itself to play a small role in maintaining equitable distribution of health care resources among provincial jurisdictions.

As indicated in the estimate by Chen Chunhui et al., the central government's share of the expenditure for health care enterprises remained mostly within a narrow range between the lowest, 1.49 percent in 2000, and the highest, 2.84 percent in 2003, while as a whole the provincial governments' share of the expenditure for health care enterprises consisted of more than 97 percent throughout the period of 1993–2003 (Huang & Fang 2008). It is not expected that, given a very small budget for health care, the central government was in a position to address the issue of disparity across regions or among provinces within the annual financial appropriation (Ge & Gong 2007; Chen & Zhou 2009a; Chen & Li 2010). From a comparative perspective, the Chinese local governments assume an exceedingly large role in public health. The nearest country cases were in Australia, whose regional governments (equivalent to provinces in China) contributed 45.42 percent of the national total in public health expenditure in 1997, and the USA, whose regional governments (i.e., states, equivalent to provinces in China) contributed 33.59 percent of the national total of the same in 1997 (Ge & Gong 2007).

There was a severe shortage of funding to public health care services and curative care services at the macro level during the reform era (Li 2007). Three features deserve close observation as follows: first, during several watershed years, namely 1985, 1988, and 1994, the financial reform resulted not only in dwindling share of revenue to the provincial/local government, but also in fragmentation and inequality among various jurisdictions; second, the role of higher level governments, especially the central government, in the transfer of payments across jurisdictions was considerably weakened, leaving public and preventive care of those underdeveloped jurisdictions poorly financed. For example, the central government had in its possession only approximately 10 percent of the total of national expenditure for health care, welfare and education, causing a shortage of funding for needed help to poor and underdeveloped regions in the realm of public health care, education, and other welfare programs; third, the shifting priority in economic growth reinforced by performance measurements pushed various jurisdictions to support pro-growth projects and thus drained the funding sources available to public health care services drastically (Qiao 2009). This led to a situation where the local governments at the county level and below were lacking needed funding support to public health care services (including both Category I pure-public health care and Category II quasi-public health care), and to considerable extent, basic curative care. In what is taken as "load shedding," through the financial reform, the responsibility of health care services was transferred down echelon by echelon to the rural county/urban district level and/or below, but the funding did not go downward accordingly (Yang & Sun 2006: 71–3).

After the introduction of RSS in 1994, how was the financial management structured at the provincial level and below? To answer the question, one finds, first of all, that there was a tendency to "pass the buck" with regard to the pressure of downward transfer of financial burden from provincial level to municipal/local level, from the bureau to the providing unit level, and even from the government to users (Du 2006: 71). Some studies suggest that the county and township level assumed heavy financial responsibility for health care services, estimated as 55 to 60 percent of the total of budgeted expenditure (Chen & Zhou 2009a: 16). Another survey of three provinces in 2003 indicates that on average the provincial government was responsible for 12.93 percent of health care expenditure while the remaining 87.07 percent is shouldered by the governments at the municipal level or below (Chen & Zhou 2009a: 16). As a rule, the local governments in low echelons were assigned with the responsibility of health care tasks but not given sufficient funds to carry them out. And, there was no consistency in the standards of personnel and fixed quota of public financing across regions. As a result, there is considerable disparity of funding of public health services among various regions (Chen & Zhou 2009a: 17).

Another issue concerns the relative shortage of funding for the operational and program-centered functions in the public health care arena. As a matter of accounting procedure, overall, the health care institutes tended to cover personnel costs and current expenditures on maintenance often at the expense of other non-recurrent expenditures for services delivery.[4] Given severe financial stringency, the lower echelons normally gave priority to personnel costs and current expenditures, often at the expense of program enforcement (Du 2006: 40–1). It was not unusual, as a consequence, that the enforcing units often find no funding to provide specific items of service, while personnel, equipment, and/or building space remain idle (Du 2005: 7).

Financial stringency in lower echelons

Questions arise among policy analysts about how the decline of the government's share of revenue affects the allocation of health care resources in lower echelons (Yang et al. 2006; Ge & Gong 2007: 28–31; Liu 2008a; Liu 2008b; Wang 2009). To deal with the issue of the provision of public health care, Wang Xiufeng argues that contrary to the original intent of the revenue sharing system (i.e., RSS as introduced in 1994), two persistent problems prevented the central government from playing an effective role in financing the provision of collective goods (e.g., especially Category I and Category II; see Chapter 2). First, one finds the delivery of collective goods exceedingly difficult because the workload was pushed downward, echelon by echelon, to local governments without adequate financial support (Chen & Zhou 2009a). Second, the central government and provincial governments were very slow to establish the rules, regulations, standards, and measures regarding the system of financial transfer and thus were not able to stop the trend of enlarging financial disparity among local jurisdictions (Li et al. 2002; Wang 2009: 12; Ding 2009: 7).

It is well known that the government's funding to the public health care programs has been proportionally curtailed ever since the inauguration of the health care reform (Li et al. 2002; Cai 2004: 12; Du 2006; 35–44). According to Du Lexun et al., there was a substantial reduction of the share of public health care expenditure in the total of the government's appropriation from 1990 to the early 2000s because of the shortage of overall funding to health care in general and budgetary and accounting considerations in particular (Du 2006: 35–44). The 2005 Report cited two national surveys indicating a visible reduction of the proportion of the government's financial input in the total revenue of the public health care providing units in urban areas, going from 46.2 percent in 1994 to 38.8 percent in 1997 and, in rural areas, going from 40.2 percent in 1994 to 34.8 percent in 1997 (Ge & Gong 2007: 30). Moreover, the expenditure on public health care in the total of financial expenditure went up in the 1980s and then followed a downward trend from the early 1990s onward: 3.2 percent in 1980, 3.7 percent in 1990, 3.5 percent in 1995, 2.7 percent in 2000, and 2.6 percent in 2002 (Ge & Gong 2007: 30).

In fact, financial support for public health care remained fluctuating and not stable, and it always fell short of the requests. As a result, many related programs could not be carried out. Overall, there registered a decline of the government's subsidies to public health from the 1990s to the early 2000s, when the government began to make effort to improve the situation. According to the data from the 2005 Report, for instance, the government appropriation to the preventive care institutes (e.g., those providing Category I pure-public health care services) consisted of 59.1 percent of the total requested sum in 1990, 38.66 percent in 2000, 39.29 percent in 2001, 42.08 percent in 2002, and 47.31 percent in 2003. In the case of health care units working with women's and children's programs (falling into Category II quasi-public health care services), the government appropriations of the total request were 56.11 percent in 1990, 37.13 in 2000, 37.01 in 2001, 38.67 in 2002, and 40.05 in 2003 (Ge & Gong 2007: 41).

Many sets of statistics available highlight the negligence of public health care up to 2003, as obviously demonstrated in the SARS (Severe Acute Respiratory Syndrome) incident, albeit the central government has, since then, taken drastic steps to beef up the funding to the public health care sector (Chen & Zhou 2009b). Minister of Health Gao Qiang admitted in July 2005 that the preventive health care system remained neglected and poorly funded.[5] He stressed, above all, that the government did not have mechanisms in place to ensure adequate funding to preventive care at the basic levels of the government. Consequently, the basic level providing units had to engage in revenue-generating activities in order to raise more than half of the funds required to sustain the existing level of public health care services (Gao 2007: 49).

Nevertheless, there has been a new trend of drastic increase of health care expenditure by the central government, which started after 2003. For example, an available group of statistics suggests that there registered a considerable increase of health care expenditure by the central government in total from 2003 onward: 5.4 percent in 2003, 6.0 percent in 2004, 8.9 percent in 2005, 9.4 percent in 2006, and 33.6 percent in 2007 (Chen & Zhou 2009a: 17). This initial increase of the central government's health care expenditure has raised the issue regarding the magnitude and consistency of policy to alleviate the financial shortage in lower echelons of provincial jurisdictions. In spite of the visible growth of health care expenditure by the central government from 2003–2007 as noted, Chen Chunhui cast doubt on how much the low echelons could receive financial help in a timely fashion in view of the lack of workable measures of financial transfer and the established priority to cover the costs of maintenance and personnel at the lower levels of the local jurisdictions (Chen & Zhou, 2009a: 17).

Focusing on the issue of commercialization, mainly of curative care, dispensary services, and medical devices, for example, the 2005 Report argues that the financial reform has resulted in the curtailment of the share of government expenditure in health care, and consequently has forced providing units to pursue "economic objectives" only. That is to say, public hospitals need to increase charges to the users (patients and insurers) in order to ensure revenue return and thus to maintain budgetary balance (Ge & Gong 2007: 153–4).

In relative terms, overall, the increase of public expenditure in health care has not been able to match economic growth in China for more than three decades. In policymakers' observation, this is attributable to the deficiency of the "compensating mechanism" to the providing unit (Chen 1992: 186–8; Gao 2007: 35–36; 51). The 2005 Report actually points to a long-term trend that formally began with the introduction of economic management in 1981 (with relevant pilot programs starting earlier in 1979) and continued up to the adoption of the financial undertaking system in 1989, through which the government was no longer responsible for revenue and loss of medical care institutes, allowing public hospitals to earn revenue through a variety of services and to tie it to remuneration and benefits of staff and workers (Ge & Gong 2007: 153). In a coherent way, Wang Xiufeng, policy analyst affiliated with the Health Care Economics Research Institute of the MOH, summarizes the situation as follows:

> The budget has become tightened because of the state's effort to concentrate capital input on economic construction; owing to the decentralization of power amidst the financial institutional reform, the health care expenditure that was originally given to the ministerial jurisdictions of the central government have been listed instead as part of the expenditure of local governments [since the reform era]; the relative weight of financial appropriation to the health care sector has been on the decline because of the strains of local finance. Moreover, the health care sector has to face the issue of how to handle fundraising in light of rising commodity prices. Therefore, the health care reform actually has evolved as

part of the strategy [of health care sector] in its fight for survival. (Wang 2009: 11) (Translation supplied.)

Above all, franchise funding mode is proven to be an effective financial tool, but it does not address its policy implications (e.g., affordability and equality) in the allocation of health care resources at the macro level. For instance, the 2005 Report takes note of several behavioral attributes of commercialization, for example, the providing unit's orientation as an entity for the pursuit of "independent interests" as well as the shift of emphasis from the concern of "social utility" to the pursuit of economic interest (Ge & Gong 2007: 153–4). In managerial terms, moreover, various authors find the increase of OPP to curative care and dispensary services warranted in order to fill the gaps created by the proportional decrease of the total of the government's health care expenditure during the same period. It is admitted that the public hospitals' revenue-generating behavior was one kind of adaptive behavior "forced" by the government's failure to provide sufficient funding for the delivery of public goods (Gao 2007: 30–1).

Concluding analysis

The foregoing analysis focues on the role of marketization in balancing among three funding sources to health care. The study specifically points out that the franchise funding mode does play an important role in improving resource management and ensuring a reliable revenue flow to finance the provision of curative care services at the providing unit level, but it produces significant consequences on the allocation of health care resources at the macro level, not only aggravating the inequality between various sectors of the population but also posing as a challenge to the fulfillment of the goal of affordable care.

The study argues that it is analytically difficulty to separate the markets from the state. In fact, commercialization does rely upon market transactions as key mechanisms, but it requires the government's intervention to be operational, for instance, franchising, user charges accompanying price control, a re-structured budgetary system among others (Chapters 7, 8, 9 and 10). Theoretically speaking, the study argues that re-engineering financial management does have bearing on affordability of medical care. Over more than three decades, the trends of two public funding sources, state subsidies and public insurances, have first experienced shrinkage, and subsequently growth, and these trends can be better explained and appreciated through the government process model rather than the government politics model, e.g., the disintegration of public insurance programs in both urban and rural areas, and the separation of policy responsibility from funding in the lower echelons within provincial/local jurisdictions. As the foregoing analysis has tackled the issue of government subsidies, re-inventing medical care insurances deserves further analysis in next chapter.

Notes

1 For example, the Development Research Center of the State Council put forth a report on China's health care reform in July 2005 (abbreviated as the 2005 Report hereafter), claiming that commercialization (or marketization) should be held responsible for "failures" of China's health care reform on the basis of an evaluation of a mix of multiple goals. Ge, Yanfeng, the principal investigator of the 2005 Report, suggests in retrospect that the view of the research team was misinterpreted with reference to their attribution of failures of health care reform only to commercialization according to the first part of their research results publicized in summer 2005 (Ge & Gong Sen 2007: 1–3).

2 The percentages about the ratios between the urban and rural residents are calculated and provided by this study.

3 The five schemes are as follows. The first scheme divided the total of the revenue pie according to a fixed rate on an annual basis, covering three directly municipalities such as Beijing, Tianjin and Shanghai. The second scheme was based upon so-called "classification of revenue and expenditure, and undertaken by governments at various echelons" (huafen shouzhi, fenjibaogan) that assigned fiscal responsibility to the central and provincial jurisdictions by categories of revenue and expenditure, covering a majority of provinces. The third scheme depended upon a calculation in accordance with a classification of revenue and expenditure in addition to a fixed quota of remittance or subsidies, including Guangdong and Fujian. The fourth scheme was an arrangement applying to remote and backward provinces such as Inner Mogolia, Xinjiang, Xizhang (Tibet), Ningxia, Guangxi, Yunnan, Qinghai, and Guizhou. The scheme concerned fixed subsidies calculated according to a classification of categories and rates of revenue and expenditure. The fifth scheme that applied to Jiangsu Provinces was a fixed quota of financial revenue determining the amount of financial remittance to the central government. See Dangdai Zhongguo Congshu Bianjibu 1988: 291–4; according to Ge and Gong, the trial implementation of financial reform led to a variety of versions, e.g. "undertaking calculated according to increments of revenue", "retained revenue based upon the total and increments", "undertaking depending upon increments of remittance", "fixed subsidies" etc. (Ge & Gong Sen, 2007: 28–31).

4 The financial appropriation to the public health sector is based upon the method of "fixed number of personnel and fixed quota," namely a fixed sum for expenditure on personnel plus a fixed quota for current expenditure (often calculated from a proportion of personnel costs) (Chen & Zhou 2009a:17).

5 According to Gao, the system was of considerable scale and complexity, being manned with the strength of 200,000 personnel and administered by the governments from the central to provincial, municipal, and county levels. He stated that the qualifications and training of personnel were less than adequate while the equipment, laboratory, testing devices, and monitoring facilities were in acute shortage. And he attributed the cause of the problem to the overall shortage of health care resources and poor allocation of health care resources (Gao, 2007: 49–50).

References

Allison, G. T. 1971. *Essence of Decision: Explaining the Cuban Missile Crisis.* Boston: Little, Brown and Company.

Allison, G., & Zelikow, P. 1999. *Essence of Decision: Explaining the Cuban Missile Crisis* (2nd ed.). New York: Longman.

Cai, R. 2004. Woguo weisheng fazhan mianlin de tiaozhan he jiyu (The challenges and opportunities of the health care development in China). *Weisheng jingji yanjiu* (Research on Health Care Economics), 12: 14.

Chen, C., & Li, S. 2010. Woguo zhongyang caizheng weisheng zhuanyi zhifu fangshi tantao (Discusion on the transfer of payment of health care in finance of the central government in China). *Zhongguo weisheng jingji (China's Health Care Economics)*, 29(1): 5–7.

Chen, C., & Zhou, J. 2009a. Woguo caizheng gonggong weisheng zhichu zhengfu jian fudan jiegou fenxi (An analysis of inter-governmental structure of financial burden of public health care expenditure in China). *Zhongguo weisheng jingji (China's Health Care Economics)*, 28(8): 15–17.

Chen, C., & Zhou, J. 2009b. Woguo caizheng gonggong weisheng zhichu zhengfujian fudang fenxi (An analysis of the structure of burdens among goverments in the expenditure of public health care in China's public finance). *Zhongguo weisheng jingji (China's Health Care Economics)*, 28(8): 15–17.

Chen, M. 1992. Chen Mingzhang buchang zai quanquo weisheng tingjuchang huiyi shang de zongjie jianghua (Minister Chen Mingzhang's concluding speech at the national conference of chiefs of bureaus/offices of health care). In R. Peng, R. Cai, & C. Zhou (Eds.), *Zhongguo gaige quanshu* (Encyclopedia of China's Reform), 184–190. Dalian: Dalian Chubanshe.

Chen, R. (Ed.). 1988. *Dandai zhongguo caizheng, shang* (Financial Administration in Modern China, volume 1). Beijing: Zhongguo shehui kexue chubanshe.

Dai, D. 1993. Shencengci weisheng gaig de gousi (Thoughts on health care reform at a deeper level). *Zhongguo weisheng jingji(China's Health Care Economics)*, 2: 26–28.

Dangdai Zhongguo Congshu Bianjibu (Ed.) 1988. *Dangdai zhongguo caizhang, shan* (Finance in Contemporary China, volume 1). Beijing: Zhongguo shehui kexue chubanshe.

Ding, Z. 2009. Woguo yiliao weisheng tizhi gaige ying zhengque chuli de jige wenti (Correctly handle several issues in medical and health care reform in China). *Zhnogguo weisheng jingji (China's Health Care Economics)*, 11: 5–8.

Du, L. 2008. Zhongguo weisheng zongfeiyong liuxian de gainei fenxi he zhengce jianyi (A preliminary analysis and policy proposal on the flowing direction of total health care expenditure). In L. Du *et al.* (Eds.), *Zhongguo yiliao weisheng fazhan baogao No. 4* (The Report of Development of China's Medical and Health Care, No. 4), 368–372. Beijing: Shehui kexue wenxian chubanshe.

Du, L. 2006. *Zhongguo weisheng yiliao weisheng fazan baoguo, No. 2* (The Report of Development of China's Medical and Health Care, No. 2). Beijing: Shehui kexue wenxian chubanshe.

Du, L. 2005. Woguo gonggong weisheng touru jiqi jixiao pingjia (Input and performance evaluation of public health care in China). *Zhongguo weisheng jingji(China's Health Care Economics)*, 24(11): 5–8.

Duckett, J. 2013. *The Chinese State's Retreat from Health*. London and New York: Routledge.

Gao, Q. 2007. Fazhan yiliao weisheng shiye, wei goujian shehui zhuyi hexie shehui zuochu gongxian (To develop medical and health care enterprises, make contributions to build a socialist and harmonious society). In Zhongguo weisheng nianjian bianji weiyuanhui (Ed.), *Zhongguo weisheng nianjian 2007* (China's Health Care Yearbook 2007), 48–56. Beijing: Renmin chubanshe.

Gao, Q. 2006. Fazhan yiliao weisheng shiye, weigoujian shehui zhuyi hexie shehui zuogongxian (To develop further the enterprises of medical and health care, contribute to building a harmonious socialist society). In Zhongguo weisheng nianjian bianji weiyuanhui (Ed.), *Zhongguo weisheng nianjian 2006* (China's Yearbook of Health Care 2006), 48–56. Beijing: Renmin weisheng chubanshe.

Gao, Q. 2007. Weishengbu buzhang Gao Qiang zai quanguo chengshi shequ weisheng gongzuo huiyi shang de zongjie jianghua (Minister of Health Gao Qiang's concluding speech at the national conference of community health care work). In Zhongguo weisheng nianjian bianji weiyuanhui (Ed.), *Zhongguo weisheng nianjian 2007* (China's Yearbook of Health Care 2007), 33–37. Beijing: Renmin chubanshe.

Ge, Y., & Gong, S. 2007. *Zhongguo yiliao gaige: Wenti, genyuan, chulu* (China's Health Care Reform: Problems, Roots and Solutions). Beijing: Zhongguo fazhen chubanshe.

Geng, Y., Pei, L., & Legge, D. 2009. Zengjia zhengfu touru tigao yiyao weisheng fuwu de gongpingxing he kejixing (Improve equality and accessibility of health care services through the increase of governmental input). *Zhongguo weisheng jingji (China's Health Care Economics)*, 28(3): 12–18.

Gu, X. 1993. Shichang jingji yu weisheng gaige (Market economy and health care reform). *Zhongguo weisheng jingji(China's Health Care Economics)*, 3: 21–24.

Gu, X. 2008. *Zouxiang quanmin yibao: Zhongguo xingyigai de zhanlue yu zhanshu* (Toward Comprehensive Medical Insurance: Strategy and Tactic of China's New Medical Care Insurance Reform). Beijing: Zhongguo laodong chubanshe.

Guangdongsheng Weishengting. 1993. Shenhua weisheng gaige, tansuo shiying shichang jingji xuyao de xintizhi (Further health care reform, in search of the new institutions to meet the needs of market economy), 4: 13–15.

Huang, X., & Fang, Q. 2008. Woguo caizheng weisheng zhichu quyu chayi yan jiu (Research on regional difference of medical expenditure in China's finance). *Zhongguo weisheng jingji (China's Health Care Economics)*, 27(4): 20–23.

Huang, Y. 2014. *Governing Health in Contemporary China*. London & New York: Routledege.

Li, S., Ma, W., & Li, S. 2002. Woguo yiliao weisheng zhichu de gonggong zhengce yanjiu (A study of public policy on the expenditure of medical and health care in China). *Zhongguo weisheng jingji (China's Health Care Economics)*, 21(7): 17–18.

Li, Y. 2007. Zhengfu dui yiyuan de touru fangxiang he yunxing jizhi de tansuo yu chuangxin (Discussion as well as innovation concerning the direction of government's input to hospitals and operating mecnanisms). In L. Du, W. Zhang, & Zhongguo Weisheng Chanye Zazhishe (Eds.), *Zhonguo yiliao weisheng fazhan baogao, No. 3* (The Report of Development of Medical and Health Care in China, No. 3), 180–193. Beijing: Shehui kexue wenxian chubanshe.

Lieberthal, K. & Oksenberg, M. 1988. *Policy Making in China: Leaders, Structures, and Process*. Princeton, NJ: Princeton University Press.

Liu, J. 2008a. Gaige kaifan sanshi nianlai woguo zhengfu weisheng touru ji zhengce huigu (The health care input and policy review of the Chinese government for the last 30 years of reform and opening up). *Weisheng jingji yanjiu* (Research on Health Care Economics), 1: 3–9.

Liu, J. 2008b. Weisheng touru de zhengfu zeren ju jiegou youhua (The government's responsibility as well as structural optimizing of health care input). *Weisheng jingji yanjiu* (Research on Health Care Economics), 6: 3–7.

Qiao, J. 2009. Gonggong weisheng fuwu jundenhua yu zhengfu zeren:Jiyu woguo fenquanhua gaige de sikao (The equalization of public health care services and responsibility of the government: Some thoughts on the basis of China's reform of decentralization). *Zhongguo weisheng jingji (China's Health Care Economics)*, 28 (7): 5–7.

Wang, M. 2002. Yiliao feiyong kongzhi youguan wenti tantao (Some discussion on the problems of control over medical care expenses). *Zhongguo shehui baozhang* (China's Social Security), 11: 15–16.

Wang, R. 2009. Zhongguo chengzhen yiliao tizhi gaige qianhou de yiliao rongzi bijiao (Comparison of medical care financing before and after the medical care reform in cities and towns in China). *Zhongguo weisheng jingji (China's Health Care Economics)*, 28 (1): 30–34.

Wang, X. 2009. Weisheng gaige 30 nian licheng huigu (To review the process of health care reform for three decades). *Weisheng jingji yanjiu* (Research on Health Care Economics), 1: 10–13.

Wang, Y. & Wang, W. 2007. Kuaishu shangzhang de yuliao feiyong yu kanbienlan kanbiengui wenti (The problem of rapid rise of medical care charges as well the difficulty to seek cure and expensiveness to seek cure). In Chen, J. & Wang, Y. *Zhongguo shehui baozhang fazhan baogao* (The Report on Development of Social Security in China). Beijing: Zhongguo shehui kexue wenxian chubanshe.

Wang, Y., Cui, X., & Li, C. 2010. Cong "kanbinggui" wenti kan woguo yiliao baozhang zhidu de biange jiqi cunzai de wenti (To examine the problem of "expensiveness in seeking cure" in light of the change and existing issues of medical care insurance system in China). *Zhongguo weisheng jingj (China's Health Care Economics)*, 29(2): 19–22.

Weishangbu. 1990. Yiyuan caiwu guanli banfa (The measures of hospital financial management). In Weishengbu Zhengce Faguisi (Ed.), *Zhonghua renimin gongheguo weisheng fagui huibian 1986–1988* (The Collection of Laws and Regulations of Health Care of the PRC, 1986–1988), 1006–1023. Beijing: Falu chubanshe.

Weishengbu. 1982. Guanyu jiaqiang zhishu ji shuangchong lingdao shiye danwei caiwu guanli gongzuo de shixing banfa (The provisional measure of the task of financial management regarding the service units of directly affiliation and under dual command). In Zhonghua Renmin Gongheguo Weishengbu Bangongting (Ed.), *Zhonghua renmin gongheguo weisheng fagui huibian 1978–1980* (The Collection of Laws and Regulations of Health care of the PRC 1978–1980), 630–634. Beijing: Falu chubanshe.

Weishengbu. 1988. Weishengbu guanyu weisheng gongzuo gaige ruogan zhengce wenti de baogao (The report of the MOH concerning several policy problems in the reform of health care tasks). In Z. Y. Weishengbu Bangongting (Ed.), *Zhonghua renmin gongheguo weisheng fagui huibian, 1984–1885* (The Collection of Laws and Regulations of Health Care of the PRC, 1984–1985), 1–6. Beijing: Falu chubanshe, Xinhua shudian.

Weishengbu, PRC. 1990. Yufang baojian sihixing youshang fuwu de huigu yu sikao (A review and observations on the implementation of paid services in preventive care). *Zhongguo weisheng jingji (China's Health Care Economics)*, 6: 26–28.

Weishengbu, PRC. 1992. Weishengbu guanyu jiaqiang jihua mianyi baochang guanli gongzuo de yijian (The opinion of the ministry of health concerning the strengthening of the managerial work of planned immunization insurance). In R. Peng, R. Cai, & C. Zhou (Eds.), *Zhongguo gaige quanshu* (Encyclopedia of China's Reform), 206–207. Dalian: Dalian chubanshe.

Weishengbu et al. 1993. Weishengbu, caizhengbu, renshibu, guojiaweijiaju, guojiaxeiwuju guanyu kuoda yiliao weisheng fuwu yaoguan wenti de yijian (The opinion of the Ministry of Health Care, Ministry of Finance, Ministry of Personnel, State General Bureau of Pricing, State General Bureau of Taxation concerning several problems in the expansion of medical and health care services). In Weishengbu Zhengce Faguisi (Ed.), *Zhonghua renmin gongheguo wiesheng fagui huibian, 1989–1991* (The Collection of Laws and Regulations of Health Care of PRC, 1989–1991), 10–11. Beijing: Falu chubanshe.

Weishengbu & Guojialaodongzhongchu. 1979. Guanyu jiaqiang yiyuan jingji guanli shihdian gongtso di yijian (Opinion concerning the strengthening of pilot work of hospital economic management). *Laodong zhengce fagui huibian* (The Collection of Policies and Laws of Labor). Beijing: Falu chubanshe.

World Bank. 1997. *Financing Health Care: Issues and Options for China.* Washington, DC: World Bank.

Xu, X. 2009. Gongli yiyuan buchang zhengce pinggu yanjiu (Research and evaluation on compensation policy of public hosptials). *Zhongguo weisheng jingj (China's Health Care Economics)*, 28(9): 35–39.

Yang, H., & Sun Naqiang. 2006. Weisheng gaige yu fazhan de pingjia yu jianyan (The evaluation and examination of health care reform and development). In L. Du (Ed.), *Zhongguo yiliao weisheng fazhan baogao No. 2* (The report of Development of Medical and Health Care in China No. 2), 47–85. Beijing: Shehui kexue wenxian chubanshe.

Yang, J., Gao, J., & Ai, P. 2006. Shilun weisheng gaige yu xingzheng tizhi,gonggong caizheng gaige (Some tentative discussions on the reforms in health care, administrative system and public finance). *Weisheng jingji yanjiu* (Research on Health Care Economics), (11): 5–8.

Zhao, You Xing, *et al.* 2008. 2006 nian woguo weisheng zongfeiyong cesuan jieguo yu jiben weisheng fuwu chouzi fangan (The results of estimate of total expenditure of health care and fundraising plans for basic health care services in the year of 2006). *Zhongguo weisheng jingji (China's Health Care Economics)*, 27(4): 5–10.

Zhongguo Caizheng Zazhishe 2012. Zhongguo caizheng nianjian (China's Yearbook on Finance). Beijing: Zhongguo caizheng zazhishe.

Zhonghua Renmin Gongheguo Weishengbu. 2012. *Zhongguo weisheng tonji nianjian 2012* (China's Health Care Statistics Yearbook 2012). Beijing: Zhongguo xiehe yiike daxue chubanshe.

5 Re-inventing medical care insurances

To study affordable medical care in China, it is germane here to dwell on the role of public insurance/funding programs in alleviating the financial burden of medical care on the people in the midst of transition from the CPE to a mixed economy. For nearly four decades since 1979, China's medical insurances have gone through different paths of transformation, and each experienced some measure of disintegration, remedial endeavors, and finally rebuilding. The chapter tries to trace the long process of change of public insurances from the phase of disintegration and weakening during the Maoist period to the rebuilding in the midst of economic reform, demonstrating how they contributed to the balancing among several funding sources from 1979 to the present. During the economic reform era, the re-inventing of the medical care insurance/funding system has been path-dependent, starting with the baseline of three conventional insurance/funding programs: Labor Insurance Medical Care (LIMC), Public Financed Medical Care (PFMC), and Rural Cooperative Medical Care (RCMC). The first endeavor in health care reform aimed at establishing a Basic Medical Care Insurance (BMCI) program for employed personnel in the planned sector. An enhanced BMCI package finally took shape with supplementary insurance added to cover catastrophic medical events; and it began full-scale implementation by the early 2000s. Meanwhile PFMC, with considerable amendments, continued to operate to provide medical care to civil servants and members of other public organizations. Among the new designs of medical care insurances there was included a new Rural Cooperative Medical Care Insurance (NRCMCI) program starting in 2003, which targeted at the vast rural population throughout China. Also, in 2007, the government made a final attempt to introduce Urban Resident Medical Care Insurance (URBMCI) programs, extending to all urban residents, either low-income residents or the unemployed, including students, retirees, redundant and unemployed workers. This chapter will be devoted to an analysis of the origins and evolution, designs and main features and implementation of these insurance/funding programs.

Legacies of public financing programs during the planned economy

As a prelude to the full-scale reform, sovereign planners concentrated on streamlining and rebuilding Public Financed Medical Care (PFMC) for public personnel (e.g., civil servants, employees of service work units, members of political parties and other public organizations) and Labor Insurance Medical Care (LIMC) programs for staff and workers employed by SOEs after the devastations during the Maoist period. Conceptually speaking, two programs represented a form of medical care benefits that constituted an integral part of the compensation package under the CPE. In China, PFMC is comparable to, and maybe better than, LIMC, with regard to the similar categories of benefits and entitlements. One may treat PFMC as a proto-insurance scheme, for it did, and still does, function as a set of mechanisms to absorb the financial risk of health issues of public personnel. Strictly speaking, however, the PFMC depends on tax revenue as a main funding source, and it does not rely on mechanisms of pooling risks through a collection of premium contributions by the multitude of enrollees. A survey indicated in the early phase of the economic reform the funding of medical care among various sectors of urban residents in the year of 1986 as follows: 16.23 percent in PFMC, 45.64 percent in LIMC, 24.18 percent in the partially subsidized category (dependents of public employees), and 13.94 in the self-paying category (Zheng 2002: 132).

Medical care benefits were formally introduced to the public sector in the early 1950s, representing a substantial part in a large package of various types of entitlements in accordance with the Regulations of Labor Insurance (hereafter, the 1951 Regulations; amended in 1953) (Dangdai Zhongguo Congshu Bianjibu 1987:302–7; Bian 1994:177–208). Here LIMC covered main category of medical care for both inpatient and outpatient services, funded by the Medical and Health Care Fund (MHCF) representing a significant portion of the welfare fund at the enterprise level (Dangdai Zhongguo Congshu Bianjibu 1988: 212–13). Also, public enterprises absorbed one half of the expenses for the dependents of staff and workers when making use of the services provided by public hospitals; and, as an option, they enjoyed coverage of expenses for diagnosis and treatments when seeking cure in enterprise-managed facilities and hospitals, as well as in contracted medical care clinics outside (Dangdai Zhongguo Congshu Bianjibu 1987: 316–17; Dangdai Zhongguo Congshu Bianjibu 1988: 235–7).

According to policy analyst Zheng Gongcheng, one may conceptually treat medical care benefits as one form of "work unit insurance" (or enterprise insurance), operating with a set of risk-pooling mechanisms on the organizational scale of an enterprise unit and supported by contributions deducted from the employees' wage fund (Zheng 2002: 126–7). Economic reform formally brought social security benefits, including medical care benefits, for collective-owned enterprises (COEs) from 1977 onward (Dangdai Zhongguo Congshu Bianjibu 1987: 329–31). By 1984, 17 million staff and workers of

COEs—or 62.9 percent of the total—had been included in social security schemes (including medical care) comparable to those of SOEs (Dangdai Zhongguo Congshu Bianjibu 1987: 330).

Parallel to LIMC, PFMC then covered expenditures for medical care for public personnel at the essential level, including clinical visits for outpatients and hospital care for inpatients (Dangdai Zhongguo Congshu Bianjibu 1987: 310–14). In September 1952, the government, for the first time, authorized funding to cover medical care for spouses and children of public personnel. Furthermore, in another policy paper promulgated in September 1955, the PFMC program offered children and dependents of personnel the option to choose either a "unified funding" scheme or a self-payment scheme, coupled with financial assistance through the welfare fund of the work unit (Dangdai Zhongguo Congshu Bianjibu 1987: 311–2).

It is noteworthy that both LIMC and PFMC were inaugurated in the 1950s, but time was too short for the said two programs to complete the follow-ups in building needed rules, procedures, and mechanisms for implementation within a short time span about one decade from the 1950s to 1960s. Major managerial problems then were entangled with the weakening of central command and coordination, the rise of a multi-centered power structure as well as the fragmentation of managerial power resulting from decentralizing financing medical and preventive care from the central level to the provincial and local levels starting from 1953 (Zheng 2002: 120–1). As of 1998, according to an overall trend, the percentages in the total of the funding for medical care in various echelons of the government were as follows: 9 percent for the central level, 18 percent for the provincial level, 27 percent for the prefecture/municipal level, 34 percent for the county level and 12 percent for the township level (Wang 2002: 104–5).

In addition, financial management was not in place while LIMC and PFMC were being implemented, producing a runaway increase in expenditure. By the early 1960s, PFMC program expenditure always exceeded budgetary limits by large margins in the absence of accountability and effective control measures.[1] Moreover, the issues of financial control over medical care spending arose due to the varying standards of pricing as well as the scope of services, catalogs of drugs, and norms for devices (Wang 2000: 104–5). According to Zheng Gongcheng, the issue of spending control was also aggravated in the midst of an expanding scope of coverage, the pressure for wage reforms, an increase in population size, and a changing economic environment during the reform era (Zheng 2002: 126).

The two programs each were confronted with challenges of a different kind after Mao. Although the PFMC program faced the pressure of over-spending despite a relatively stable funding source, namely tax revenue, the LIMC program appeared to have lacked a reliable funding source to sustain itself, often depending on the economic performances of various enterprises (Guojia Tigaiwei et al. 1999). This means that under the LIMC, a sizable number of staff and workers of SOEs might go under financially, making it considerably difficult to gain access to the BCMI benefits in the industrial sector (Zhang 1999; Peng 1999; Guojia Tigaiwei et al. 1999). The issue of PFMC was mainly spending control. For example, the expenditure for PFMC is reported in 1982 to have exceeded the budgetary limit by 3,700 million RMB (Dangdai Zhongguo Congshu Bianjibu 1988:234–5; Zheng 2002: 121–9). It is estimated that, taken together, the expenditure for medical care increased by 20 percent on average annually from the early 1980s to the late 1990s (Peng, Cai, & Zhou 1992: 16–17).

Also, a number of new factors increased pressure to overhaul public insurances. For example, the quest for better compensation and improvement in the standard of living reinforced the tendency toward an unauthorized expansion in the scope of benefits and entitlements, the broadening of parameters of reimbursement, and propelling of unfettered growth in expenditure for health care services. Furthermore, some over-charges and other financial abuses worsened as hospitals and medical personnel needed to generate revenue by taking advantage of increased medical demands in the changing health care market during the early phase of the economic reform.[2]

Spending control and risk-pooling mechanisms

Since sovereign planners did not have a master plan for establishing the basic medical care insurance (BMCI) program, it ended up evolving over a long stretch of time with key components added to the designs bit by bit. It started to cover the main body of the labor force employed in the public sector, and then extended to the periphery of urban residents who are dependents, retirees, partially employed, and unemployed. Under the circumstances, sovereign planners had to explore first the measures of spending control and then new funding options to meet the rapidly growing expenditure. Long before launching pilot programs for medical care insurances during 1994–1998, policymakers had been able to accumulate considerable hands-on experience with spending control issues (Liu & Liu 1999:87; Song & Liu 2001: 89–90; Zheng 2002: 131–9; Yang 2004: 106; Zheng 2011: 17–20). One may identify a number of policy precedents and early designs of organizational, managerial and financial tools proposed, tried and employed by various government units as follows:

- Establishing a PFMC office or managing committee each separate from the respective bureaus of various jurisdictions (Peng, Cai, & Zhou 1992: 17–18);[3]
- Experimenting with financial accountability systems, e.g., the "undertaking" (baogan) system to hold the work unit, hospital management and funding unit accountable for expenditures (Song & Liu 2001: 90; Zheng 2002: 134–5);
- Listing and categorizing methods for the control of the rapid increase in demand and thus spending pressure for basic medical care (Dangdai

Zhongguo Congshu Bianjibu 1988; 233–5; Cheng 1999: 397; Cheng et al. 2002: 120–33; Zheng, Gao & Yu 2010: 17–18); and

- Launching pilot experiments for spending control measures such as deductibles, co-payment, and ceilings in both the PFMC and LIMC programs (Song & Liu 2001: 89; Zheng et al. 2002: 133).

As one of the most remarkable policy initiatives, sovereign planners made use of an insurance design, namely, risk-pooling mechanisms, to establish a funding system with two distinct features: first, a conceptual distinction from ordinary government revenue, and second, building institutional and managerial autonomy separate from the government. Taken as "social unified funding" (shehui tongchou; hereafter, SUF), public insurances represented risk-pooling mechanisms operating through a collection of contributions from a multitude of employers and employees in a mixed economy.[4] However, the organizational design of the public insurances fund does not follow a corporate form in China today; and it nonetheless represents a non-governmental public body characterized as a "quasi-foundation" (benjijin) by policy analyst Zheng Gongcheng (Zheng et al. 2002: 122).

During the late 1980s and early 1990s, there were two policy precedents regarding funding design leading to experiments in and establishment of risk-pooling mechanisms at later stages of reform (Zheng, Gao, & Yu 2010: 18–19). First, there were reform initiatives to build up the SUF providing medical care expenditure for retired personnel (including those retirees on the "leave for recuperation" program, known as liuxiu) in such places as the municipality of Mushi in Shantong Province and the municipality of Jingxi in Liaoning Province.[5] Second, the often-cited case of the Vegetable Company of the East City District in Beijing represented an embryonic design of risk-pooling mechanisms for funding catastrophic medical events (Zheng 2002: 136). In 1992, the Ministry of Labor started to solicit opinions on medical care social insurance at the enterprise level and to authorize the trial implementation of SUF for major illnesses.[6] Subsequently, Dandong, Shiping, Huangshi, Zhuzhou, and other cities adopted SUF pilot programs, extending further to 20 municipal jurisdictions, covering 3,746,000 staff and workers by the end of 1994 (Zheng 2002: 133).

In order to promote SUF pilot programs for a "major illness," policymakers had to come to terms with the issues of conceptualizing and defining operationally "major illness," placing emphasis on spending control. Here the term, "major illness" (dabing) refers to a medical event involving high expenditure, literally "medical care for large sum expenditure" (dae feiyong yiliao), underscoring the concern of cost containment (Liu & Liu 1999: 62–4; 87). An early classification scheme of medical care services with three zones emerged amidst the experiments with the SUF programs as follows:

- Zone I: clinical care that involves a relatively small expenditure;
- Zone II: hospital care that requires a relatively large expenditure; and

- Zone III: catastrophic medical events pertaining to potentially uncontrollable expenditure.

Falling in Zone II and III mentioned above, both the insurance program for retired personnel and the SUF program for "major illnesses" among staff and workers grew in their enrollments from 1993 to 1996. On the basis of a compiled statistical set, the results for both programs were impressive: for example, enrollees for the former enjoyed rapid growth from 225,182 in 1993 to 664,715 in 1996, and those for the latter from 2,679,094 in 1993 to 7,911,835 in 1996 (Zheng 2002: 137–8). By the early 1990s, moreover, policymakers had accumulated a considerable number of policy precedents for spending control and funding modes, laying the foundation for a draft program of basic medical care insurance for working people in the planned sector.

Basic medical care insurance in the planned sector

Tracing the origin of the basic medical care insurance (BMCI) package, one discovers that short of a master plan, the early BMCI design for staff and workers only evolved through a series of pilot programs and policy experiments (Zheng et al. 2002: 119–59; Deng 2008: 106–10; 2002; Zheng 2010: 18–20; Chen & Yi 2011: 1–56). In the final form, an enhanced BMCI package was offered to all eligible enrollees at a later stage, with supplementary insurance added, in order to cover Zone II hospital care and Zone III catastrophic medical events. It was for full-scale implementation beginning in 2001 through to the present.

Seen from a broad perspective, policy advocates for the BMCI package position themselves within a spectrum of opinions ranging from the pro-market view to the pro-state position, as they address issues regarding the choice of type of medical benefits, modes of funding, and ways of management (Du 2008: 72–96; Du et al. 2008: 1–31). The pro-state position enjoyed considerable saliency in the drafting of the BMCI package. For example, Guan Zhiqiang, Cui Bin, and Don Chaohui underscore the importance of the state in dealing with both the positive and negative "externality," minimizing "market failure" and maximizing the utility of public health policy (Guan, Cui & Don. 2007: 48–51). As noted by Gu Xin, the role of the state is prominent in the field of basic medical care insurance from the angle of public finance (Gu 2010: 1–36).

The present study argues that rather than "retreat," the state has actually reasserted its active role not only in public policy in general but also in public finance in particular through the health care insurance reform during the era of economic reform. To a certain extent, nonetheless, policymakers have incorporated market mechanisms into the institutional apparatus and managerial system of public insurances subsumed under the state hierarchy. By design, the BMCI reform intended to lend the state a prominent role not only to fulfill health care policy goals but also to produce "collective goods"—enhance labor mobility, maintain a healthy, productive labor force, and control risks while competing in expanding markets, and absorbing the spillover social costs of economic growth in China (Song & Liu 2001: 114–16).

It is evident that the state addressed the choice of what kind of insurance entitlements ought to be made available to people while re-engineering affordable medical care policy. As mentioned in the 1994 Opinion, sovereign planners took a stand on four major policy goals to guide drafting of the BMCI. First, in terms of type of service, they opted for a "basic" (or essential) medical care insurance. Second, they aimed at broadening the scope of insurance enrollment to go beyond the CPE, by including initially all employees in both public and non-public sectors rather than only the public sector, and eventually even the unemployed, retirees, students and children, and low-income earners. Third, they intended to adopt co-insurance for both employers and employees to substitute for the "work unit insurance" (or taken as enterprise insurance) the premium of which was paid for solely by the work unit. Fourth, they chose a combination of personal account (PA) and unified social funding account (USFA), integrating a personal saving scheme with a risk-pooling mechanism while covering both outpatient and inpatient services.[7]

To policymakers, affordable health care means an essential level of services funded by public medical care insurances. As there were several ways to define "essential" (i.e., basic) medical care covered by BMCI as noted in Chapter 2, sovereign planners became practical, giving considerable weight to the financial consideration of the state.[8] A basic level amounts to a "low level." Wu Ritu and Chen Jinfu, ranking officials of the Ministry of Labor and Social Security, advocated for the "low level" curative care insurance, simply meaning to treat the financial capacity of all parties involved in realistic terms. Wu and Chen added that benefits and entitlements for essential curative care should be set at a low level in light of the burden of public enterprises regardless of their financial status.[9]

Furthermore, the volume of premium contributions and expenditure ought to be compatible with the overall financial capacity of the country, which must take precedence over user demands in light of the level of productivity at a given stage of economic development in China. Some policy analysts cited Hainan Province as an illustration for the operational definition of "low level." For instance, the newly proposed medical care insurance was committed to the target of being lower than then exiting PFMC and LIMC in three areas: the level of premium contributions, the level of expenditure, and the growth rate of the revenue of the providing unit (compatible with the ability of the insured to pay) (Gao 1999: 383).

In light of both medical and financial considerations, policymakers at the central and provincial/local levels followed an interpretative scheme with regard to the three types of services that bore on the choices of various insurance packages as just noted. They included clinical care (outpatient services) in Zone I, hospital care (inpatient services) in Zone II, and catastrophic medical events in Zone III (Wu 2013: 61). In policy papers issued in 1994 and 1996, Zone I and Zone II were included in the funding scheme, but not Zone III. In financial terms, Zone I and Zone II combined were equivalent to the package of services covered originally by the early designs of PA-USFA, while Zone III was optional—subject to availability of funding and approval of the head of the work unit in charge—on an ad hoc basis. In accounting term, Zone III covers expenditure that exceeds the ceiling of payment of the early designs of PA-USFA.

For purposes of financial management, sovereign planners decided to install two accounts in the BMCI package, by adopting a combination of PA and USFA. In accordance with the 1994 Opinion, the amount of funding for BMCI should not exceed 10 percent of the total wage bill, beyond which approval from the respective financial department of the government would be required. As sovereign planners could not entirely rule out financial crises involving the BMCI, the 1994 Opinion recommended preparing for contingencies by making use of other funding sources as needed, including: first, tax revenue for BMCI benefits for civil servants and members of public organizations such as the personnel of service units, political parties and associations, etc.; and second, retained revenue (part of which was often converted into "welfare fund") to support insurance for staff and workers employed by public enterprises (Guojia Tigaiwei et al. 1999).

Proponents of BMCI saw five merits in insurance funding: first, it was "social," meaning a larger scale of funding than that had previously been made available through work unit insurance. The BMCI represented a set of risk-pooling mechanisms on a relatively large scale, going beyond enterprise insurance and making it possible to absorb a large financial burden. And, it intended to maintain balance among numerous enterprise units, and to coordinate mutual assistance among the multitude of enrollees in a time of need. Second, it was a co-insurance scheme allowing both the employer and employees to make their respective financial contributions. For the PA-USFA design, both the individual user and the employing work unit, in principle, had to pay a share of the contribution; as a rule, the work unit was required to pay at least 50 percent (Guojia Tigaiwei et al. 1999: 101). As in the pilot programs of Jiujiang and Zhenjiang municipalities, contributions for the PA-USFA followed the guideline of setting aside 10 percent of the total average annual wage as well as funding for retirement payment (Guowuyuan 1995). Third, PA-USFA represented a set of risk-pooling mechanisms allowing not only a pool of financial resources for mutual sharing on the horizontal level, but also a reservoir of funding based upon personal savings on the vertical level. Through the BMCI, not only did USFA build a large-scale funding reservoir to meet expenditures for hospital care and other costly services (which remained undefined then), but also PA provided savings to prepare for the aging of the population (Wu & Chen 1999: 364–6). The funding sources still followed existing channels of financial appropriation depending on the status of the public organization.[10] Fourth, the PA-USFA incorporated mechanisms for saving not only to ensure the stability of the insurance fund but also to forestall the crashing financial burden of an aging society. As PA design relied heavily on personal savings, USFA required premium contributions for long years, say, 10 or 15 years, prior to eligibility for insurance entitlements. Fifth, BMCI included payment schemes connecting the funding system tightly to spending control measures and to enhancing the effective operation of the funding design. For example, a patient was required, as a spending control measure, to pay a fixed portion at each step in the payment schedule (i.e., co-payment, deductible, and ceiling), meanwhile ensuring the insured would pay less progressively while moving from small and less costly items to larger, more expensive items.

For the first time, the 1998 Decision put on the policy agenda the establishment of supplementary medical care insurance (SMCI) programs in public enterprises originally under LIMC to cover Zone III, and coupled them with a comparable subsidy scheme for civil servants and members of some other public organizations under the PFMC, in accordance with a policy paper subsequently circulated in 2000 (Guowuyuan 1999). With this enhanced BMCI package (armed with SMCI) in its final shape and ready for implementation, Zone I was covered mainly through PA and user charges, while Zone II and Zone III relied heavily on USFA with its mechanisms of financial risk-pooling on a relatively large scale.

Catastrophic medical events and the enhanced BMCI package

During the drafting process from 1994 to 1998, sovereign planners confronted a dilemma when having to choose between the early BMCI package on the one hand and catastrophic medical events on the other hand. The former represented one brand of affordable care, focusing on common and frequent illnesses while addressing the medical demands of outpatients for clinical visits in Zone I and inpatients for hospital care in Zone II (Wu & Chen 1999: 364–7). The latter mainly addressed expensive catastrophic illness in Zone III (Guojia Tigaiwei et al. 1999). In terms of premium contributions, the former was considered more costly than the latter. Prior to the policy experiments of the BMCI starting in 1994, various jurisdictions were only able to focus on a design to help public enterprises cope with financial crises caused by rapid growth of medical care expenditure and uncontrollable amount of catastrophic medical cases. As policymakers began their pilot programs concerning the early BMCI, they instead focused on Zone I and Zone II, the areas originally covered by PFMC and LIMC.

Overall, policy analysts suggested that in the early BMCI package, the PA-USFA design financially embraced Zones I and II, and it was less costly than the entire range of medical care services provided by either the PFMC or LIMC program (Cheng et al. 2002: 153–9). According to an estimate made in 1996, the total premium payment of the proposed version of BMCI would amount to only 70 percent of the total expenditure of the then-existing PFMC and LIMC programs combined, meaning that the level of the PFMC and LIMC exceeded the level of BMCI by 30 percent, equivalent to 20 billion RMB (Zhang 1999; Wu & Chen 1999: 369; Wang 2000: 132–5). In accordance with the 1994 Opinion, however, the early BMCI package did not address the most expensive catastrophic medical care cases in view of the insufficient funding for the said gap (e.g. the 30 percent just noted).

As soon as the economic reform commenced, in fact, there were enterprises facing financial ruin when encountering—even with a very small number of staff and workers—exceedingly expensive catastrophic medical care cases. Although cases of catastrophic illness were small in percentage, they involved relatively high costs when all expenditures were added up. As cited by Wang Dongjin, a survey from the late 1990s era indicates that expenditures of 696,000 users for medical care insurance exceeded the ceiling of pilot programs in various jurisdictions, and this was 0.5 percent of the total of the patients in the survey (Wang 2000: 132). It was also noted that, on average, the expenditure of these users for medical care services exceeding the ceiling of payment amounted to an average 10 percent of the total expenditure, ranging between 6 to 16 percent across jurisdictions, a margin posing as significant financial risks to the stability and continuity of the proposed BMCI (Wang 2000: 132).

Accordingly, policymakers entertained four proposed types of supplementary medical care funding. The first type was concerned with the "large medical care expenditure subsidy" (daer yiliao feiyong buzhu; hereafter, LMCES), which was targeted for catastrophic medical care events, often covering expensive items exceeding the ceiling of USFA (Wang 2000: 129). The idea of LMCES was tested in a policy experiment in two cases. One was Xiamen municipality, which the author was able to visit personally, where LMCES was entrusted to a commercial insurance company on a contractual basis (Liu 2004: 160–86; Interview 2002a; Interview 2002b; Interview 2002c). The other was the pilot program of Zhenjiang, which represented the majority of jurisdictions across the nation, where a social insurance institute (a non-departmental public entity) took charge of LMCES (Wang 2000: 129). After 2001, many jurisdictions began to introduce LMCES in conjunction with the early BMCI design. Cited in a set of internal references, 76.67 percent of the 30 municipal jurisdictions surveyed adopted LMCES up to 2002 (Deng 2008: 119). As reported in early 2002, each user's annual premium contribution to LMCES, on average, was about 60 RMB in full, paid either by enrollees themselves or by employing work units or, in some cases, by both (Deng 2008: 119). The LMCES absorbed about 85 percent of the "large amount expenditure" exceeding the USFA ceiling while enrollees paid for the rest (Deng 2008: 119).

The second type of SMCI pertains to supplementary enterprise medical care insurance (qiye buchong yiliao baoxian; hereafter, SEMCI), which aims at filling the gap between the lower standards of BMCI and the existing, higher standards of enterprise-managed medical care of well-to-do enterprises. The SEMCI follows the same consideration of the medical care subsidy to public personnel (gongwu renyuan yiliao buzhu; hereafter, MCSPP) since the existing level of medical care insurance for public employees is to be maintained regardless of the lower level of basic medical care services prescribed by the BMCI reform. To put it plainly, sovereign planners choose to recognize and perpetuate the privileged benefits and entitlements of this generation of staff and workers who have already worked under CPE. According to the 1998 Decision: "as a transitional measure, enterprises are permitted to establish supplementary enterprise medical care insurance (SEMCI) in order not to lower the level of consumption of medical care by staff and workers in some specific trades, provided that they participate in the basic medical care insurance (BMCI)." (Guowuyuan 1998). The 1998 Decision further states that SEMCI was allowed to charge to the welfare fund account up to 4 percent of the supplementary wage. However, if 4 percent of the supplementary wage was found to be inadequate, the remaining amount would be charged to production costs upon approval by the bureau of finance at the respective administrative level within the jurisdiction (Guowuyuan 1998; Deng 2008: 119–200).

As just mentioned, the third type has to do with the medical care subsidy to public personnel (gongwu renyuan yiliao buzhu; hereafter, MCSPP) established early on and reconfirmed in accordance with the 2000 Opinion issued by the Office of State Council. The 2000 Opinion underscored the need to maintain medical care entitlements to public personnel at the existing level of compensation in the respective jurisdiction, compatible with economic development and financial capacity (Laodong Baozhangbu & Caizhengbu 2000). In a timely fashion, the policy of MCSPP enjoyed enthusiastic responses from various jurisdictions throughout China. For example, 43.3 percent had adopted and implemented MCSPP as of the year 2002, according to the statistics of 30 municipalities (Deng 2008: 119). Various jurisdictions tried to make better, creative use of MCSSP to stretch it to cover some defined benefits. In Hunan Province, for example, MCSPP covers cases bordering on catastrophic nature: clinical treatments for selected cases of serious diseases, part of the co-payment for drug prescriptions, and special treatments and uses of medical devices, among other types of coverage (Deng 2008: 119).

As a general principle, the 2000 Opinion also detailed the conditions for implementing MCSSP, addressing the issue of catastrophic medical care events with the explicit purpose of controlling, if not minimizing, expenses exceeding the USFA payment ceiling for public personnel across various jurisdictions (Laodong Baozhangbu & Caizhengbu 2000). Meanwhile, in operational terms, sovereign planners enforced spending controls with the introduction of MCSSP, for example, in the listing of each item of expenditure required in the relevant prescription catalogs, in the lists of medical care services, and in the criteria for using medical devices, in addition to well-designed payment schemes, featuring deductible, co-payment, and ceiling of spending, etc. (Laodong Baozhangbu & Caizhengbu 2000). Of course, there is the fourth type of SMCI which provides extra protection to enrollees, and, it is funded through commercial insurance programs so long the enrollees and employing work units find it financially feasible.

In retrospect, as policymakers were in search of an insurance option less costly than conventional public insurances such as LIMC and PFMC, they could have chosen between two packages: *either* the early design of BMCI *or* an insurance package for catastrophic medical cases only. As it turned out, they chose both for the employed in the planned sector. In fact, they found themselves unable to retreat from the high level of expenditure set by the preceding programs. For the full-scale, country-wide implementation starting in 2001, they settled on an enhanced BMCI package incorporating PA-USFA plus SMCI. In contrast, they chose an insurance package for catastrophic medical cases only, a less expensive option, for those insured enrollees belonging to the non-planned sector, a topic to be tackled immediately below.

Basic medical care insurances for the non-planned sector

As soon as sovereign planners had successfully dealt with the enhanced BMCI package for employees in the planned sector by the early 2000s, they lost no time addressing medical care insurance for two other groups of people belonging to the non-planned sector. Accordingly, they put forth two health care insurance plans as follows: the New Rural Cooperative Medical Care Insurance (NRCMCI) for peasants introduced in 2003 and the Urban Resident Basic Medical Care Insurance (URBMCI) for unemployed and low-income personnel beginning in 2007. Both represent a state building process—the advance of the state to the health care sector. In policy terms, one may consider these insurance plans as ones for the residual categories of people not covered by the enhanced BMCI. Some authors even take the enhanced BMCI, NRCMCI and URBMCI together as the three key components of China's medical care insurance system. These insurance plans accompanied the building of primary care services in health care centers at the urban community level and in health care stations at the rural village level (Ma & Gui 2012).

Furthermore, the said two insurance plans share a number of commonalities with the enhanced BMCI version, for example, the funding mode using a risk-pooling mechanism, the standard spending control measures and the managerial and operational tools associated with marketization within the public hospital system. However, they differ from the enhanced BMCI version in that they do not intend to cover the comprehensive range of services (including Zone I, II and III) as covered by the enhanced BMCI package. The two plans instead place emphasis on "large expenditure" cases such as hospital care in Zone II and catastrophic medical events in Zone III. Overall, they are more affordable, as enrollees are required only to pay a smaller premium for these insurance plans in view of the stress of catastrophic medical events, characteristic of its narrow coverage albeit prohibitively high expenditure for each case.

After introducing NRCMCI in 2003 and URBMCI in 2007 respectively, sovereign planners endeavored to clarify and reaffirm the policy priority of major illness in the implementation of two medical care insurances in the 2012 Advisory Opinion.[11] In this document, for instance, the State Development and Reform Commission (SDRC) and another five ministerial units address the need for major illness insurance in the entire system of national medical care insurance, and underscore the policy concern of impoverishment due to the inadequate design of major illness insurance.[12] Sun Zhigang, Director of the Medical Care Office of the State Council, urged the government to accelerate the introduction of major illness insurances for both urban and rural residents for the period of the 12th Five Year plan up to 2020 (Sun 2013. 3: 49). In addition to its medical and professional dimensions, Sun defines catastrophic medical illness in financial terms, referring to an expenditure for a medical care event that exceeds the total of disposable average annual income of a resident in a rural or urban area, coupled with the consequence leading to impoverishment (Sun 2013. 3:51).

Sovereign planners began to inaugurate the NRCMCI in 2003, taking into consideration not only the need of a viable and effective funding mode for health care after the collapse of Rural Cooperative Medical Care (RCMC), but also the problem of impoverishment caused by the increasing burden of medical expenditure on peasants (Qin & Jiang 2013. 4: 28–9). NRCMCI has its historical roots. One may trace its origin to the first RCMC station in 1955 in the midst of the agricultural collectivization movement. RCMC grew rapidly for more than a decade, reaching its climax while covering 90 percent of the production brigades and 80 percent of the peasants in rural China in the late 1970s when the MOH with other five ministerial units promulgated the "Regulations of Rural Cooperative Medical Care" in December 1979 (Yu, 2018). RCMC formed an integral part of rural China's collective economy that went beyond the reach of the state, with RCMC operating at health care facilities at the township level and health care stations at the village level. It suffered a setback starting in the 1980s when the People's Communes collapsed and the agricultural joint responsibility system assumed dominance (Yu 2018).

As indicated in a series of policy papers, NRCMCI appeared on the policy agenda of central policymakers as soon as the enhanced BMCI package was underway for full-scale implementation in the early 2000s. The General Office of the State Council issued the 2003 Circular concerning the establishment of NRCMCI in January 2003 explicitly addressing the issue of accessibility and affordability of medical care for the peasantry (Wu 2013: 5: 60). Accordingly, the MOH and other ministerial units authorized pilot programs for NRCMCI throughout the country in 2003, followed by the 2004 Advisory Opinion on further extension of pilot programs for NRCMCI issued by the MOH and other 11 ministerial units (Wu 2013: 5: 60).

Assuming "new" in its title, NRCMCI is markedly different from the RCMC of early years, as noted by Yu (Yu 2018). First, the former operates at the county level, the organizational status of which is elevated to the state level, representing the lowest reach of the Party-state hierarchy, whereas the latter represents a form of voluntary organization in the collective economy in the non-state sector. Second, the former involves a major institutional metamorphosis in the sense that the insurance fund is managed by a new form of public organization, operating independently, and separating itself institutionally and managerially from the state in resource management (i.e. personnel and financial management). Third, in terms of types of benefits and entitlements, the former focuses on "major illness," but does not exclude outpatient services, meaning cases of large expenditure, hospital care, and catastrophic medical events, with the explicit policy goal of preventing impoverishment caused by illness. The RCMC of early years addressed less serious illness and injuries. Fourth, the former organizes insurance at the county level, entailing a considerable scale of risk-pooling mechanisms, while the latter worked with too small a scale to function effectively as a funding mode at the village level. In principle, the former sets aside a larger portion of funds for "major illness" and a smaller portion devoted to minor cases, while the latter covered all reimbursement applications, most of which were small items of expenditure, on a first-come-first-serve basis. Additionally, the former is a form of co-insurance requiring enrollees to pay for their own share of premium, normally one quarter of it, as the government and the collective chip in their shares.

NRCMCI intended to alleviate the financial burden of peasants mainly for catastrophic medical care events while introducing spending control measures similar to what the enhanced BMCI had already adopted. For instance, NRCMCI copied from BMCI spending control measures for staff and workers, featuring standard schemes for deductible, co-payment, and ceiling of expenditure. Explicitly it set the ceiling of reimbursement at six times of the average annual income of peasants. Through NRCMCI, sovereign planners endeavored to deal with the excess of exorbitantly high user charges (especially for medicine and medical devises) coupled with government subsidies for medical care in the early 2000s (Wu 2013. 5: 59–62).

Not only did NRCMCI intend to make health care more affordable to the peasantry, but also it tried to correct the phenomenon of "reverse pyramid" by shifting more health care resources to the lower echelons of the state hierarchy. Accompanying NRCMCI, the government injected funding to strengthen the three-tier health care system, incorporating health care centers at the village level, health care facilities at the township, and county hospital level into one integrated health care system, allowing lower level health care centers/stations to play the role of "gatekeeper" primary care, linked to the first level hospitals at the county level and/or above through a refurbished referral system.

Sovereign planners introduced URBMCI in 2007 as most of the municipal/county jurisdictions had already made considerable progress in implementing the enhanced BMCI program. In 2007 the State Council took a major step in building a new but different brand of BMCI for urban residents to embrace the unemployed and all low-income residents in urban area such as students, dependents, children, and retirees. It is noteworthy that the enhanced BMCI package does not cover dependents of employed personnel who were covered by conventional funding schemes such as LIMC and PFMC in urban China. In accordance with the 2007 Advisory Opinion, the State Council authorized various provincial jurisdictions to conduct pilot programs for URBMCI, and worked out the operational details focusing on hospital care as well as specific major illness cases in clinical care (Peng, Lei, & Liu 2013: 7:44).

While both URBMCI and an enhanced BMCI cater mainly to the medical demands of those with an established household registration in urban areas, they differ somewhat from each other. In the former, enrollees join URBMCI as members of a family unit. Financially speaking, under the former, enrollees mainly depend on the support of family income in addition to government subsidies. The former works with risk-pooling mechanisms with tax revenue representing the other funding sources to help subsidize payment for premiums for needy and low-income enrollees, while the latter covers employees whose insurance benefit constitutes an integral part of a total wage bill. And while in the former, tax revenue covers indirectly the government subsidies to help enrollees pay their insurance premium, it differs from PFMC where tax revenue went directly into a medical care benefits account for public personnel.

Furthermore, sovereign planners endeavored to build an organizational framework and to apply managerial mechanisms pertaining to URBMCI by addressing the policy concern of optimal allocation and deployment of health care resources. URBMCI drew a division of labor between primary care services in community health care centers and more advanced services in the hospitals at the first, second and even third tier. Again, URBMCI adopted spending control mechanisms similar to BMCI, for instance, the listing/catalog of services, drugs and devices, as well as payment schemes featuring deductible, co-payment and an upper-ceiling for expenditure. Also, URBMCI adopted a sliding payment scale to allow a smaller co-payment for lower tier hospitals, and a bigger co-payment for higher tier hospitals. For instance, patients paid 25 percent of a medical care bill at the lowest tier health care facilities (including first tier hospitals and community health care centers/clinics), 40 percent at the second tier and 50 percent at the third tier (Wu 2013. 5: 60–1).

Issues of implementation

Since the foregoing analysis has dwelled so far on policymaking, it is appropriate here to deal with the issues of implementation. In fact, three medical care insurance programs were inaugurated at different times, and each made progress with its own pace. With regard to the growth of enrollments in each of the three, an estimate indicates that by 2011, enrollees in public insurances reached 1,295 million in total, the breakdowns of which are: 832 million peasants had enrolled in NRCMCI, 216 million urban residents had subscribed to URBMCI. 216 million and 247 million employed personnel had joined the enhanced BMCI package (Li & Gui 2012: 76–7; Qin & Jiang 2013. 4:9). In addition, an estimated 100 million people had not been protected by any medical care insurance; most of these had retirees from bankrupt COEs and SOEs, flexibly employed personnel, agricultural laborers and dependents (Li & Gui 2012: 76–7). It is noteworthy that regardless of reforms, PFMC retained its separate organizational status claiming not only a considerable number of enrollees but also a substantial share of public finance.[13]

Both NRCMCI and URBMCI moved fast along the process of implementation, resembling the so-called "bandwagon" phenomenon as mentioned by Huang Yanzhong (Huang 2014). Chou Yulin and Huang Guowu cited a set of statistics regarding an increase in enrollment in NRCMCI for a short time span of six years, from 179 million in 2005 to 832 million in 2011 (Cou & Huang 2013. 11: 44). According to a set of statistics cited by Peng, Lei & Liu, URBMCI made quick progress in enrollment within four years, from 43 million in 2007 to 195 million in 2010 (Peng, Lei, & Liu 2013. 7: 44). Policy analysts suggest that local jurisdictions endeavored to move fast to expand enrollment in NRCMCI, as they tried to take advantage of matching funds from higher echelons of the central, provincial and local governments. Another possible explanation for the very short period required for introducing NRCMCI and URBMCI has to do with the small scale of funding required for each, and therefore a lighter financial burden imposed on the government units in various echelons. In contrast, the enhanced BMCI package took a longer time to implement than did NRCMCI and URBMCI. According to Gu's statistical analysis, the percentage of enrollees in the enhanced BMCI package in urban China climbed slowly, from 7.8 percent of the employed population in 1998 to 56.3 percent in 2008. This means that for the whole decade from 1998 to 2008, a little more than half of the targeted insured was only able to be enrolled in the enhanced BMCI (Gu 2010: 51).

Not entirely expected, the accumulation of relatively large deposits of insurance funds occurred invariably in all three programs. According to Gu Xin, all three insurance programs showed considerable savings by 2008. In the case of NRCMCI, for example, the accumulated deposit reached 19,890 million RMB by 2008, representing an accumulation rate of saving at 25.5 percent for five years from 2004 to 2008 (Gu 2010: 75). With reference to URBMCI starting in 2007, the accumulated deposit was 12,810 million RMB by 2008, with an 82.7 percent rate of saving (Gu 2010: 78). In case of the enhanced BMCI, the accumulated deposit was 330, 600 million RMB by 2008, with an accumulation rate of 114.5 percent (Gu 2010: 80–1). As mentioned by Ma & Gui, the deposit for the enhanced BMCI and URBMCI was equivalent to 19.6 months and 24.1 months of insurance payments respectively in the year 2008, while NRCMCI remained basically balanced within the policy guideline (meaning within the range between 15 to 25 percent) (Ma & Gui 2012: 4. 78).[14]

Since a deposit is necessary for any insurance program designed to absorb risk and meet obligations for payments, policymakers have to address the issue of the appropriate scale of deposit. Various central authorities tried to set up guidelines about the scale of the insurance fund deposit. For example, the MOF, the MOH and the State Chinese Herbal Medicine Bureau issued a policy paper in July 2007, requiring all jurisdictions to observe the 15 percent ceiling for insurance deposits to NRCMCI (Gu 2010: 75–6). The 2009 Implementation Plan, promulgated by the State Council on April 6, 2009, requires the enhanced BMCI and URBMCI to adhere to a fixed annual saving rate and to an accumulation rate of the total of deposited funds, while scaling down the total of existing deposit funds to a reasonable level, that is, the range between 15 percent and 25 percent (Gu 2010: 73). Gu Xin diagnosed the reasons behind the high accumulation rates of the enhanced BMCI: an effective, but tight control of spending; insurance funds set aside for the staff and workers of bankrupt and closed enterprises; insurance funds set aside for the retirees of enterprises; personal saving in PA; funds set aside for paying for the low-income ensured; and a matter involving the calculation formula (Gu 2010: 83–8). Among many issues regarding the accumulation of insurance funds, insurance for retirees stands out as one of the most salient issues in China in anticipation of the arrival of a large cohort of elderly around the 2030s, a topic to be tackled in future studies.

Furthermore, there exist some gaps between expectation and performance with regard to newly introduced public insurance programs. First of all, the re-engineering endeavor has *not* been able to put forth insurance programs at a "basic" spending level—such as in the early BMCI—lower than the spending level of conventional public insurances. In drafting the early BMCI in 1994, policymakers began with a design the overall level of expenditure of which was lower than the level of expenditure of LIMC and PFMC. When this was found unacceptable in view of political considerations and costs of implementation, they needed to add supplementary insurances in order not to reduce the spending level of the enhanced BMCI to a level lower than what employed personnel had already enjoyed under pre-reform arrangements.

Besides, disparities between the enhanced BMCI and URBMCI, and between the enhanced BMCI and NRCMCI with regard to coverage and level of spending resulted in creating two classes of people, thereby privileging those who worked in the planned sector. Moreover, the government has to treat public personnel as a separate but unequal category in light of their privileges in the reformed PFMC package. An attempted explanation is two-fold: administrative and political. In administrative terms, policymakers are reluctant to scale down any benefits schemes that could amount to compensation reduction, since medical care and other entitlements are conceptually treated as components of compensation in view of the low-pay policy practiced under the CPE. In addition, administrative costs arise when existing employees in the planned sector are asked to opt for lower standards in a benefit package, while it is feasible to offer a new package to those who join the benefit program for the first time in the later periods. In fact, it has been an established practice in policy implementation in China not to lower standards for an existing group of beneficiaries, while any new adjustments of benefits, especially lower ones, take effect with a fresh group of users. In political terms, moreover, one may treat such disparities as a manifestation of corporatism in the sense that, as a legacy of the CPE, employees of the planned sector enjoy better compensation packages than other social strata (such as dependents and low-income employees) and a vast number of peasants in light of the former's sacrifices and contributions during the forced modernization through the CPE.

Concluding remarks

The transformation from LMCI and PFMC to a new system of public insurances involves great complexity, which is largely institutional and managerial in its characteristics. The entire policymaking process takes a long time from policy experiments, policy designing, to implementation. The case of the enhanced BMCI took more than two decades from 1994 to the 2010s. For a shorter time-span, either NRCMCI or URMCI need more than one decade for full implementation. In contrast to the image of a singular rational actor who was omnisicient and omnipotent in making a decision for a quick change, the restructuring of public insurances could be better characterized as a loosely coordinated process by multiple policymakers institutionally positioned in various echelons of Party-state hierarchy. And they initiated the change with constraints of resources and in shortage of needed information. Moreover, a keen observer would detect hints of politics, for instance, the privileges and vested interest of the employed personnel in the planned sector, albeit it can be interpreted as policy-oriented, for example, compensation policy for those who had endured the low-pay policy of the CPE era.

Notes

1 For instance, there was an actual expenditure of 24.6 RMB on average for each individual public employee over the budgeted sum of 18 RMB in 1960 and 34.4 RMB over the budgeted sum of 26 RMB in 1965 (Zheng 2002: 120–1).
2 In the early 1980s, the health care markets were marked by increasing costs of medically related materials, rapid aging of the population, higher life expectancy, higher percentage of senior residents in the population, change in the profile of illness, and advancement in medical technology and equipment (Zheng 2002: 131).
3 It is noteworthy that the establishment of the PFMC office or committee only represented a pre-requisite to a financial accountability system. The PFMC program held neither the work unit nor individual enrollee accountable for spending, while the state treasury acted as the payer, and the hospital unit as the payee. Accordingly, the central government urged various jurisdictions to adopt mechanisms for spending control based on multiple-level management, multiple-function

management, integration of responsibility with incentive, and components connecting well-financed allocation, management, and expenditure (Zheng 2002: 134).

4 Policy analysts and practitioners choose the wording "social" (shehui) to highlight
   institutional independence from the government, while "unified funding" refers to
   a reservoir of funds maintaining a measure of financial autonomy against
   encroachment by the government.

5 This scheme required participant enterprises to pay an annual premium in full to SUF
   for the enrollees in order to cover the expenditure of retired personnel and "lixiu" personnel for clinical care, hospital care, physical check-ups, and transportation costs for
   referrals. In addition, it incorporated the feature of co-payment that followed the principle of a three-way sharing of medical care expenses among government, work unit,
   and patient with or without a ceiling for spending. In some cases, the design gave "lixiu"
   personnel leeway in claiming reimbursement according to actual expenses, meaning no
   ceiling for expenditure. On November 28, 1990, the Ministry of Labor endorsed the
   policy initiatives of SUF for retirees at a work conference attended by participants from
   various provinces and municipalities. In 1994, an estimated 14,000 enterprises, with
   357,000 subscribers, in fourteen jurisdictions adopted SUF programs in one form or
   another, representing a 26.1 percent increase over the one-year period from 1993. . In the
   same year, the total collection amounted to 60 million RMB with outgoing payments of
   more than 70 million (meaning a shortfall of about 10 million). Despite difficulties at the
   initial stage, the accumulated savings reached 6.72 million in 1993, albeit with a decrease
   of 12.31 million from that of the preceding year. Also, some insurance institutes experimented with building clinics and hospitals for retirees, which also proved effective in
   containing cost increases (Song & Liu 2001: 89; Zheng et al. 2002: 135–6).

6 As one of its first steps during the early 1990s, the Ministry of Labor drafted the
   "Opinion regarding the Trial Implementation of Unified Social Funding for
   Expenditures for Major Illness" on March 19, 1992 (Zheng 2002: 137).

7 These four operational goals are literally: "low level, wide coverage, shared financial responsibility by two parties, and the combination of personal accounts with a
   unified social funding account" (dishuiping; guanfugai; shuangfan fudan; tongz-
   hang jiehe). (Guojia Tigaiwei et al. 1999; Song & Liu 2001)

8 For alternative operational definitions, the "basic level" refers to the following. (1)
   a bare minimum but adequate level of services in medical and technical terms; (2)
   the kinds, levels, and standards of curative care services mandated by the state and
   often funded by public finance, including tax revenue, (3) a "reasonable" level of
   medical care provision in accordance with the scope and standards of the state, (4)
   a low-level medical care, equivalent to a form of social security whose funding
   design differs from that of insurance, and (5) the criteria and norms of social
   acceptability among residents of a community (Peng 1999: 8; Cheng & Dong 1999;
   Guowuyuan 1999; Guojia Tigaiwei et al. 1999; Lee 2013).

9 It is therefore recommended, in the view of Wu and Chen, that contributions to
   essential curative care be set at 6 percent of total wages in light of the actual
   financial capacity of enterprises and local financial units. Given the 6 percent as a
   controlling indicator, each jurisdiction could make necessary adjustments according to actual situations (Wu & Chen 1999: 366).

10 For state organizations, fully budgeted service units and partially budgeted (also
    called "differential quota budgeted") work units (e.g., service work units such as hos-
    pitals), contributions to the PA-USFA were to be charged to the budgeted fund of the
    work unit concerned. For partially budgeted service units and self-financed and
    entrepreneurially oriented service units, contributions to the PA-USFA would come
    from the medical care fund. In those enterprises, contributions for staff and workers to
    the PA-USFA had to be charged to the welfare fund for staff and workers; and in the
    case of retirees, their contributions had to be charged to the labor insurance expendi-
    ture account at the enterprise level (Guojia Tigaiwei et al. 1999: 101).

11 According to Wu, the 2012 Advisory Opinion was a clarification and reaffirmation of the established policy priority on major illness insurance pertaining to NRCMC and URCM from the very beginning, namely, 2003 and 2007, respectively (Wu 2013).
12 The full title of the 2012 Advisory Opinion is: Guanyu kaizhan chengxiang jumin dabing baoxian gongzuo de zhidao yijian (The advisory opinion regarding the inauguration the task of major illness insurance for urban and rural residents), issued by the State Development and Reform Commission and other five ministerial units in August, 2012. (Sun 2013.3: 49–52).
13 For illustration, the total of enrollees in PFMC was estimated at 34.2 million, while its expenditure was 41,410 million RMB in 2007 (Gu 2010: 51; 57–62).
14 Ma & Gui (2012). 4: 78; A set of statistical figures cited by Gu Xin indicates that the saving in the BMCI for the ensured increased over time, from 4.5 months in 1998, 12.4 months in 2001, 14.3 months in 2005 to 19.6 months in 2008 (Gu 2010: 81).

References

Bian, Y. 1994. *Work and Inequality in China*. Albany, NY: State University of New York Press.
Chen, W., & Yi, L. 2011. *2011 nian Zhongguo yiyao weisheng tizhi gaige baogao* (The Report of Medical and Health Care Reform in China in the Year of 2011). Beijing: Zhongguo xiehe yike daxue.
Cheng, L., & Dong, S. 1999. Guanyu yiliao baoxian feiyong kongzhi wenti de yanjiu (A study regarding spending control of medical insurance). In D. Zheng, D. Liu, & B. Zhang (Eds.), *Shehui baozhang zhidu gaige zhinan* (The Guide for the Reform of Social Security System). Beijing: Gaige chubanshe.
Cou, Y. & Huang, G. 2013. Woguo yiliao baozhang zhidu zhuanxian yanjiu (A study on transformation of medical care insurance system in China). *Shehui baozhang zhidu* (Social Security System), 11: 44.
Dangdai Zhongguo Congshu Bianjibu. 1987. *Dangdai zhongguo zigong gongzhi fuli he shehui baoxian* (The Wage, Welfare and Social Insurance for Staff and Workers in Contemporary China). Beijing: Zhongguo shehui kexue chubanshe.
Dangdai Zhongguo Congshu Bianjibu. 1988. *Dangdai zhongguo caizheng, xia* (Finance in Contemporary China, volume 2). Beijing: Zhongguo shehui kexue chubanshe.
Deng, D (ed.). 2008. *2006–2007 Zhongguo shehui baozhang gaige yu fazhan baogao* (The Report of Reform and Development of Social Security in China in Year of 2006–2007). Beijing: Remin chubanshe.
Du, L. 2008. Zhongguo tese gongli yiyuan rongzi luzai hefang? Zaijiaoxia (Where is the avenue for public hospitals with Chinese characteristics? Right here). In L. Du *et al.* (Eds.), *Zhongguo yiliao waisheng fazhan baogao, No. 4*. (The Report of Developlment in Health and Medical Care in China, No. 4), 72–96. Beijing: Shehui kexue wenxian chubanshe.
Du, L. *et al.* 2008. Lun zhongguo tese shehui zhuyi yiliao weisheng gaige fazhan daolu (On the road of reform and development of Socialist medical and health care in China). In L. Du *et al.* (Eds.), *Zhongguo weisheng fazhan bao, No. 4* (The Report of Medical Care Development in China, No. 4) 1–31. Beijing: Shehui kexue wenxian chubanshe.
Gao, R. 1999. Tansuo geren zhangfu yu gongji zhangfu fenbie yunzuo moshi, goujian kongzhi yiliao feiyong guokuai zenzhang de yaoxiao jizhi (Exploring the

operational model of separation between individual accounts and collective acconts, building effective mechanisms for control of rapid growth of medical care expenses). In D. Zheng, D. Liu, & B. Zhang (Eds.), *Shehui baozhang zhidu gaige zhinan* (The Guide for the Reform of Social Security System). Beijing: Gaige chubanshe.

Gu, X. 2010. *Quanmin yibao de xintansuo* (New Exploration of National Medical Insurance). Beijing: Shehui kexue wenxian chubanshe.

Guan, Z., Cui, B., & Don, C. 2007. Zhongguo weisheng gaige yu yiliao baozhang tixi jianshe de zhongsilu (Overall consideration of health care reform and construction of medical care system in China). In J. Chen, & Y. Wang (Eds.) *Zhongguo shehui baoxian fazhan baogao* (The Report of Social Insurance Development). Beijing: Shehui kexue wenxian chubanshe.

Guojia Tigaiwei *et al.* 1999. Guanyu yiliao zhidu gaige shidian yijian (Opinions concerning the reform of medical care system of staff and workers). In D. Zheng, D. Liu, & B. Zhang (Eds.), *Shehui baozhang zhidu gaige zhinan* (The Guide for the Reform of Social Security System), 100–103. Beijing: Gaige chubanshe.

Guowuyuan. 1995. Guanyu Jiangsu Sheng Zhengjiangshi Jiangxi Sheng Jiujiangshi zhigong yiliao baozhang zhidu gaige shidian fangan de pifu (The reply to the proposal of pilot programs of medical care security system of staff and workers in Zhengjiangshi, Jiangsu Province, and Jiujiangshi Municipality, Jiangxi Province). *Renshi zhengce fagui zhuankan* (Journal of Personnel Policy and Law), 6: 4–12.

Interview 2002a (Two interviewee 23/01/2002).

Interview 2002b (One interviewee morning 25/01/2002).

Interview 2002c (One interviewee afternoon 25/01/2002).

Laodong Baozhangbu & Caizhengbu. 2000. Guanyu shixing guojia gongwuyuan yiliao buzhu de yijian (The opinion concerning the implementation of medical care subsidy to public personnel). *Guowuyuan gongbao* (Bulletin of State Council), 21:13–14.

Lee, P. 2013. China's Health Care in Perspective. In F. Cheung, J. Woo, & C. Law (Eds.), *Health Systems: Challenges, Visions, and Reform from a Comparative-Global Perspective*. Hong Kong: The Chinese University of Hong Kong.

Liu, G., & Liu, X. 1999. *Zuixin shiyong yiliao baoxian zhengce huida* (The Most Recent and Practical Book for Q & A of Medical Care Insurance). Beijing: Jingji kexue chubanshe.

Liu, Z. 2004. *Zhongguo yiliao gaige de zhidu fenxi* (A systems analysis of China's medical care reform). Jiayi, Taiwan: National Chung Cheng University.

Ma, L., & Gui, J. 2012. Wanshan jiben yiliao baozhang zhidu yanjiu (Perfect research on basic medical care insurance system). *Tizhi gaige* (System Reform), 4: 73–87.

Peng, P. 1999. Zai quanquo zhigong yiliao baozhang gaige shidian kuada huiyi shang kaimushi de jianghua (Speech at the opening of the national work conference for the expansion of pilot programs of medical care insurance reform of staff and workers). In Guojia tigai fenpei he shehui baozhangsi (Ed.), *Zhigong yiliao baozhang zhidu gaige* (The Reform of Medical Care Insurance for Staff and Workers). Beijing: Gaige chubanshe.

Peng, J., Lei, X., & Liu, G. 2013. Yiliao baoxian cujin jiankan ma? Jiyu zhongguo chengchen jumin jiben yiliao baoxian de shizheng yanjiu (Would medical care insurance promote health? Empirical research on basic urban resident medical care insurance). *Shehui baozhang zhidu* (Social Security System), 7: 44–45.

Peng, R., Cai, R., & Zhou, C. 1992. *Zhongguo Gaige Quanshu* (Encyclopedia of China's Reform). Dalian: Dalian chubanshe.

Qin, L., & Jiang, Z. 2013. Xinxing noncu hezuo yiliao yu chengzhen jumin yiliao baoxian heping yanjiu (A study on combining New Rural Cooperative Medical Care Insurance with Urban Resident Medical Care Insurance). *Shehui baozhang zhidu* (Social Security System), 4: 29–32.

Song, X., & Liu, H. 2001. Yiliao baoxian zhidu gaige ji peitao cuoshi (The reform and measures of coordination in medical care insurance reform). In Song Xiaowu (Ed.), *Zhongguo shehui baozhang tizhi gaige yu fazhan baogao* (The Report of Reform and Development of Social Security System in China). Beijing: Zhonguo remin daxue chubanshe.

Sun, Z. 2013. Shishi dabing baoxian shi jianqing remin jiu fudan de guanjian (Implementation of major illness insurance is key to alleviating the people's medical burden). *Shehui baozhang zhidu* (Social Security System), 3: 49–52.

Wang, D. 2000. *Zhongguo shehui baozhang zhidu yu fazhan* (The Reform and Development of Social Security System in China). Beijing: Falu chubanshe.

Wu, R., & Chen, J. 1999. Jianli chengzhen zhigongn jiben baoxian zhidu, quanmian tujin woguo yiliao baoxian zhidu gaige (Build basic medical care insurance of staff and workers in cities and towns, and propel reform of insurance system). In D. Zheng, D. Liu, & B. Zhang (Eds.), *Shehui baozhang zhidu gaige zhinan* (The Guide for Social Security System Reform). Beijing: Gaige chubanshe.

Wu, R. 2013. Guanyu dabing baoxian de sikao (Some considerations on insurance of major illness). *Shehui baozhang zhidu* (Social Security System), 5: 61.

Yang, T. 2004. Wanshan yiliao baozhang zhidu de silu he duice (The thought and proposal on how to perfect medical care insurance system). In J.Chen, & Y. Wang, *Zhongguo shehui baozhang fazhan baogao* (The Report on the Development of Social Insurance in China). Beijing: shehui kexue webxian chubanshe.

Yu, Shaoxiang. 2018. Xinnonghe: shi dachan? haishi jile? Xinnong chunhezuo yiliao fazhan baogao (Banquet or junk food? The research report on the development of new rural cooperative medical care). Zhongguo faxuewan (China's Legal Study Net). www.iolaw.org.cn/showNews.asp?id=22842.

Zhang, Z. 1999. Laodong shehui baozhangbu buzhang Zhang Zuoyi zai quanguo chengzhen zigong yiliao baoxian zhidu gaige gongzuo huiyi shang de jianghua (The speech of Minister of Labor and Social Security Zhang Zuoyi at the national work conference on the reform of medical care insurance system for staff and workers in cities and towns). In Laodong he Shehui Baozhang Bu Shehui Baozhang Baoxiansi (Ed.), *Zhonguo baoxian zhidu gaige zhengce yu guanli* (The Reform of Policy and Management of Medical Care Insurance in China). Beijing: Zhongguo shehui baozhang chubanshe.

Zheng, B., Gao, Q. & Yu, H. 2010. Xinzhongguo shehui baozhang zhidu de bianqian yu fazhan (The change and development of social security system in new China). In D. Zou (Ed.), *Zhongguo shehui baozhang fazhan baogao* (The Report of Development of Social Security in China). Beijing: Shehui kexue wenxian chubanse.

Zheng, D. 2010. Gongli yiyuan chengben hesuan yu qiye chengben hesuan de bijiao fenxi (A comparative analysis of costs accounting between public hospitals and enterprises). *Zhongguo weisheng jingji* (China's Health Care Economics) 29 (11): 66–68.

Zheng, G. 2002. Zhongguo zhigog yiliao baozhang zhidu bianqian yu binggu (The change and assessment of medical care insurance of staff and workers in China). In G. Zheng *et al.* (Eds.), *Zhonguo shehui baozhang zhidu bianqian yu pinggu* (The

Change and Assessment of Medical Care Insurance System in China). Beijing: Remin chubanshe

Zheng, G. *et al.* 2002. *Zhongguo shehui baozhang zhidu bianqian yu pinggu* (The transformation of China's social insurance system and its evalution). Beijing: Remin daxue chubanshe.

Zheng, G. 2011. *Zhongguo shehui baozhang gaige yu fazhan zhanlue* (The Strategy of Reform and Development of Social Security in China). Beijing: Zhongguo remin chubanshe.

6 Price control amid the rise of regulated markets

Starting in the 1950s, the government adopted the low-price policy for medical care services in order to provide affordable medical care to all, and this policy has remained intact throughout the reform era, which started in 1979. Price control is required as an instrument to implement the low-price policy to the extent that it directly affects user charges for various items of health care services and how much each patient has to pay out of pocket. As a regulatory instrument wielded by the government, price control has become increasingly demanding and complex in the midst of changing task environment during the period of economic reform.[1]

This chapter is devoted to an analysis on price control in the wake of the repackaging and expansion of health care provision during economic reform. It will try to assess how successful the government has been in solving the issues of price control at the providing unit level by highlighting the role conflict of providing unit in dealing with the government's policy price control as follows: on the one hand, the providing unit is required to carry out the low-price policy of certain categories of medical care services on behalf of the government, and on the other hand, it is expected to address the issue of its budgetary balance, revenue concerns, and resource management. While the former often means a smaller revenue for the providing unit, the latter entails a quest for more revenue. And this role conflict is often manifested in the tendency of financial irregularities and legal violations on the part of providing units and medical personnel. Moreover, it becomes even more complex that some government units such as the price bureau try to impose control, while the other departments are inclined to support the providing unit, and to be relaxed on the pricing issue. The study will be able to have a close look at various episodes relevant to operational and managerial side of policy implementation in the health care sector during the economic reform period.

The changing style of policymaking: the case of pricing

China's health care system was first built and incorporated into the centrally planned economy (CPE) starting in the 1950s when both the providing unit and drug industry were subject to central planning and public management. Not only did sovereign planners impose tight control over the delivery of health care services and the production and distribution of drugs, but also they handled the revenue of work units and compensation of staff and workers through plan. Public hospitals and drug enterprises were treated as enforcing vehicles at the bottom of the Party-state hierarchy and at the receiving end of the pricing policy from the top policymakers (Zhou 2008:120–1). Policy analysts and authors describe the institutional framework of pricing in the health care as "restrictive, bureaucratic, and highly centralized" prior to economic reform (Wang 1994a; Xu & Qiu 1993).

By and large, the restructuring of price control system had begun well before the eve of formal inauguration of the basic medical care insurance reform in 2001. Arising from this early phase of the medical care reform were two salient themes of pricing policy: one regarding decentralization and the other concerning market-oriented perspective. From 1978 to the mid-1990s, there was an overall tendency of decentralization of pricing power from the ministerial level to the provincial level and further down to the municipal/prefectural level, expectedly resulting in greater regional diversity as well as fragmentation of the policymaking process (Chen 2000a). Sovereign planners started to adopt the policy of "unified policy and management by various echelons," meaning to assign responsibility for pricing policy and control measures to each echelon of the government from the central level down to the provincial, and finally municipal level. Also, in 1996, the State Planning Commission (SPC) issued a circular to entrust responsibility to each level of the government for handling concrete issues of implementation and even the schedules of user charges of medical care services (Guojia Jihua Weiyuanhui, Weishengbu, Caizhengbu 1998). In 1997, sovereign planners promulgated a major policy paper to propose the new policy guidelines of pricing and modes of price management.[2] Furthermore, in 2000, they initiated some major changes of pricing policy in concrete terms, including the forms of management and the readjustment of unreasonable prices of medical care services.[3]

According to Chu Jinhua and Yu Baorong, the ministerial units were normally in charge of policy and regulations, while the concrete tasks of price setting were delegated to the governments at the provincial and municipal levels, including the formulating of policy proposals and setting of prices. The provincial and municipal governments were also given powers concerning organizational and managerial matters during the economic reform. At the provincial level or below, for example, there were three forms of implementation: (1) centralized management by the provincial jurisdictions, (2) managerial power divided up and shared between the provincial and municipal echelons, and (3) division of labor among relevant bureaus in both provincial and municipal governments (Chu & Yu 2010: 64–5).

Facing the rise of market economy, moreover, SPC and Ministry of Health (MOH) put forth a policy paper (known as the 2000 Opinion) in 2000, intending to adopt a new pricing system which consisted of both government-guided pricing and market-adjusted pricing at the various ministerial units, provincial level, and further down to the municipal level.[4] Accordingly, public hospitals gained autonomy to mark up the prices of medical care services within a "floating range" in line with the standards made by the bureaus of price in charge. Non-public profit-oriented hospital units were permitted to adopt market-adjusted prices according to market situation (Luo 2006). In October 2000, moreover, SPC, together with other ministerial authorities, took one step further to provide a unified listing of items, contents, and titles of standard prices of medical care services throughout the country. And meanwhile, the provincial and municipal jurisdictions acquired autonomy to mark up prices on the basis of calculation by respective price bureaus and bureaus of health care at the municipal/local level (Luo 2006).

In broad outline, the ministerial units were responsible for making policy guidelines and plans of pricing, creating principles of marking-up and price adjustments, and formulating proposals and schedules for implementation (Wang 1994a). The exercises of pricing and management of fees/charges were to be governed by a unified set of policy papers, regulations, and measures, for instance, the guide of prices of services, the schedule of standard charges/fees, the wage system of public hospitals, the system of public subsidies, and lists of market prices (Wang 2008: 253–4). In general, the State Price Bureau (SPB) assumed the main responsibility over pricing policy, in collaboration with other ministerial units.[5]

The government continued to maintain its price control over the basic medical care services during the economic reform, while the autonomy of pricing over non-basic medical care services (e.g., special care services) was delegated downward to the providing unit level. That is to say, the markets played a salient role over the non-basic medical care services, albeit the government still retained a say over the scope of services, principles of pricing, levels of revenues, specific marking-up of items, financial management, and compensation packages (Wang 1994a).

As a result of a series of efforts at reform, it was very much up to the government at the provincial and municipal level to build specific organizational structure in order to undertake the task of pricing (Wang 2008: 253–4; Chu & Yu 2010: 64–5). Often it was divided and shared among several overlapping and functionally interdependent bureaus (e.g., the price bureau, food and drug administration, health care bureau, and finance bureau, among others) at the provincial and municipal levels. They worked jointly in charge of prices and fees/charges of the providing units throughout the country in accordance with relevant policies, regulations, and systems by the central government (Wang 2008).

At the provincial/municipal level, various bureaus were organized in correspondence with their counterparts at the central level, though adapted to the local situation. For illustration, a survey of 42 public hospitals during 2002 to 2004 shows that in 15 out of 42, the pricing bureau was solely in charge of price-regulating exercises; in nine, price-regulating work was divided up and assigned to three relevant units, such as the bureau of pricing, health care bureau, and food and drug administration; in another nine, price control was handled jointly by the bureau of pricing and food and drug administration. There were other combinations in the remaining nine cases: the food and drug administration only, the bureau of pricing working with the health care bureau, and a team formed by the finance bureau, bureau of pricing, health care bureau, and food and drug administration (Luo 2006).

In accordance with the 1997 Decision since 1997, there has been delegation of price-regulating power to lower echelons in each jurisdiction, but the policy has been found contradictory to itself in some cases. On the one hand, the central government urged the provincial jurisdictions to initiate a process of decentralization and liberalization in the midst of rapid market growth coupled with new mechanisms for timely price adjustments in order to allow greater discretion and flexibility at each level of the hierarchy.[6] The 1997 Decision also encouraged indirect management in relations with the providing units through working on planning, criteria, standards, and methodical approach. It further advised the provincial jurisdictions to avoid making price changes unilaterally on an ad hoc basis. In addition, it recommended adopting "cost-based price" (a price deducting the cost of regular subsidy) in its calculation of pricing for non-basic medical care services (Zhonggongzhongyang 1997).

On the other hand, it started new cycles of bureaucratic control in order to cope with such unintended and undesirable policy consequences as over-provision and "excessively high charges" in the health care sector (Chen 1999; Liu 2008). All the proposed changes of pricing policy have been further elaborated and confirmed in a series of policy papers, including two major ones in 2000, and resulted in a series of new legislation (Guowuyuan tigaiban, Guojia Jiwei, Guojia jinmaowei et al. 2000; Guojia Jiwei 2001: 27–8). This includes: (1) a new feature regarding the separation of accounting/management between curative care services and pharmaceutical retail, and (2) the centralized control of revenue of pharmaceutical franchise of dispensary services at the bureau level. According to Zhu Hongbiao et al., this has pointed in an untenable direction of diluting or even taking away the franchise of pharmaceutical retail from the public hospitals without a clear idea of its managerial implications (Zhu 1999). Gu Xin criticizes this as another round of bureaucratization, a retreat backward to the CPE (Gu 2008: 285). As the foregoing analysis has covered rebuilding of the institutional structure, installing of regulatory means, and re-inventing managerial tools regarding the issue of pricing, the study moves into concrete tasks and operations in price control.

Two approaches to price-regulating tasks

Throughout the medical care reform, the government entertained two different approaches to price-regulating tasks: the market-oriented approach and policy-oriented approach, depending upon various categories of health care services, characteristics of the providing units, proportions of government funding, and different policy purposes (Wang 1994b: 18). By and large, the former endeavored to determine prices of the medical care services strictly according to the considerations of market transactions, such as supply and demand, bargaining and competition, value of services in question, cost accounting, and revenue/profit and loss. And it often applied to those private goods (or marketable benefits) in those non-basic medical care services, such as special care services catering to the demands of high-income users. Also, it was necessary to use the former to handle pricing when the providing units were privately owned, corporate owned, and cooperatively owned. Definitely the providing unit had a say in such cases where price was determined through the market.

The latter, the policy-oriented approach, pertained to the authoritative allocation of values through attempts to attain policy objectives (not necessarily excluding revenue targets in some cases), meanwhile applying mandatory power to maintain the proper balance of interests among strata, sectors, and groups of people, coupled with other political implications. In some concrete cases, for examples, the government often adopted mandatory pricing through pricing plans in the interest of "social utility" at the providing unit level (Wang 1999). Throughout the reform period, the government adopted the policy-oriented approach in exercising price control in order to address the issue of inequality as well as protection of the needy, weak and marginal sector of population. For instance, the ministerial officials reaffirmed in the early 1990s the long-established policy of "three assurances and three flexibilities," namely, the assurance of priority given to the tasks of price control of health care in rural areas, for preventive care, and basic curative care services, but for more flexibility of discretion for pricing in urban areas, non-basic curative services, and non-essential care (Hong 1993).

It is apparent in the policy-oriented approach that the government was often confronted with the task to maintain a measure of balance between revenue targets and other public policy concerns. As the government applied the policy-oriented approach to pricing of health care services, it invariably encountered divergent interpretations of "social utility" and often deviation from market reality. Besides, that the government was not represented by one actor but by several departments acting on behalf of the government. And yet each interpreted public policy in its own right. According to policy analyst Meng Qingyao, for instance, the various departments of finance would stress that they intended to alleviate the burden of the people, as they succeeded to reduce the financial burden of the government; the health care departments would argue that they served the best interest of the people by maintaining the good operation of health care providing units and the effective provision of health care services; the departments of pricing would argue that they actually served the people well by making medical care affordable when they control the price level of medical care services (Meng, 2000: 6–7). Some authors noted that the price bureau was often biased against the people who work in the medical profession in so far as the upward adjustment of price was made at the expenses of a low-price policy of basic medical care services.

In many other instances, the MOH tended to defend and even advocate the interests of the providing unit and medical personnel (Liu & Gao 2009).

In a telling example in price control during the early phase of economic reform, the government employed the policy-oriented approach in the case of policy experiment with the "system of two charge schemes" (liangzong feiyong zhidu), making the enrollees of the PFMC and LIMC program pay more than those uninsured residents in urban areas for more than one decade from 1979 to 1992 (Weishengbu 1984a: 482–4). The said system was intended to create an additional revenue source for the providing units and to "compensate" their loss resulting from excessively low charges/fees of curative care services as well as runaway medical inflation after the Maoist era (Xia 1990). It meant to alleviate the inequality among the populace in the transitional economy, specifically addressing the issue of disparity between two classes of users, namely insured and non-insured (Wong, Lo, & Tang 2006; Peng, Cai, & Zhou, 1992: 36–40; Zhou, Qu, & Li 2003:11–35).

However, the respective work units (including the government work units, service work units, and public enterprises) shouldered the costs of additional charges to the users of PFMI and LIMC programs respectively. As a result, an estimated 20 percent in the total revenue growth of the health care sector was derived from the PFMI program to be absorbed by the state budget and 80 percent from the LIMC program to be charged to the accounts of revenue retention and the welfare fund at the enterprise level, but not as production costs (Weishengbu 1984b: 495–7). In 1992, the two charge schemes were subsequently abolished, returning to the one singular charge scheme once again, because of complaints from insured patients, arguing that the enrollees of public insurances actually had to subsidize non-insured patients by shouldering a heavier financial burden. Besides, some of those SOEs that were supposed to provide insurance funding were in financial hardship, and found difficult even to honor their own obligations to enrollees to LIMC programs.[7]

The task of price control had encountered great challenges in the wake of the increasing weight of the market-oriented approach relative to the policy-oriented approach in midst of health care reform. They were manifested in several issues of price-regulating task as follows. First, the price bureau and providing unit had to redefine their respective roles and to work out division of labor to share the pricing job. As a rule of thumb, funding sources rather than other factors determined who ought to have greater discretion over pricing. For instance, when the services were commercialized, relying on user charges entirely, the providing unit has more say. Under the circumstance, "production price" would apply, namely, cost-based price plus average profit of society in technical terms (Weishengbu 1984b: 495–7). By contrast, the government might have more say about those services depending upon the extent of each service's financial support from the government.[8] The policymakers often adopted cost-based pricing (normally excluding the government's subsidies and profit/revenue) for those basic curative care services which were seen with considerable externality, for instance, for maintaining the quality of the labor force and enhancing labor productivity of the economy. With or without subsidies, they also applied cost-based pricing to those quasi-public health services such as paid immunization packages and insurance programs for children and women (Weishengbu 1984b: 495–7).

Second, from the perspective of administrative rationality, it has been an established practice to apply different pricing schedules for different classes of public hospitals. For example, those public hospitals that were professionally and technically advanced would normally adopt a portion of adjustment charges (meaning higher charges) to recognize and reward their investment, as well as extra work on difficult and complex cases of diseases, while those average hospitals applied the standard charge schedules for dealing with common and frequently found cases of illness. The schedules of user charges, based upon technical appraisals, were found helpful in making better use of health care resources, for instance, in the case of applying lower charges to encourage those patients with common and frequent illnesses to go to average-class hospitals (e.g., Tier 1 hospitals) and community health care centers, and in other cases of higher charges to those patients with difficult and complicated cases to seek cure in the technically sophisticated hospitals (e.g., Tier 3 hospitals) (Weishengbu 1984b: 495–7).

Third, there often existed the gap between the expectation and performance with regard to the price-regulating job of the price bureau. Many analysts considered that the price bureau did not have adequate information and competence to assume such a role as an adjudicator of diverse interests and as an effective price controller in market transactions in view of the increasing complexity of the job contents as well as the task environment. Examples include the rapid improvement of living standards, the increase of inflation, the advent of medical technology, rapid development of medicine, increasing costs for upgraded facilities, demographic change, the aging of population, the changing profile of illness, and the arrival of new insurance programs (Li 2000; Liu, 2008; Wang 2006; Wang & Wang 2007; Wang 2008b; Zou & Zheng 2010). Moreover, relevant price bureaus were often insensitive to quality differences and not infrequently delayed in making timely price adjustments due to a shortage of knowledge and information (Luo 2006; Wang 2008b). As claimed, a "full-fledged" market-oriented approach was not yet in place to carry out the pricing task for a long period after 1979 (Wang 1994a; Zhang 2011). Even up to 2006, for example, some relevant departments still admitted that the system of information collection and mechanisms of price adjustments were not in place (Luo 2006).

Fourth, it appears that the market-oriented approach was preferable to the policy-oriented approach in order to gauge the real contribution of medical personnel in curative care service and to lend fair recognition to the demands of the providing unit for appropriate increase of charges and fees in the midst of expanding markets (Ge 2000). The medical care profession circle often complained that there were made losers in sharing the fruits of the expansion of market economy because the government did not have sufficient knowledge and information in place to act upon changing market situations (Chen 1992a; Wang 1994a). According to Du Lexuan, voices from the medical care sector registered grievances that the government missed the prime time of price adjustment at the expenses of the medical care profession circle, as it failed to consult indexes of high inflation rates of medical material during the early 1990s (Du 2005: 6). In addition to medical personnel, users played an increasing important role in pricing because of introduction of user charges, an issue to be tackled next.

Pricing issues and the repackaging of health care services

The price-regulating task had to face changes and restructuring arising from the repackaging and expanding of various categories of health care services throughout the reform era (Chapter 2). During the early phase of the reform, first of all, a new set of user charges was formulated and added to the Category II quasi-public health services when it was first differentiated from the conventional Category I pure-public health services, and user charges were also introduced to Category IV, the non-basic curative care services as it was separated from Category III, the basic care services in accordance with the 1985 Report and the 1988 Opinion.[9] Moreover, the paid public health services was made one of the main policy initiatives of health care reform in accordance with the policy paper entitled the Outline of China's Health Care Development and Reform, 1991–2000. (Weishengbu, PRC 1990; Cui 1992; Peng, Cai, & Zhou 1992: 211–20).

The said repackaging is inseparable from the affordable care policy that ensures the provision of a floor of basic health services to all through provision of Category I, purely public health care, Category II, quasi-public health care, and Category III basic medical care. And three are subsidized by the government to varying extents. Category II, Category III, and Category IV are supported by user charges in varying degrees according to charge schedules. The repackaging was intended to answer not only revenue concern but also meet the growing diversity of demands for health care services. As mentioned previously, the revenue-generating endeavor remains controversial, and nonetheless justifiable from sovereign planners' financial strategy (Chapter 4). In other word, revenue-generating is not necessarily in contradiction to the affordable care policy, but it is only intended to reduce the government's financial input to support the same policy. Also, it is warranted to meet the rising demands for upgrading and diverse types of health care in the midst of improvement of income, purchasing power, and living standards, changing profile of illness and aging of the population, the use of new drugs and advanced medical technology, among others in transition to the mixed economy. According to Wang Bozhen, this marked a significant change by officially giving more choices and a greater share of financial responsibility to users overall in order to encourage careful use of health care resources (Wang 1994a:10–11).

In fact, the policymakers at both the ministerial and provincial levels pushed another round of commercialization of special care services in accordance with the 1992 Decision.[10] It advocates treating and managing health care services as a tertiary industry, urging provincial policymakers to promote the "entrepreneurial orientation" of the public hospitals and to underscore the "commodity value" of health care services (Dai 1993; Gu 1993). Various provincial jurisdictions argued invariably that since it was not feasible to rely only upon the financial input of the government, it was necessary to explore the full revenue-generating potential of health care services (Dai 1993). To go beyond the 1985 Report, for example, they promoted the further expansion of special care services into four types: the time-oriented type, such as services provided with an overtime schedule or extended hours of home services; the personnel-oriented type in terms of appointments with specialists; the devices/facilities-oriented type regarding upgraded wards or imported devices for examination; and the contents-oriented type concerning cosmetic surgery, dental services, recuperation, and hospice facilities, among others (Dai 1993). As an example, in Guangdong Province, the 1992 Circular recommended a new schedule of charges for special care services.[11]

The repackaging of health care services created new issues of pricing and charges in the perspective of regulatory control, that highlights the advantages of medical profession in the revenue-seeking game at the providing unit level (Chapter 1). There witnessed, for instance, a tendency of the providing unit working closely with medical personnel in over-provision for non-basic care services at the expense of the curtailment of basic medical care services. The providing unit and medical personnel are often motivated to induce/persuade the patients to use more of non-basic medical care services for revenue seeking considerations, albeit this might appear advisable on pure medical ground (Meng 2000). Due to "asymmetric information", it is by no means easy for the insurer and the patients to say "no" to expensive options of non-basic care services, and to stick only to basic medical care services. It is equally difficult for the supervisory bureaus to adopt and enforce an appropriate operational definition of basic medical care and to ensure the delivery of affordable care to all, as noted previously (Chapter 2).

In addition, patients might play an active role in opting for the non-basic care category in pursuit of the least risk and better quality of medical care services, given the rapid improvement of living standards and rising expectations (Chen & Lo 2011; Li, 2006). According to ministerial ranking official He Jiesheng, it was justifiable for various social strata of people who were riding on the prosperity of the commodity economy to demand "multiple layers of medical needs" in both the basic and non-basic types of medical care (He 1992:169). In view of Li Huaiyong et al., patients themselves were willing to accept "over-provision" because of their increasing demand for better services and improving purchasing power (Li 2006: 66).

Theoretically speaking, the providing unit operates with two budgetary modes: Mode One and Mode Two are found relevant here. In Mode One, being dominant prior to 1979, the providing unit was not held accountable to budgetary balance, as the government was expected to maintain adequate financial input, coupled with low user charges (Peng, Cai, & Zhou 1992: 5; Chu & Yu 2010: 64–5). It was much easier to enforce price-regulating requirements in Mode One because the providing unit often complied with pricing schedules, and normally was not held financial accountable for revenue and loss. Mode Two pertained to the situation where public hospitals had to work with accountability, wrestling between the pressure of earning main portion of revenue from user charges (i.e. OPP) and the tight price control policy during the reform era after 1979. In Mode Two, it became difficult for the supervising bureaus to implement price-regulating measures because price control often adversely affected the revenue flow and thus budgetary balance at the providing unit level.

In the financial strategy of health care reform, there are several policy and managerial options based upon the mix of the tools of the government subsidies and price-regulating measures, entailing choices among several policy options.[12] In practical terms, the government was confronted with the dilemma to reduce proportionally its financial appropriation to the providing unit on the one hand, and it had to maintain low user charges for health care services on the other hand, in light of the concern of social utility (for instance, covering Category I pure-public health, Category II quasi-public health, and Category III basic health care).[13] In other cases, as the public funding dwindled in proportion, the providing unit was still not allowed to seek compensation by earning adequately from medical care services. Chen and Yin treat this as a "distorted pricing system," becoming the fundamental cause for all kinds of financial irregularities and legal violations at the providing unit level during the reform era (Chen & Yin: 1989).

Price control and cost shifting

Here the notion of cost shifting means to shift the real cost of lowly priced items of service to better priced ones in order to compensate the loss of the former, and thus to maintain the budgetary balance at the providing unit level. And cost shifting practice is closely related to price control in health care sector since price control determines costs of services and the volume of revenue at the providing unit level. Conceptually speaking, Wang Yanzhong proposes the "double-track" pricing system to analyze various types of health care services in connection with the issue of cost shifting during the health care reform. One is a restrictive pricing track where price control is normally imposed from above, coupled with the government's "hidden subsidy" e.g., appropriation to fund investment in infrastructure, facilities and equipment, management and operation, and pay to medical personnel. Here "restrictive" means working within the framework of bureaucracy, and limited exposure to the market forces. The other pertains to an open track, allowing the providing unit to operate with accountability for its own revenue and loss in the market situation, and, therefore, to have room of discretion in fixing charges/fees, such as user charges to non-basic curative care, prescription drugs, and advanced medical devices. In the former, the providing unit was made to render the basic medical services at regulated and in fact low price, but the actual amount of "hidden subsidy" might not be adequate to cover costs. In shortage of the government's funding, as a rule, the cost of the basic medical care is expected to shift to non-basic medical care, which allowed the providing unit to generate revenue from the latter against total cost (Wang 2008: 37–8).

As an integral part of commercialization, the repackaging and expansion of franchises have resulted in a pattern of cost shifting among four major types of medical care services: basic technical-medical care services (e.g., diagnosis and treatments), non-basic services such as special care services, advanced medical devices, and expensive type of prescription drugs. In general, the basic technical-medical care services were priced lower than their real cost, while the remaining three might be priced higher than their real cost. Logically speaking, the basic technical-medical care services were supposed to be "cross subsidized" financially by the remaining three that are priced at a higher level reflecting the real cost generated through market transactions.

In conceptual terms, moreover, curative care services include three related components: diagnosis and treatments, medical devices, and drug prescriptions. Each is covered by a set of franchise, and each adopts a different way of pricing. It is always within the discretion of medical personnel to make use of medical devices and drug prescriptions medically as tools for diagnosis and treatments (Zhu 1999: 6). In pricing management, one finds it difficult to segregate diagnosis and treatments from the remaining two, namely, medical devices and prescription drugs. At the end of the day, not only doctors have a say over pricing of diagnosis and treatments, but also that of prescription drugs and medical devices.

Throughout the reform, the government followed the restrictive pricing track by providing basic technical-medical care services (e.g., diagnosis and treatments) at tightly regulated prices, while, ideally, allowing "hidden subsidies" to be passed on to the patient. With the restrictive pricing track, price management tended to suppress the true costs of diagnosis and treatment, but, through the open pricing track, it gave the providing unit more discretion over pricing of the other two components (medical devices and prescription drugs) to fetch better revenue. As the reform policy to move toward the open pricing track, the providing unit was allowed flexibility to make schedules of charges for the tests and examinations with advanced medical devices. Besides that, the providing unit was allowed to continue to make use of the franchise of pharmaceutical retails to generate revenue to fund curative care services, normally at 15 percent for Western medicine, 16 percent for manufactured folk medicine, and 25–30 percent for folk herb medicine, according to doctors' prescriptions during the reform era (Yang & Sun 2006: 71–80;

Zhou, Qu, & Li 2003: 137–67; Sun & Du 2006; Zhu 2006; Wu 2002; Hu, Gong, & Xu 2000; Zhu, 1999).

The government found it difficult to monitor and control medical personnel who wielded considerable discretion over the process of making decisions of technical-medical care services (Chapter 1). Also, it was up to medical personnel to choose among several options of diagnosis and treatments in a range of prices—more or less expensive. Moreover, curative care services were operationally inseparable from the drugs and devices. As a consequence, medical personnel, in collaboration with the providing unit, could often prescribe the kinds of drugs and order medical devices at the high end of the price range for cost shifting purpose in order to generate revenue and compensate for the financial shortfall (Chu & Yu 2010: 66).

The issue of excessively low fees in the categories of medical-technical labor input, namely, the fees for medical doctors and nurses, was first attributed to the ultra-leftist influence of Mao's era in terms of one-sidedly emphasizing the low-price package of basic curative care. During this early phase of health care reform, the top policymakers took initiatives to address the issue of meager pay to medical personnel (Peng, Cai, & Zhou 1992: 5–6). However, they did not seem to make the effort to find remedies to the issue of low-priced curative care. Furthermore, no method of cost calculation of the value of health care services had developed until 2010, meaning that to a considerable extent, the pricing of a job is still dictated by subjectivity and arbitrariness.

MOH did make a pledge to improve the unreasonably low charges to technical-medical care services gradually.[14] To make price adjustment upward, moreover, it proposed to follow the principle of "old prices for old items and new prices for new items" to remain sensitive administratively and managerially to the price levels of curative medical care services that had already built a client base. The 1985 Report did recommend price hikes in broad categories of new items—except for the basic curative care—including the diagnoses and treatments that relied upon new medical devices and facilities. The new price schedules adopted a cost-based formula of calculation. As just noted, some new charges schemes were introduced for "special care services," e.g. upgraded wards and appointments with specialists. Also, those hospitals that had been newly built, rebuilt, or renovated were permitted to shift to new schedules of charges in order to fetch better revenue (Weishengbu 1985a).

Building upon MOH's endeavors to forge a consensus on pricing policy since the mid-1980s, the 1988 Opinion (known as Document Guofa No. 10, 1989) drew the conclusion that "the current price schedules of registration, hospital beds, and surgical operation are on the low side, requiring reasonable adjustments" (Weishengbu et al. 1993b: 11–13; Guowuyuan 1993: 1–2). It urged, furthermore, that the price bureaus and the health care bureaus at the provincial and municipal/local levels to work out systematically the new pricing schedules, standards, methods of calculation, and the scope and range of price adjustments in the categories of basic curative care in collaboration with the ministerial units of Finance, Health Care, and Pricing under the unified arrangement of national price reform by the State Council, seemingly putting pricing adjustment on the policy agenda (Weishengbu, PRC 1993). To what extent is the effort to adjust prices in health care services successful? This is a question to be answered in the remaining sections.

Policy issues of price adjustment

In theoretical terms, the total volume of cost shifting can be diminished if the policy on pricing is able to narrow down the gaps between the price of a service and its real cost, an issue remaining controversial for more than a decade from the mid-1980s to mid-1990s. Meanwhile some jurisdictions were allowed to introduce a number of pilot programs concerning price adjustments of medical care services and pharmaceutical reform.[15] And some other provincial and municipal jurisdictions subsequently took the initiative to enact price reform, for example, in the cases of Guangdong, Shandong, Zhejiang, and Henan, among others (Dai 1993; Gu 1993; Guangtongsheng weishengting, jicaiju 1993; Xu & Qiu 1993).

Three issues of price control have remained unsolved throughout the medical care reform since the mid-1980s. First, the policymakers wrestled with the issue of pricing of prescription drugs which was in cost shifting from low-priced "medical-technical labor." In a new trend as shown Table 6-1, sovereign planners have endeavored to curtail further price growth of prescription drugs, but tried to balance this with upward adjustments of charges for curative care services and medical devices from 1990 to 2008.[16] The policymakers ought to be credited for their vigorous efforts to bring down the payments for prescription drugs from 67.9 percent in 1990 to 50.5 percent in 2008 for outpatients and from 55.1 percent for inpatients in 1990 to 43.3 percent in 2008 respectively. As of 2010, sovereign planners had made 26 cuts of prices in various categories of pharmaceuticals, contributing to the further lowering of the expenses of pharmaceutical products for patients (Huang 2014).

The policymakers appeared making effort to recognize the contribution of medical personnel and lend greater weight of real cost of "medical-technical input" in pricing the curative care services. And Table 6.1 demonstrates a growth of "examination and treatment" from 19.3 percent for outpatients in 1990 to 30.9 percent in 2008, and from 25.7 percent for inpatients in 1990 to 34.5 percent in 2008 respectively, indicating some visible improvement of the fees for the services of medical personnel.

The second issue of price control is concerned with the component of medical devices that have modernized and upgraded the curative medical care services in China. And this has reflected on the policy change of pricing. For example, it is stated in the 1985 Report that all of those newly introduced services of diagnoses and treatments with advanced medical devices may adopt the new standards of charges, which are based on costs

Table 6.1 Average medical care expenses in China: outpatients and inpatients, 1990–2008

Year	Outpatient Expenses					Inpatient Expenses				
	Expenses in RMB			% of Total outpatient expenses		Expenses in RMB			% of Total inpatient Expenses	
	Average outpatient expenses	Prescription expenses	Exam & treatment expenses	Prescription expenses	Exam & treatment expenses	Average inpatient expenses	Prescription expenses	Exam & treatment expenses	Prescription expenses	Exam & treatment expense
1990	10.9	7.4	2.1	67.9%	19.3%	473.3	260.6	121.5	55.1%	25.7%
1995	39.9	25.6	9.1	64.2%	22.8%	1,667.8	880.3	507.3	52.8%	30.4%
2000	85.8	50.3	16.8	58.6%	19.6%	3,083.7	1,421.9	978.5	46.1%	31.7%
2002	99.6	55.2	27.9	55.4%	28.0%	3,597.7	1,598.4	1,320.7	44.4%	36.7%
2003	108.2	59.2	30.8	54.7%	28.4%	3,910.7	1,748.3	1,411.6	44.7%	36.1%
2004	118	62	35.1	52.5%	29.8%	4,284.8	1,872.9	1,566.3	43.7%	36.6%
2005	126.9	66	37.8	52.1%	29.8%	4,661.5	2,045.6	1,678.1	43.9%	36.0%
2006	128.7	65	39.9	50.5%	31.0%	4,668.9	1,992	1,691.1	42.9%	36.2%
2007	139.1	68	42.4	50.5%	31%	4,973.8	2,148.9	1,734.6	43.2%	34.9%
2008	146.5	74	45.3	50.5%	30.9%	5,463.8	2,400.4	1,887	43.9%	34.5%

Source: Zhongguo Tongji Nianjian Bianji Weiyuanhui (Ed.). 2009. Zhongguo tongji nianjian 2009 (China's Statistics Yearbook 2009), 96. Beijing: Zhongguo xiehe yike daxue chubanshe.

(Weishengbu1985a: 5). Accordingly, public hospitals enjoyed considerable discretion over pricing of new medical devices prior to 2004. However, this did not mean that the government adopted a hand off policy regarding the pricing of medical devices (Chapter 7).

From time to time, the government still seeks to play an active role in the market of medical devices on top of drugs. For example, the government began to experiment with collective bidding and procurement of drugs in 2004, subsequently extending to medical devices. In June 2007, the government encouraged all public hospitals and non-public hospitals to take part in collective-bidding procurement programs, including all large-scale, expensive, and advanced medical devices.[17] However, it was found that the policy would be difficult to implement price control over medical devices, given the wide variety of high-end products in the markets that were often non-standardized with multiple technical specifications. These products were not entirely amenable to price-regulating in view of franchise and rigidity of prices. It is suggested that the government has never been able to develop effective price management over the links of production and circulation of these high-end medical devices (Zou & Zheng 2010: 5I)

Third, as a whole, the policymakers have been lagging behind in addressing the pricing of "medical-technical input" in spite of some relevant departments' sympathy with and support to the demands of medical personnel for reasonable price adjustments of curative care service in order to improve their compensation. With reference to the total charges in the mid-1990s, Chinese policy analyst Xu Guanwei gave an estimate: prescription drugs normally commanded a price range at 55–70 percent, fees for medical devices at 15–30 percent, medical-technical services (nursing and diagnosis and treatments by doctors) at 7–10 percent, and the non-technical services at 20 percent (Xu 1995: 36–7). In collaboration with the price structure noted above, the ratios of the four parts remained relatively stable over time in light of available statistics and various surveys conducted during the reform era.[18] Xu suggests that overall, medical-technical services charges are deemed at the low side compared with those of the West, often at 50–5 percent for items such as surgery, diagnosis and treatment, clinical visits, and medical devices (Xu 1995: 36–7).

Sovereign planners were able to forge a coherent view on price policy and strategy belatedly in accordance with the 1996 Circular promulgated on October 15, 1996 (Guojia jihua weiyuanhui, Weishengbu & Caizhengbu 1998: 919–21). The 1996 Circular addresses the issue of the low price of the "highly graded medical-technical component" (i.e., work of medical personnel) in curative care services and posits that it needs to be adjusted in a timely fashion. The 1996 Circular highlights the overall problem of the pricing policy that arose from the health care reform: very low charges for the medical-technical component coupled with excessively high charges for prescription drugs and relatively high charges for medical devices (Guojia jihua weiyuanhui, Weishengbu & Caizhengbu 1998: 919–21). This view has dominated the price policy for the coming two decades up to the present.

Concluding remarks

It is understood on the basis of the foregoing analysis that in price-regulating matters, the government is the principal actor in the tightly regulated markets of medical care services in China today (Zou & Zheng 2010). However, the government often failed to address the issue of budgetary balance and revenue concerns at the providing unit level, creating the tug of war between the government and the providing unit. Above all, professional expertise and access to first-hand information lent the providing unit and medical personnel considerable weight in countering the price-regulating measures imposed from above, as previously mentioned (Chapter 1). Moreover, the medical care reform saw the increasing salience of the market-oriented approach because price-regulating allows flexibility of price adjustments by taking cues from the market.

Among several issues of public management, the providing unit developed a strategy of cost shifting under the circumstances of tight price control and drastic shrinkage of state appropriation in order to meet the shortfall caused by lowly priced curative care services throughout the health care reform.[19] In the process of policy evolution, the mechanisms of cost shifting concerning prescription drugs had been in existence prior to the reform, and it has perpetuated since 1979 and gained considerable strength from the early 1990s onward (Liu, 2012: 16–18; Zhou et al. 2003: 136–53; Guojia jihua weiyuanhui 1998). Also, a new dimension of franchising has to do with expanded services involving upgraded laboratory tests with expensive medical devices whose charges are often determined with broad discretion at the providing unit level (Yang & Sun 2006: 74). Overall, this study argues that the emerging pattern of cost shifting is a function of the price control imposed on the providing unit by the government. As to the question how active and powerful is the state in its newfound roles in the growth of regulated markets of curative care services, drugs and medical devices during economic reform, one needs to treat it in a relative term by examining the part played by the providing unit in succeeding chapters as given in Part III.

Notes

1 During the economic reform, the choices of policy instruments have interacted with a changing task environment, raising new issues of health care services such as a greater variety of health care services introduced, upgrading of quality of medical care, introduction of novel technology, new drugs and medical devices, new demands derived from improvement of income and purchasing power, new profile of illness and aging of the population, uncompromising professional

requirements for the quality of services, safety of drugs, right treatment and minimal risks, just to name a few.

2 The Party Center, CCP, and State Council promulgated the Decision of Health Care Reform and Development in early 1997 (Zhonggong Zhongyan, Guowuyuan 1999; Chu & Yu 2010).

3 The Party Center, CCP, and the State Council promulgated the Advisory Opinion of Institutional Reform of Medical Care and Dispensary Services in Cities and Towns in 2000 (Chu & Yu 2010; Chen, 2000b: 457–70).

4 As endorsed by the State Council, on July 20, 2000, the State Planning Commission and the Ministry of Health Care promulgated the Opinion of the Reform of Price Management in Health Care Services (abbreviated as the 2000 Opinion hereafter) (Luo 2006).

5 For example, they include the Ministry of Health, Ministry of Human Resources and Social Security, Ministry of Finance, the Reform and Development Commission, the Bureau of Supervision of Foods and Drugs, and Chinese Herbal Medicine Bureau (Wang 2008: 253–4).

6 In January 1997, the Central Committee, CCP, and the State Council erected a new landmark by making the Decision Concerning Health Care Reform and Development (abbreviated as the 1997 Decision). (Zhonggongzhongyang 1997).

7 According to the author's interview in Guangzhou, furthermore, it did not appear reasonable to impose extra burden on industrial enterprises as well as their employees while many poorly performing enterprises could not even provide adequate funding to the LIMC program; and as a result, a considerable number of insured patients could not even get the reimbursement of their medical bills, in part or in full, letting along to pay higher user charges for the basic curative care services that they had received. Personal interview with (three interviewees), 11/05/2000, Guangzhou.

8 In descending order, for example, more say in cases about welfare price than cost-based price and more say about cost-based prices than production prices. (Weishengbu 1984b: 495–7).

9 The two policy papers are: the Report of the Several Policy Problems of Health Care Work in 1985 (abbreviated as the 1985 Report hereafter) and the Opinion Concerning the Problems of Expansion of Medical and Health Care Services in 1988 (abbreviated as the 1988 Opinion hereafter) (Weishengbu et al. 1993a; Weishengbu 1985b)

10 The title of the policy paper is as follows: the Decision Concerning the Accelerating of the Development of Tertiary Industry (abbreviated as the 1992 Decision hereafter) promulgated by the Party Center and the State Council in 1992.

11 In November 1992, the Health Care Office, the Price Office, and the Finance Office jointly promulgated the Circular on Several Issues of the Price Reform in Medical Care Services (abbreviated as the 1992 Circular in November 1992 (Guangdongsheng Weishengting 1993).

12 Theoretically speaking, there might at least be four policy options as follows: (1) stringent subsidies and tight price regulating measures, (2) generous subsidies and relaxed price measures, (3) stringent subsidies but relaxed price control, and (4) generous subsidies and tight price measures.

13 Chen Jijiang and Yin Yungong characterize this as follows: "We [policymakers] control funding to the health care institutes on the one hand; [we] regulate the prices of medical care services on the other hand" (Chen & Yin 1989). And the same observation was also made by other policy analysts later (Peng, Cai, & Zhou 1992: 36).

14 The Ministry of Health openly pledged "to reform the unreasonable charge system gradually" in the 1985 Report, and this position was further affirmed by Minister Chen Mingzhang in 1986 (Chen 1992b: 152–3).

15 For example, Wenzhou municipality began a pilot program to spearhead a comprehensive medical care and pharmaceutical price reform in July 1988 (Gu & Chen 1990: 39–43).
16 It was confirmed by interview sources at the ministerial level and bureau level that as an overall policy during the late 1990s, the price of curative treatment and examination was to be adjusted upward. See Interview (one interviewee), 17/08/1995, Beijing; see interview (three interviewees), 01/06/2000, Guangzhou. The interviewee in Beijing suggested that in order to control inflation, the State Council would withhold specific approvals on the upward adjustment of labor costs until an appropriate time, in spite of overall policy direction pointing to this upward adjustment.
17 The Ministry of Health promulgated the Circular Concerning the Strengthening of Management of Concentrated Procurement of Medical Devices (abbreviated as the 2007 Circular hereafter) (Zou & Zheng, 2010: 5).
18 According to a survey of hospitals in 1988, in the total of income from registration consists of 1.6 percent, hospital services 4.9 percent, devices and treatment 25.1 percent and medicine 61.6 percent. (Peng, Cai & Zhou 1992: 37); The annual accounting report of those comprehensive and large hospitals affiliated with the Ministry of Health in 1991 gives break downs of charges/fees as follows: in the total of clinical services, registration fee consists only of 2.2 percent, devices and treatment 18.9 percent, and prescription drugs 68.7 percent. In the total of hospital services, bed charges consist of 8.7 percent, surgery 3.9 percent, examination and treatment 21.8 percent and medicine 54.8 percent (Dai 1993: 27–8). As cited by Li Huaiyong, another illustration of a hospital chosen in Beijing of the mid 2000s shows that on average the patient spent 43 percent for drugs, 7 percent for laboratory tests, 13 percent for examinations, 8 percent for treatment, 4 percent for surgery, 10 percent for medical material, 6 percent for hospital bed and 9 percent for others. In Li's view, the charge to surgery (only calculated as 4 percent) is considered far too low in view of its true medical-technical value (Li 2006).
19 This is often thought of as "classics" in financial management at the providing unit level: the loss of curative care service to be cross-subsidized by drug sale; the revenue flow of drug sale, if constrained, to be compensated by laboratory tests; and the deficit of core services to be compensated by auxiliary services and affiliated services. (Peng, Cai, & Zhou 1992: 36).

References

Chen, B., & Lo, W. 2011. 2008 niandu woguo yiliao fuwu feiyong jiegou fenxi (An analysis of the structure of charges of medical care services in China in 2008). *Zhongguo weisheng jingji (China's Health Care Economics)*, 30(1): 27–29.
Chen, J., & Yin, Y. 1989. Weisheng gaige de kunhuo yu chulu (Puzzles and solutions of health reform). *Jingji yanjiu cankao zhiliao (References of Economic Research)*, 102: 29–38.
Chen, M. 1992a. Chen Mingzhang buchang zai quanquo weisheng tingjuchang huiyi shang de zongjie jianghua (Minister Chen Mingzhang's concluding speech at the national conference of chiefs of bureaus/offices of health care). In R. Peng, R. Cai, & C. Zhou (Eds.), *Zhongguo gaige quanshu (Encyclopedia of China's Reform)*, 184–190. Dalian: Dalian chubanshe.
Chen, M. 1992b. Chen Mingzhang tongchi zai yijiu balu nian quanguo weisheng tingjuchang huiyi shang de zongjie jianghua (Comrade Chen Mingzhang's concluding speech at the 1986 national conference of chiefs of bureaus/offices of health

care). In R. Peng, R. Cai, & C. Zhou (Eds.), *Zhongguo gaige quanshu (Encyclopedia of China's Reform)*, 152–153. Dalian: Dalian chubanshe.

Chen, M. 1999. Chen Minzhang buzhang zai 1998 nian quanguo weisheng tingjuzhang huiyi shang de baogao (The report of Minister Chen Minzhang at the 1998 national conference of office/bureau chiefs of health care). In Zhongguo weisheng nianjian bianji weiyuanhui (Ed.), *Zhongguo weisheng nianjian 1999* (China's Yearbook of Health Care 1999), 7–10. Beijing: Renmin weisheng chubanshe.

Chen, Y. 2000a. Diwupian, diyizhang: Yiliao fuwu jiage de gaige yu guanli (part five, chapter one: The reform and management of pricing of medical care services). In Y. Chen, (Ed.), *Zhongguo chengzhan yiyao weisheng tizhi gaige chitao quanshu, shanqun* (Encyclopedia for the Guides of Institutional Reform of Medicine and Health Care in Towns and Cities in China, volume 1), 457–487. Beijing: Zhongguo wujia chubanshe.

Chen, Y. (Ed.). 2000b. *Zhongguo chengzhen yiyao weisheng tizhi gaige zhidao quanshu* (Encyclopedia of Medical and Health Reform in Urban China). Beijing: Zhonguo wujia chubanshe.

Chu, J., & Yu, B. 2010. Woguo yiliao fuwu jiage guanli tizhi yanjiu zongshu (A general observation on the pricing management of health care services in China). *Zhongguo weisheng jingji (China's Health Care Economics)*, 29(4): 64–66.

Cui, Y. 1992. Cui Yueli tongchi zai yijiu bawu nian quanguo weisheng tingjuchang huiyi shang de jianghua (Comrade Cui Yueli's speech at the national conference of chiefs of bureaus/offices of health care). In R. Peng, R. Cai, & C. Zhou (Eds.), *Zhongguo gaige quanshu, yiliao weisheng tizhi gaige juan (Encyclopedia of China's Reform)*, 129–134. Dalian: Dalian chubanshe.

Dai, D. 1993. Shencengci weisheng gaig de gousi (Thoughts on health care reform at a deeper level). *Zhongguo weisheng jingji(China's Health Care Economics)*, 2: 26–28.

Du, L. 2005. Woguo gonggong weisheng touru jiqi jixiao pingjia (Input and performance evaluation of public health care in China). *Zhongguo weisheng jingji(China's Health Care Economics)*, 24(11): 5–8.

Ge, P. 2000. Shilun shenhua weisheng gaige mianling de maodun (A tentative discussion on the contradiction confronting the further reform in health care). *Weisheng jingji yanjiu(Research on Health Care)*, 1: 22–23.

Gu, X. 1993. Shichang jingji yu weisheng gaige (Market economy and health care reform). *Zhongguo weisheng jingji(China's Health Care Economics)*, 3: 21–24.

Gu, X., Chen Xientan. 1990. Wenzhou weisheng gaige de huigu yu sikou (Retrospect and thoughts on health care reform in Wenzhou). *Zhnogguo weisheng jingji(China's Health Care Economics)*, 1: 39–43.

Gu, X. 2008. *Zouxiang quanmin yibao: Zhongguo xingyigai de zhanlue yu zhanshu* (Toward Comprehensive Medical Insurance: Strategy and Tactic of China's New Medical Care Reform). Beijing: Zhongguo laodong chubanshe.

Guangdongsheng Weishengting. 1993. Shenhua weisheng gaige, tansuo shiying shichang jingji xuyao de xintizhi (Further health care reform, in search of the new institutions to meet the needs of market economy), 4:13–15.

Guojia Jihua Weiyuanhui, Weishengbu, Caizhengbu. 1998. Guanyu jiaqiang he gaijinyiliao fuwu shoufei guanli de tongzhi (The circular concerning the strengthening and improvement of the management of charges of medical care services). In Weishengbu Zhengce Faguisi (Ed.), *Zhonghua remin gongheguo weisheng fagui huibian, 1995–1997* (The Collection of Laws and Regulations of Health Care of the PRC, 1995–1997), 919–921. Beijing: Falu chubanshe.

Guojia Jiwei, W. 2001. Guanyu gaige yiliao fuwu jiage guanli de yijian (The opinion on the reform of price management of medical care services). In Weishengbu Fazhi yu Jiandusi (Ed.), *Zhonghua renmin gongheguo weisheng fagui huibian: 1998–2000 (The Collection of Laws and Regulations of Health Care of the PRC)*, 26–28. Beijing: Falu chubanshe.

Guowuyuan. 1993. Guowuyuan pizhuan guojiajiaowei de bumen guanyu shenhua gaige guli jiaoyu keyan weisheng danwei zengjia shehui funwu yijian de tongzhi (The circular of the state council on the opinion of the state education commission and other units regarding the further reform of and encouragement to the increase of social services of educational, scientific research and health care units). In Weishengbu Fazhi yu Jiandusi (Ed.), *Zhonghua renmin gongheguo weisheng fagui huibian, 1989–1991* (The Collection of Laws and Regulations of the Ministry of Health of the PRC, 1989–1991), 1–2. Beijing: Falu chubanshe.

Guowuyuan Tigaiban, Guojia Jiwei, Guogji Jingmaowei *et al.* 2000. Guanyu chengzheng yiyao weisheng tizhi gaige zhidao yijian (The advisory opinion concerning the reform of medical and health care system in cities and towns). *Guowuyuan gongbao* (Bulletin of the State Council), 11:10–13.

He, J. 1992. He Jiesheng tongzhi zai yijiu baba nian quanguo weisheng tingjuchang huiyi shang de zongjie jianghua (Comrade He Jiesheng's concluding speech at the 1988 national conference of chiefs of bureaus/offices of health care). In R. Peng, R. Cai, & C. Zhou (Eds.), *Zhongguo gaige quanshu (Encyclopedia of China's Reform)*, 168–173. Dalian: Dalian chubanshe.

Henan Sheng Weishengding Jicaichu. 1993. Yiliao fuwu jiage guanli xianzhuang ji gaige (The current state and reform of the pricing management of medical care services and its reform). *Zhongguo weisheng jingji(China's Health Care Economics)*, 2: 33–34.

Hong, N. & Yang, Z. 1993. Shi shiying shichang, haishi shichanghua? (To adapt to market or to marketize?). *Zhongguo nongcun weisheng shiye guanli* (The Management of Rural Health Care Enterprises in China), 11: 8–10.

Hu, S., Gong, X., & Xu, K. 2002. Quanguo yiliao jigou yaopin piling chajia shouru yanjiu (Research on the revenue of price differential between wholesale and retail of pharmaceutic products in health care institutes throughout the country). *Zhongguo weisheng jingji (China's Health Care Economics)*, 19(6):5–7.

Huang, C. 2011. Yiliao weisheng lingyu de jiage guanzhi wenti zhiyi: Guanzhi chengyin yu guanzhi danwei (The issue of price control in the health care sector: The origins and units, no. 1). *Zhongguo weisheng jingji (China's Health Care Economics)*, 30(2): 5–6.

Interview (one interviewee, 17/08/1995).

Interview (three interviewees, 01/06/2000).

Li, H. 2006. Gaige jizhi, jiaqiang guanli, yizhi yiliao feiyong guokuai zengzhang (The reform of mechanisms, strengthening of management, checking of fast growth of medical care expenditure). *Zhongguo weisheng jingji (China's Health Care Economics)*, 25 (11): 65–67.

Li, W. 2000. Zhongguo jingji tizhi gaige yu weisheng gaige (The reform of eocnomic system and health care reform). *Weisheng jingji yanjiu (Research on Health Care Economics)*, 1: 4–6.

Liu, G. 2008. Yiliao fuwu shoufei jiage gaige (Reform on the charges and fees of medical care services). In L. Du. (Ed.), *Zhongguo yiliao weisheng fazhan baoguo No. 4* (Annual Report on China's Health Care No. 4), 175–196. Beijing: Shehui kexue wenxian chubanshe.

Liu, J. 2012. *Zhongguo yigai xiangguan zhengce yanji* (Study on Policies related to China's Medical Care Reform). Beijing: Jingji kexue chubanshe.

Liu, J., & Gao, L. 2006. Woguo gongli yiyuan jianguan moshi yuanjiu (A study on the model of supervision of public hospitals in China). *Zhongfuo weisheng jingji (China's Health Care Economics)*, 8:12.

Luo, L. 2006. Dui woguo yiliao jigou fuwu jiage jiandu guanli de sikao (Some considerations on the supervision and management of pricing of health care services in China). *Zhongguo weisheng jingji (China's Health Care Economics)*, 25(11): 56–58.

Meng, Q. 2000. Woguo yiliao fuwu jiage chengce de gongneng, wenti he zhengce xuanze (The functions, problems and policy options of price policy of medical care services in China). *Zhongguo weisheng jingji (China's Health Care Economics)*, 19 (8): 5–7.

Peng, R., Cai, R., & Zhou, C. (Eds.). 1992. *Zhongguo gaige quanshu* (Encyclopedia of China's Reform). Dalian: Dalian chubanshe.

Sun, N. & Du, L. 2006. Jiankang yu yiyao baojiian de fazhan (The development of health and drug services). In L. Du, *et al.* (Eds.), *Zhongguo yiliao weisheng fazhan baogao, No. 2* (The Report of Development of Medical and Health Care in China, No. 2), 145–179. Beijing: Shehui kexue wenxian chubanshe.

Wang, B. 1994a. Yiliao fuwu jiage gaige de shaugcheng hanyi, (1) (Double implication of price reform of medical care services, part 1). *Zhongguo weisheng zhengce (China's Health Care Policy)*, 5.

Wang, B. 1994b. Yiliao fuwu jiage gaige de shuangcheng hanyi, (2) (Double implication of price reform of medical care services, part 2). *Zhongguo weisheng zhengce (China's Health Care Policy)*, 7.

Wang, B. 2008. *Zhengfu yiliao guamzhi moshi ghonggou yanjiu* (Research on the Restructuring of Mode of Governmental Control). Beijing: Renmin chubanshe.

Wang, L. 2006. "kanbinggui" de chengyin jiqi duiche (The causes of and solution to "the expensiveness of seeking a cure"). *Weisheng jingji yanjiu(Research on Health Care Economics)*, 11: 13–15.

Wang, L. Yiliao fuwu jiage de xingchen jizhi yu zhengce tiaozheng (The mechanisms in the formation of prices as well as policy adjustment of medical care services). *Zhongguo weisheng jingji (China's Health Care Economics)*, 18(6): 17–18.

Wang, Y. & Wang, W. 2007. Kaishu shangzhang de yiliao feiyong yu kanbienlan kanbiengui wenti (The problems of rise of medical care charges as well as the difficulty to seek cure of illness and expensiveness to seek cure). In J. Chen & Y. Wang (Eds.), *Zhonggui shehui baozhang fazhan baoguo* (The Report of Development of Social Insurance in China), 17–36. Beijing: Zhongguo shehui kexue wenxian chubanshe.

Wang, Y. 2008a. *Zhongguo weisheng gaige yu fazhan shizheng yanjiu* (An Emperical Research on the Reform and Devolopment of Health Care). Beijing: Zhonguo laodong shehui baozhang chubanshe.

Wang, Y. 2008b. Lun yiliao feiyong kongzhizhong de tanxing yu jili zhidu (On the flexible system and incentive system regarding the control of medical care charges). *Zhongguo weisheng jingji (China's Health Care Economics)*, 27(3): 12–15.

Weishengbu. 1984a.Weishengbu guanyu jiejue yiyuan peiben wenti de baogao (The report of the ministry of health concerning how to solve the problem of deficit). In Weishengbu bangongting (Ed.), *Zhonghui Renmin Gongheguo weishengsheng fagui huibian (The Collection of Laws of Ministry of Health, PRC, 1981–1983)*, 482–484. Beijing: Falu chubanshe, Xinhua shudian.

Weishengbu. 1984b. Weishengbu, caizhengbu guanyu yiyuan shixing an chengben shoufei shidian qingkuan ji jinhou yijian de qingshi baogao (The report for the request for advice and the state of pilot implementation for cost based charges of hospitals of the Ministry of Health and Ministry of Finance). In Weishengbu ban-gongting (Ed.), *Zhonghui Renmin Gongheguo weishengsheng fagui huibian (The Collection of Laws of Ministry of Health, PRC, 1981–1983)*, 495–497. Beijing: Falu chubanshe, Xinhua shudian.

Weishengbu. 1985a. Guanyu jiejue yiyuan peiban wenti de baogao (The report of the Ministry of Health concerning how to solve the loss of hospitals). In Weishengbu Bangongting (Ed.), *Zhonghua renmin gongheguo weisheng fagui huibian, 1981–1983* (The Collection of Laws and Regulations of Health Care, 1981–1983), 482–484. Beijing: Falu chubanshe.

Weishengbu. 1985b. Guanyu weisheng gongzuo gaige ruogan zhengce wenti baogao (The report concerning several policy problems in the reform of health care work). In R. Peng, R. Cai, & C. Zhou (Eds.), *Zhongguo gaige quanshu (Encyclopedia of China's Reform)*, 139–142. Dalian: Dalian chubanshe

Weishengbu. 1988. Weishengbu guanyu weisheng gongzuo gaige ruogan zhengce wenti de baogao (The report of the MOH concerning several policy problems in the reform of health care tasks). In Weishengbu Bangongting (Ed.), *Zhonghua renmin gongheguo weisheng fagui huibian, 1984–1885* (The Collection of Laws and Reg-ulations of Health Care of the PRC, 1984–1985), 1–6. Beijing: Falu chubanshe, xinhua shudian.

Weishengbu, PRC. 1990. Yufang baojian sihixing youshang fuwu de huigu yu sikao (A review and observations on the implementation of paid services in preventive care). *Zhongguo weisheng jingji(China's Health Care Economics)*, 6: 26–28.

Weishengbu, PRC. (1992). Weishengbu guanyu tuixing fuyou baojian baochang zer-enzhi de yijian (The opinion of the Ministry of Health Care concerning the intro-duction of insured responsibilty system of health). In Peng, R., Cai, R. & Zhou, C. (Eds.), *Zhongguo gaige quanshu (Encyclopedia of China's Reform)*, 201–202. Dalain: Dalian chubanshe.

Weishengbu *et al.*1993b. Guanyu kuoda yiliao weisheng fuwu yaoguan wenti de yijian (The opinion concerning the related problems of expansion of medical and health care services). In Weishengbu Zhengce Faguisi (Ed.), *Zhonghua renmin gongheguo weisheng fagui huibian, 1989–1991* (The Collection of Laws and Regulations of the Ministry of Health of the PRC, 1989–1991), 10–12. Beijing: Falu chubanshe.

Wong, C., Lo, V. I., & Tang, K.L. 2006. *China's Urban Health Care Reform: From State Protection to Individual Responsibility*. Lanham, Boulder, and New York: Lexington Books.

Wu, M. 2002. Yaopin fuwu tigong gecheng zhong xunzu xingwei chansheng yuanyin fenxi (Analysis on the cause of rent-seeking behavior in the provision of dispensary services). *Zhongguo weisheng jingji (China's Health Care Economics)*, 21(11): 4–6.

Xia, H., & Meng, W. 1990. Xianxing yiliao jiage gaige fangxiang de tantao (Discus-sion on the direction of the current medical care price reform). *Zhongguo weisheng jingji* (China's Health Care Economics), 45–47.

Xu, G. 1995. Shishui taigao le yiliafei? (Who has raised medical care charges?). *Gaige neican* (Internal Reference on Reform), 7: 36–39.

Xu, L., & Qiu Fenglin. 1993. Shenhua yiliao fuwu jiage gaige de sikao (Thoughts on further reform of charges to medical care services). *Zhongguo weisheng jingji (China's Health Care Economics)*, 5:12–20.

Yang, H., & Sun, N. 2006. Weisheng gaige yu fazhan de pingjia yu jianyan (The evaluation and examination of health care reform and development). In L. Du (Ed.), *Zhongguo Yiliao Weisheng Fazhan Baogao no. 2* (The Report of Reform and Development of Medical and Health care in China no. 2), 47–85. Beijing: Shehui kexue wenxian chubanshe.

Zhang, S. 2011. Gongli yiyuan jianqi gongyixin yeying zhongshi heli shouru (Public hospitals should insist on not only their public welfare orientation but also reasonable revenue). *Weisheng jingji yanjiu (Research on Health Care Economics)*, 2: 7–8.

Zhonggong Zhongyang & Guowuyuan. 1999. Guanyu weisheng gaige yu fazhan de jueding (The decision concerning the reform and development of health care). In D. Zheng, D. Liu, & B. Zhang (Eds.), *Shehui baozhang zhidu gaige zhinan* (The Guide for the Reform of Social Security System). Beijing: 43–51. Beijing: Gaige chubanshe.

Zhonggongzhongyang & Guowuyuan. 1997. Zhonggongzhongyang, guowuyuan guanyu weisheng gaige yu fazhan de jueding (The decision of CC, CCP and State Council concerning health care reform and development). In Weishengbu Weisheng Fazhi Yu Jiandusi (Ed.), *Zhonghua renmin gongheguo weisheng fagui huibian (The Collection of Laws and Regulations of Health Care of the PRC)*, 1–10. Beijing: Beijing: Falu chubanshe.

Zhou, L., Qu, Q., & Li, G. 2003. *Jujiao weisheng gaige* (Focusing on the Health Care Reform). Beijing: Zhongguo shehue chubanshe.

Zhou, X. 2008. *Zhongguo yiliao jiage de zhengfu guanzhi yanjiu* (A Study on the Government Control of Medical Care Pricing in China). Beijing: Zhongguo shehui kexue chubanshe.

Zhu, H. 1999. Guanyu chengzhen yiyao weisheng tizhi gaige de jidian sikao (Some considerations concerning the reform of medical care and pharmacy in towns and cities). *Zhongguo weisheng jingji(China's Health Care Economics)*, 11: 5–7.

Zhu, Y. 2006. Woguo yaopin jiage xugao liyi zhuti de liyi fenbu ji chengyin fenxi (Analysis on interest configuration among interest entities as well as its causes in case of artificial high prices of pharmaceutic products). *Zhongguo weisheng jingji (China's Health Care Economics)*, 25(11): 15–18.

Zou, L., & Zheng, P. 2010. Gongli yiyuan jiage huayuquan yanjiu (A research on the right of say over pricing in public hospitals). *Zhongguo weisheng jingji (China's Health Care Economics)*, 29(9): 38–40.

Part III
Re-making China's medical care delivery

7 Learning from the enterprise style of management

Health care reform has focused on the theme of commercialization of medical care services, a subject matter provoking heated debates amongst the policy circle, the medical profession, and the public for more than a whole decade since 2005 (Ge & Gong 2005). These debates within the health care circle and in the media led to another round of discussions for the policymaking group on health care, coupled with extensive consultation with experts and scholars in the field, laying down the foundation for a "new health care reform" launched in 2009 (Du 2009: 1–59). The issue of commercialization did not start in 2005, for its roots lie much deeper than what the ongoing debates suggest. In fact, it can be traced back more than three decades to the very beginning of health care reform in 1979. Accordingly, the study will first undertake to lend a brief review on the origin and evolution of commercialization from its very start.

The study proposes to examine the introduction and development of commercialization in terms of two installments of restructuring of financial management of medical care services. The first installment focuses on internal dimension of commercialization, namely restructuring within the organization, while the second installment deals with external dimension pertaining to the organization's outside relationship with task environment. This chapter provides an account of the first installment that is concerned with the so-called "learning from the enterprise style of management" lasting from 1979 to the late 1980s. And the following examines the second installment that pertains to repackaging franchises, coupled with the introduction of user charges in curative care services, drugs and medical devices covering the mid-1980s to early 1990s. In view of the importance of drugs in financial management at the providing unit level, moreover, two separate chapters (9 and 10) will be devoted to extensive discussion of sale of drugs and regulatory control respectively.

In its first installment, China's health care reform featured managerial restructuring copied from the "enterprise style of management" (qiye guanli fanshi; hereafter, ESM), consisting of economic management, budgetary reform, an undertaking responsibility system (hereafter, URS), retained revenue schemes, performance appraisals, material incentives, inter alia. The first installment marked a trend parallel to the rise of New Public Management (hereafter, NPM) in the West for a long period from the 1980s to the present. This gives rise to a cluster of questions: To what extent is it fruitful for public organizations to borrow from business/industrial management? How does Chinese public management differ from its counterparts in the West in learning from the managerial experience of a firm/enterprise in a market-oriented economy often located in the West? What are the common challenges that a firm/enterprise faces in a similar learning process? This chapter tries to provide some answers to these questions.

Shifting toward resource management in the public sector

Health care reform started in the midst of economic reform in China, when sovereign planners went through a major review of the ideology, policy-making style and approaches of implementation within the CPE framework as previously noted (Chapters 1 and 2). The review led to some new policy orientation that placed considerable weight on resource management in the production sector as much as the distribution sector. With reference to the latter, the main concern of this study, they began to overhaul spending programs and experiment with some new approaches to transplant business/industrial management and to make use of market-oriented instruments to render health care services. By and large, production sectors and distribution sectors within the CPE involve the issues of resource management in a conventional sense, for instance, known as three Es (economy, effectiveness and efficiency) in the West.

In conceptual and theoretical terms, overall, the re-engineering endeavors represent the movement towards transaction-oriented management, underscoring resource management (Chapters 1 and 2). In the realm of public policy within the conventional framework of the CPE, as a rule, the production side lends weight to revenue tasks, while the main emphasis of distribution sector lies on so-called spending programs that are normally funded by tax revenue. In economic reform in China, however, the re-engineering of the distribution sector is not limited to the conventional emphasis of a spending program, but priority is given to the revenue task as well, characteristic of adoption of franchise funding mode together with user charges as being incorporated into the programs of commercialization.

In operational terms, it is useful to trace how Chinese policy participants originally defined resource management and investigate what is subjectively meaningful to them in the health care sector during the earliest phase of health care reform. Economic management (jingji guanli; hereafter, EM) was first introduced by the Ministry of Health (MOH) in line with the national policy platform of "adjustment, rectification, reform, and upgrading" as put forth by the 3rd Plenum of the 11th National Congress of the CCP at the end of 1978 and beginning of 1979.[1] Incorporated into EM are the core ideas of resource management in the health care sector in China as noted in the policy paper, the 1979 Opinion: "The application of economic instruments to ensure the rational use of human, material, and financial resources to perform such tasks as curative and preventive care, research, and teaching and to gain better medical care and economic results" (Weishengbu, PRC 1985).

In a broad conceptual sense, EM embraces two distinctive components of resource management in the Chinese health care sector: one is a generic design and the other is a particular design, often known as the "undertaking responsibility system" (chengbao zerenzhi; hereafter, URS).[2] In fact, there is a considerable overlap between the two designs, for both tackle the issues of how to make better use of resources, except that each has a different emphasis (Wu 1992: 448).

The former, the generic design of resources management, attempts to move toward transaction-oriented management by strengthening financial accountability, improving efficiency and effectiveness of task performance, upgrading the quality of health care services, minimizing costs, and generating more revenue (Weishengbu 1982). Conceptually speaking, top policymakers treat the generic design in a very similar vein to the NPM of the West (e.g., highlighting financial accountability, performance appraisal, incentive packages, and economic utility in the public sector) (Mintzberg 1983; Rainey 1991; Carter et al. 1992; Messy 1993; Pollitt 1993; Ferlie, Ashburner, Fitzgerald & Pettigrew 1997; Pollit & Bouchaert 2004). Similar to its Western counterparts, the generic design of resource management is output-centered, being organized on the basis of measurable performance and results. It was introduced as a prioritized task beginning in 1979 (Weishengbu & Guojialaodongzongju 1979; Weishengbu & Guojialaodongzongju 1980). Starting with a focus on managerial restructuring anchored in a budgetary reform featuring revenue retention system, it became increasingly fused with the market-oriented reform, shifting to an emphasis on the revenue-generating undertaking policy from 1985 onward.

Here the generic design of resource management deals with both economic and non-economic policy goals in the health care service sector: the standards of efficiency regarding the input-output ratio in a pure economic and financial sense, an emphasis on effectiveness in attaining public policy goals, and the implementation financed by public revenue and handled by appointed public employees. For example, on March 22, 1979, Minister of Health Qian Xinzhong explained the guiding principle of health care reform, to meet a mix of policy goals, in his own words: "[We] should follow the principle to get business done in accordance with the law of economy, strengthen economic management, and stress economic results. [We] should make sure to gain maximum or better preventive and curative care results with minimum labor input."[3] In line with the generic design, overall, the "1979 Opinion" recommended that providing units adopt economic methods to manage delivery of services, expenditures, and financial return in order to ensure the fulfillment of missions (meaning both economic and non-economic policy goals) as given (Weishengbu & Guojialaodongzongju 1979).

Although the notion of accountability is found relevant to both generic and particular versions of resource management, accountability refers to different things. In the Chinese context, many policy analysts and policy participants use the concept of "responsibility" (as used in "responsibility system," for example) in the realm of resource management (Cui 1992). The concept "ziren" (often translated as responsibility) is broader than "keze" (accountability). The notion of accountability places emphasis on a specific and concrete practice in resource management, as in the case of financial accountability based on quantifiable and measurable results handled through methods of accounting and auditing, calculation and statistics (Weishengbu, PRC 1985). It permeates all jobs of resource management, for instance, the management of liquid assets (such as current expenditure accounts), earnings and deficit, saving and revenue, management of fixed capital, and material inventory (Weishengbu, PRC 1985).

In the generic design of resource management in the health care sector in China, the providing unit is, as a rule, chosen as a legal entity to be held accountable to the state budget, performance and results, management of liquid assets, use of retained revenue, various disposable funds, inventory control, and property management in the health care sector (Weishengbu, PRC 1985). The hospital director, assisted by headquarters, acts on behalf of the providing unit and is normally held accountable to the state. Under command of the hospital director, the department/office, which is a sub-unit in the hierarchy, does not enjoy independent legal status to claim a share of revenue and savings. To put it simply, a department/office is neither a "legal person" (work unit) nor an accounting unit in the budgetary process (Weishengbu & Guojialaodongzongju 1979; Weishengbu, PRC 1985; Li, Zeng & He 1988). It is considered undesirable, moreover, to introduce a revenue retention scheme centered on the department/office because of the possibility of breeding department-centered rivalry based on vested interests, causing systematic distortion in the provision of medical services, thereby thwarting public policy (Qian 1990: 40; Zhang & Lin 1998: 17). Nonetheless, in practice, the department/office is often allowed to adopt and manage revenue retention for its own personnel.

It appears from an interpretative scheme of policy actors in the health care sector in the early 1980s that ESM represents a systematic endeavor from the delineating of categories of resources, introducing various of performance indicators, to ensuring that participant work units be evaluated and compared scientifically and fairly. And this enabled participant works units to compete with one another on a comparable basis. From the perspective of public management, a close examination of various categories of health care resources in the health care sector suggests that administrative instruments are often used no less than pure economic tools in the generic design of resource management (Weishengbu 1982). In China's health care sector, resource management includes four categories of resources as follows:

- First, the management of "liquid assets," e.g., the issues of current expenditure accounts, revenue and expenditures, charges and fees, etc. (Weishengbu, PRC 1985: 488–9);
- Second, the management of property and material, including book-keeping and accounting, rates of depreciation, repairs and maintenance (Weishengbu, PRC 1985: 488–9);
- Third, the management of medicine and pharmaceutical products and inventory (Weishengbu, PRC 1985: 488–9);
- Fourth, human resource management, comprising an integral part of the public personnel system and a unified wage schedule under CPE (Weishengbu, PRC 1985: 488:9).

Among these four categories of resources, the first and third categories (liquid assets and drugs, respectively) are handled through market transactions to a considerable extent, and the remaining two categories (property and material, manpower) are basically appropriated through administrative channels, i.e., the exercise of command.

The top policymakers made best use of the generic design—borrowed from the industrial sector—by encouraging various jurisdictions to adopt a brand of "managed competition" among providing units in conjunction with the introduction of EM, meaning to pit one providing unit against another to achieve better performance on the basis of comparable workloads and resource endowments.[4] Beginning in the early 1980s, for instance, ministerial policymakers took steps to carry out the task of "five fixes" (wuding,), namely to "fix" (1) missions, (2) the number of beds, (3) established the size of personnel, (4) services and technical indicators, and (5) subsidy to current expenditure (Weishengbu & Guojialaodongzongju 1979; Weishengbu & Guojialaodongzongju 1980; Weishengbu et al. 1982). Subsumed under planning management and norms management, in other words, the five fixes tried to strike a balance between capability and resource endowment (e.g., hospital beds, number of personnel, and current expenditure) one the one hand, and goals and workloads (i.e., relative to the mission, norms, and performance indicators) on the other hand (Weishengbu & Guojialaodongzongju 1979; Weishengbu 1985).

Among five "fixes", two "fixes", namely, mission and service and technical indicators, are concerned with the articulation and choices of policy goals at the providing unit level. Typical of existing managerial practices in the public sector, "mission" refers to a plurality of policy goals concerning a variety of tasks such as curative care, preventive medical care, medical education, and scientific research (Weishengbu, PRC 1985). Beyond general instructions, however, EM goes a step further in requiring the providing unit to work out services and technical indicators as much as possible through a realistic assessment of the concrete conditions, the best historical records, and a "better than the average" level for a given jurisdiction in order to assess the potential and capacity of providing units to meet indicators and satisfy work norms (Weishengbu, PRC 1985). The remaining three "fixes" have to do with the supply of input variables, which often depends upon the exercise of command rather than market transactions, for instance, the number of hospital beds and established size of personnel.[5] In the category of fixed liquid assets, a fixed subsidy by the government to current expenditure helps partly to absorb costs of wages and salary, benefits and welfare, and retirement funds (Weishengbu, PRC 1985: 487). Above all, the clear delineation of various categories of health care resources is inseparable from performance appraisal, assignment of comparable workloads to all participant work units, as well as mechanisms of competition among the providing units in the same jurisdiction. In addition, it is closely associated with the notion of accountability to be tackled in next passages.

Financial accountability and retained revenue schemes

Understood as an integral part of ESM, EM is indicative of a major shift in financial strategy from reliance on tax revenue and public insurances to user charges and revenue-generating endeavors at the providing unit level. Among reformers in the post-Mao era, Vice Premier of the State Council Li Xiennian made history by first advocating the application of ESM to the health care sector, stating on October 5, 1979: "It should be taken as a policy guideline to ensure that all service units that have the potential to generate their own revenue follow the enterprise style [of management] and be held accountable for their own earning and loss."[6] Li Xiennian had a kick-off with the undertaking responsibility system (URS), a particular design of resource management, featuring revenue-generating activities in all service units, including providing units in health care, throughout the country.

ESM represents a budgetary reform featuring performance appraisal and an incentive scheme, among other things; and it has subsequently been linked to the repackaging and expansion of franchising, creating an opportunity for the providing unit to earn revenue through market transactions (Sun & Du 2006: 124–5; Du 2007: 32; Liu 2012: 15–18). In other words, the introduction of financial accountability is often strengthened through some built-in incentive to the participant work units. In its early origin, the built-in incentive centered on the proportion of saving the providing unit had been able to realize in the implementation of the budget. For instance, an innovation was introduced during the early 1980s, allowing the providing unit to retain a portion of savings out of a fixed subsidy in the "budgetary undertaking system (BUS)" whenever medical personnel could economize; however, it would not receive additional subsidy beyond the approved budgetary provision whenever new positions were added, meaning that the providing unit was allowed to retain saving from any cut of personnel cost (Weishengbu et al. 1982; Weishengbu, PRC, 1985). As an alternative, the built-in incentive, taken as "revenue retention system," was normally attached to total revenue realized by the participant providing unit.

Building upon policy experiments and pilot programs in various jurisdictions, the ministerial leadership for health care began to push for the undertaking responsibility system (hereafter, URS) in the early 1980s, formally in 1985, and then again in 1988. As a particular design of resource management, URS is a key feature of ESM. By 1990, it was estimated on the basis of a survey of 26 provinces, autonomous regions, and directly administered municipalities that about 51 percent of providing units at the county level or above had established a variety of URS, and approximately 64 percent of providing units at the level of township and towns had implemented some kind of URS. The remaining units had implemented a variety of revenue retention schemes under the budgetary reforms (Peng, Cai, & Zhou 1992: 35).

The introduction of URS was also an integral part of a re-engineering of budgetary systems in the public sector by transferring the "budgetary undertaking" (yusuan chengbao) system into the "current expenditure undertaking" (jingfei chengbao) system.[7] The two systems differ from each other in terms of funding sources. The former pertains to the budgetary system, which holds the providing unit accountable for funds from the state, mainly in terms of saving out of the subsidies appropriated by the government. In the latter case, the service unit is held accountable to revenue that it has generated through market transactions. That is to say, the service unit (namely, the providing unit here) is partially subsidized and held accountable for the management and use of a current expenditure account—an increasing portion of which stems from user charges—in order to practice saving and to generate surplus on an annual basis. Bearing a close resemblance to the practice of the industrial sector, once the revenue target is reached, the work unit is allowed to retain an agreed portion of surplus, called "retained revenue" (lirun liuchen).[8]

In fact, Gu Xin argues that the early phase of health care reform was no more than a few small steps within budgetary reform (Gu 2008: 276). To put it simply, URS represents a budgetary reform packaged with an "undertaking agreement" (chengbao xieyi; abbreviated as UA).[9] Cui Yueli, a ministerial ranking official, stated that health care reform should follow the direction illuminated by "Document Zhongyang No. 1" (1983) with regard to implementing various forms of "responsibility system" (zerenzhi; abbreviated as RS) and "undertaking system" (chengbaozhi; abbreviated as US) in agriculture, commerce, supply and sale corps, and commune enterprises (Cui 1992).

Some policy analysts have attempted to trace the origin and evolution of the revenue retention system, a main component of the budgetary system at the providing unit level preceding 1979 and thereafter. For example, Liu Junmin observes that, owing to the welfare-oriented policy packages of medical care services that took shape from 1960 to 1979, the government ended up assuming a heavy financial burden, while development of providing units remained stagnant.[10] In accordance with the general circular jointly promulgated by the MOH and Ministry of Finance (MOF) in February 1960, the government started to cover all basic wages and supplementary wages (e.g., payment in kinds, such as benefits, insurance and welfare) while the hospital undertook responsibility for the remaining expenditures and was allowed to retain the surplus and savings so generated. Part of the savings could be used for procurement of medical devices at the discretion of the hospital (Liu 2012: 15–20). From 1958 to 1979, moreover, the government took the responsibility of absorbing all loss created by cuts to charges under the budgetary system called "full-quota budget, subsidy by special funding, and savings to be remitted to the upper echelon." (Liu 2012: 16). Through the budgetary reform starting in 1979, retention of savings was permitted at the providing unit level. Meanwhile the providing unit was authorized to keep revenue earned from its drug franchise at a wholesale/retail ratio (piling chajia; hereafter, W/R ratio) (Liu 2012: 15–20).

Although the revenue retention system enhanced providing units' revenue motivation, this did not necessarily result in a revenue-maximizing orientation, as the government was able to absorb the major costs for the provision of medical care services. From 1979 onward, providing units which chose to take part in URS pilot programs began to enter into a new budgetary and financial game centered on retained revenue in what was understood as "full-quota [budgetary] management, fixed-quota appropriation, savings retained for use" in accordance with the provisions of EM, as previously noted (Liu 2012: 15–20). Here in the notion of "fixed-quota appropriation," "fixed" always means less than the total amount of appropriation, that is, partial subsidy only, thus entailing a large shortfall in government funding for curative care services at the providing unit level. This represents a critical shift that has defined the direction of health care reform since 1979. Pivotal to URS, financial accountability builds on quantifiable and measurable results obtained through methods of accounting and auditing, and through calculation and statistics. In the Chinese case, URS serves as a constructive managerial tool to build and maintain the connection of the performance appraisal system with incentive schemes; and the latter is tied to the revenue generated through franchising. Subsequently, URS was anchored to the franchise system in the legacy of the CPE.

After the introduction of URS, retained revenue was no longer the retained portion of savings as in the previous case of "full-quota appropriation" (quane bokuan), through which the providing unit had been funded in full by the government regardless of earning or loss. To be precise, it stemmed from two other sources: first, the market, including revenue from user charges through curative care service franchise, the dispensary and medical device franchise, and the auxiliary service franchise and affiliated enterprises (often accompanying the franchise or tax exemption or both); and second, partial state appropriation, albeit considerably reduced in the form of a "differential-quota appropriation" (chae bokuan), or a "fixed-quota appropriation" (dinger bokuan) expended mostly for infrastructure through conventional channels (Song 1990).

Issues arising from URS

How did URS impact the medical care system in China? To begin with, it is claimed that the URS was intended to "push the providing unit to the markets" through the policy of "the amalgamation of power [autonomy], accountability, and incentives (quanzeli de jiehe)." (Wang 1992: 118; Cui 1992:121). Under such a reform policy, basically, the providing unit was expected to improve its "rate of self-sufficiency" through the generation of revenue from the further expansion of health care services (Cai 1988; Ren 1988). As Sun and Du put it, after the government started to promote the policy of "differential-quota appropriation and revenue retention" in the 1980s, the share of state appropriation to providing units was substantially reduced in relative terms in the 1990s.[11] According to Du, the revenue-maximizing orientation of the providing unit was attributed to budgetary reform that put pressure on the providing unit to earn more revenue.[12] As noted previously, this is known as load shedding—shifting the financial burden of health and medical care from higher echelons of the government to lower ones, and from various echelons of municipal/local government to providing units, and finally to patients themselves (Yang & Sun 2006: 71).

This budgetary reform required providing units to increase user charges to patients to generate revenue and thus maintain budgetary balance. The reform was first introduced on an experimental basis in 1979 and in a full-fledged form in 1985, continuing from that time (Peng, Cai, & Zhou 1992: 38; Sun & Du 2006: 124). As a result, patients had to pay more and more out of pocket proportionally for seeking treatment. Hard pressed by substantially reduced percentages of state appropriation, on the whole, providing units operated within tightly regulated markets, which granted units minimal pricing power especially in the realm of curative care services (Cao 1988; Peng, Cai, & Zhou 1992: 36–8, 64–7).

In Mode C commercialization of medical care provision, the resemblance between the revenue-maximizing orientation of the providing unit in the Chinese CPE structure and the profit-pursuing firm in a Western market economy is only superficial. In the case of URS, conceptually speaking, a providing unit is not comparable to a private firm or even a charitable organization in a market economy, in that a Chinese public hospital is nothing but a component of the Party-state hierarchy; nor does it have the status of a property-owning corporate entity as found in a free market economy (Li 1990; Peng, Cai, & Zhou 1992: 37). While highlighting key characteristics of URS, it is noteworthy that the size of retained revenue represents a portion of "earnings" calculated on the basis of "current expenditure," meaning that the providing unit is not held accountable for any loss in its property value (Li 1990). In other words, "revenue" is actually a kind of financial surplus in the budgetary and accounting system, and it is not something that can be taken as profit relative to investments and property ownership in the context of a market economy.[13] Nor it is often tied to the size of endowments or to a fixed quota appropriation (e.g., special grant for infrastructure and devices) (Weishengbu & Guojialaodongzongju 1979).

As a legacy of CPE, the economic-financial system often made the revenue source for providing units inseparable from the large financial pool in the country in general and in each local jurisdiction in particular. In fact, the so-called soft budget constraints worked in a double-edged fashion: on the one hand, the state provided an easy exit for the work unit to let itself off the hook financially when it was in deficit; and, on the other hand, the state permitted supervising bureaus to encroach upon financial reservoirs at the work unit level as a matter of administrative discretion. This often entangled providing units in fights for a share of the revenue pie in complicated situations either within a jurisdiction or within the country at large.[14] For example, in the long-term trend of load shedding taking shape from the mid-1980s onward, sovereign planners curtailed the share of state appropriation to providing units, making the health care sector shoulder considerable financial burden, not only with regard to the provision of basic medical care and preventive care but also in the overall expansion and growth of health care services into the early 2000s.[15]

Although URS was thought of as a success with regard to the fulfillment of revenue targets, the issue of dilution of social utility was subsequently raised by the late 1980s, calling for a major shift in policy priorities. In managerial terms, this entailed change from a revenue-centered mode of performance appraisal to a multi-goal mode. In response to Premier Li Pang's comment on an article regarding the "comprehensive undertaking responsibility system" (hereafter, CURS) published in *Wenhui Daily* in August 1989, Minister of Health Chen Mingzhang, took the initiative to organize a joint investigation team with more than seven government units and put forth a proposal on the change from URS to CURS (Chen 1992: 194).

Beginning in 1990, Minister Chen advocated CURS, not only extending performance appraisals (e.g., focusing on revenue) to the functional realm where policy purposes become less definable, quantifiable, and measurable, but also proliferating performance indicators coupled with an ever-broadening scope of bureaucratic control, a trend continuing from the 1990s to the present (Chen 1992: 191–200). Minister Chen made three points. First, URS in the health care sector differs from its counterpart adopted by the industrial sector in terms of meaning, contents, and objectives. Second, URS ought not to include economic goals only, but also comprehensive contents including "tasks and missions, technical quality, organization and management, professional ethic, economy and accounting, and appraisal and penalty." Third, there was no need to follow the common terminology of URS, and it is permissible to adopt any name whenever appropriate (Chen 1992: 197). It is true that then Party Chairman Jiang Zemin did later register his reservations about URS by requesting the MOH and other ministerial units to refrain from further use of the term URS (Sun & Du 2006: 125). Nonetheless, the application of URS and the like have continued in light of the heavy reliance of jurisdictions and providing units upon revenue retention systems such as this throughout the country.

As noted in the analysis in Chapter 1, performance appraisal tends to lose its effectiveness when the policy goals in question are less definable, quantifiable and measurable. As the government held providing units accountable to the implementation of less definable, quantifiable, and measurable policy goals such as "social utility," it does not appear in theoretical terms that CURS could make use of performance appraisal as an effective policy tool any longer. Above all, the shift of emphasis from URS to CURS attests to the diminishing effects of market-oriented tools as they move away from tasks of resource management. The policy episode concerning the shift from URS to CURS proves that performance appraisal fits business/industrial management better than public management because of the scenario of multiple, but less measurable goals operating in the latter.

Performance appraisals and incentive packages

Conducting performance appraisals was one of the most striking features in management's output-centered design at the providing unit level (Chapter 1). By and large, supervising bureaus often tied performance indicators to some form of evaluation system as well as incentive schemes at the providing unit level. In the Chinese context, "indicators" (zhibiao) and "fixed norms" (dinger) are often used interchangeably in connection with performance appraisals, albeit, strictly speaking, the two concepts are not identical.[16] As a salient feature of transaction-oriented management, the design of performance appraisals was intended to provide a common starting point for an objective and "scientific" evaluation of performance among organizational members as well as managed competition between the providing units. However, questions are raised with reference to the usefulness and limitations of transaction-oriented management to the health care sector, and more fundamentally, the farthest reach of "market paradigm" to the public sector.

First of all, how measurable are the jobs in the public sector? It appears that in extension of performance appraisal from the business/industrial sector to public sector, one often finds that some jobs are more measurable than others. In applying performance appraisal to the health care sector, for example, hospital management and medical staff often worked with a difference between "hard" and "soft" indicators in order to distinguish how closely each was tied to a material advantage at stake. For example, among the "soft" indicators were tasks whose utility was diffuse, social, long-term by nature, and, above all, it means less definable, quantifiable, and measurable, for example, maintenance work, utilization of fixed assets, preventive care, and teaching and research. Such indicators tended to receive low priority whenever they were not directly related to the immediate concerns of curative care services, and thus to receive even less attention when they were not relevant to revenue targets.

In addition, it is apparent that financial indicators were in general "harder" than non-financial indicators; and measurable indicators concerning current expenditure and revenue targets were "harder" than less measurable indictors of fixed assets, facilities, and equipment under the circumstances where neither performance was tied to revenue targets and compensation of medical staff, nor the evaluation of the providing unit's performance reflects the appreciation of property value (Luo 1990; Chang, Zhou, & Wang 1990). The 1979 Opinion, for instance, lists performance indicators to monitor and assess the extent of "mission completion," including non-financial performance indicators, such as clinical visit workload, utilization rates and circulation rates of hospital beds, cases of accurate diagnosis, success rates of curative care, infection rates from surgery, incident rates, and the ratio of family/informal caregiver.

Also, the performance appraisal is often inseparable from the career considerations of hospital directors. Under the pressure of fixed terms of appointment in some versions of URS, a director had to concentrate his/her efforts on revenue targets of the providing units and immediate interests of staff and workers within a short period (normally a term of three years), for example, bonus payments and material goods to individuals rather than for group-oriented collective welfare (Zhang 1990).

Furthermore, performance appraisal is closely linked to overall endeavor in introducing transaction-oriented management at the providing unit level, often subject to abuses. One may characterize URS as output-centered to the extent that hospital units employed output as a cornerstone in building various managerial mechanisms, e.g., monitoring and supervision, gauging of performance and results, and incentive and motivational behavior. As the providing unit and its members often took part in designing and choosing performance appraisals, distortion likely occurs when their material interests are involved. For example, the creation of the undertaking agreement (UA) was directly related to formulating and selecting performance indicators, a process entailing a conflict of material interests.[17] Likely, many providing units found it in their interest to propose a set of indicators with the expected level of attainment (called "fixed norms") as low as possible, making it easier to fulfill the plan and therefore maximize revenue retention (Chen 1990). To counter this tendency, supervising bureaus borrowed from ESM by employing a three-year rolling average of revenue targets and using historical records of performance to prevent providing units from sliding down to a less challenging set of performance indicators (Zhang & Cui 1990). To maintain some measure of neutrality among organizational units, the application of "scientific methods" was recommended, coupled with the principle of a "comprehensive set of norms and reasonably advanced targets" (Li, Zeng, & He 1988). For instance, Hebei Province introduced pilot programs featuring, through open competition, the recruitment and appointment of hospital directors on the basis of their pledges for targets, coupled with evaluation by the Committee of Experts (Li, Zeng, & He 1988).

The application of performance appraisal hinges on how it is tied to the incentive schemes to the providing unit. By and large, the providing unit is less inclined to cooperate in the adoption of performance appraisal if it often infringes upon the providing unit's financial interest. For example, policymakers employed UA as a managerial tool in order to motivate providing units to comply voluntarily with agreed upon revenue targets, while minimizing arbitrary use of power by the supervising bureaus. However, it was not unusual that a supervising unit might unilaterally and/or even arbitrarily reduce its agreed amount of subsidy to a providing unit in a following financially stringent year, thus creating uncertainty in financial planning at the providing unit level.[18] Also when a supervising unit perceived that a hospital unit had earned handsomely in a particular year, for example, it might, in the next year, unilaterally reduce the amount of revenue to be retained at the providing unit level or even impose excessive and unfair demands on better performing units in what is called "whipping the buffalo which runs even faster" (Chen 1990).

Starting in 1979, for instance, the design of EM was intended to make sure that hospital units could compete with one another on an equal footing. Providing units were then grouped on the basis of their comparability regarding assigned targets, financial indicators, workload, established size of personnel, and resource endowment (i.e. the five fixes previously mentioned) in a given jurisdiction. With a shortage of effective economic leverages that would give providing units a common starting point for competition, the supervising bureaus had to adopt some administrative approaches to ensure comparability, albeit in a rough way. The 1979 Opinion recommends, for example, that the creation of performance indicators should fellow some kind of rule of thumb approach rather than a more precise scientific method in order to maintain a measure of fairness and to minimize any arbitrariness by supervising bureaus. Examples include the best historical records of the hospital unit and the highest average standards among all providing units in a given jurisdiction (Weishengbu & Guojialaodongzongju 1979; Weishengbu, PRC 1985).

It is assumed, theoretically, that the application of performance appraisals is effective as a tool in forging consensus within an organization and minimizing disputes among members due to the "scientific," standardized nature of measuring yardsticks in hospital management. In practice, however, performance appraisal was not really as scientific and objective as expected, as a providing unit had to work with multiple, less measurable goals in the health care sector. Therefore, hospital management was encouraged to build consensus among rank and file, and to seek support from supervising authorities when performance indicators were not sufficiently scientific and effective (Weishengbu & Guojialaodongzongju 1979; Weishengbu, PRC 1985). Neither colleagues' consensus nor superiors' support can really substitute for scientific measurements, however.

Funding for bonus payments, benefits and welfare (including health care) stemmed largely from retained revenue, the amount of which was set aside in accordance with the relevant rules and regulations of each jurisdiction. In the design of EM, moreover, the funding source for incentive schemes invariably depended on a financial surplus calculated according to the balance between revenue and expenditure (Weishengbu et al. 1982; Weishengbu, PRC 1985). In the midst of the first round of pilot programs, the MOH promulgated the "1981 Provisional Measure," requiring the actual amount of funding for various remunerative and incentive schemes to follow the relevant regulations in various jurisdictions. Once the portion of retained revenue was decided and set aside, it was the responsibility of hospital management headed by the director, to devise various schemes on the basis of a performance appraisal to determine the size of a bonus and awards going to each individual, office, or department within the work unit in accordance with imposed policies and regulations.[19]

Hospital management normally adopted two sets of criteria to divide savings and retained revenue. The first set had to do with rules to divide retained revenue into three portions: a development fund (e.g. 40 percent at the minimum), a welfare fund, and a bonus fund (e.g. these last two at about 60 percent taken together). The welfare fund was group-oriented, normally going into a special account handled jointly by the hospital director, the Congress of the Representatives of Staff and Workers (CRSW), and the Trade Union (hereafter, TU) at the work unit level. The second set of criteria pertained to monetary rewards, including the following two types: comprehensive awards for overall performance and singular awards for selected items of achievement. Both types of award were given according to task performance as measured and evaluated in terms of performance indicators. Payment for each type required review and approval by higher supervising units in charge. In practice it was expected that, in the case of comprehensive awards, the aggregate of points in all categories of indicators (e.g., routine functions and medical care quality) had to exceed 60 percent of the total points, with the remaining money going to singular awards (Weishengbu, PRC 1985).

Owing to the three-way division of retained revenue among development funds, welfare funds, and bonus funds, many SOEs were presented an option to set aside portions of welfare fund to finance enterprise-managed medical facilities/hospitals, under the tight control of wage policy during the early phase of economic reform (Chapter 2). This amounts to the hoarding of health care resources by the enterprise-managed providing unit, denying its sharing with the residents in local community. That is to say, above all, the generic design of resource management, which features financial accountability, performance appraisal, revenue retention system and incentive schemes, tends to produce sub-optimal results in the allocation of health care resources. In addition, the increase of enterprise-managed providing unit was indicative of an expansion of "collective welfare" facilities at the SOE level, a by-product of tight wage control during the early phase of economic reform.

Concluding remarks

The foregoing analysis has examined the endeavor of transplanting ESM to the health care sector, demonstrating an endeavor in rebuilding financial management at the providing unit level. It has dealt with two policy episodes, EM and URS, in some depth. Students of China's industrial management would find EM and URS surprisingly similar with the basic tenets of ESM, as it was being introduced to the health care sector (Shurmann 1968; Lee 1987). While both contributed considerably to improving resource management at the providing unit level, they encountered substantial obstacles to move into functional territories pertaining to non-economic goals, proving that the so-called market paradigm enjoys diminishing utility in the functional territory other than resource management.

From the perspective of public management, the study argues that as policy tools, the state and markets each find their respective strengths as much as weaknesses in the public sector. For the curative care services, especially non-basic care category, the markets find room in resource management including revenue generating activities, but not far beyond the economic arena. There is no solid managerial grounding for the markets to move into functional territories where social utility takes precedent over economic utility, and where command-oriented management can fare better than transaction-oriented management.

Notes

1 One of the earliest policies on health care reform is based upon the policy paper promulgated by the Ministry of Health, Ministry of Finance and State General Bureau of Labor on April 28, 1979. It full title reads as the follows: "Opinion Concerning the Task of the Pilot Program for Strengthening Hospital Management" (hereafter, the 1979 Opinion) (Weishengbu & Guojialaodongzhongchu: 1979).

2 The undertaking responsibility system (chengbao zerenzhi) is often translated as "contractual responsibility system." It is appropriate to use the term "undertaking" as it stresses obligation of subordinate units to supervising authorities in an administrative context, whereas "contractual" is misleading, for it highlights market transactions.

3 In his report to the first National Health Conference of Bureau Chiefs on March 22, 1979, Minister of Health Qian explained the idea of "economic management" (Qian 1983a).

4 The overall framework of managed competition is summarized in "Provisional Measure for In-hospital Economic Management," issued in early 1983 (Weishengbu, PRC 1985).

5 In managerial terms, the number of hospital beds represents a composite indicator, pertaining to building space, technical capability, medical care equipment, and facilities; and it is fixed or made available to the providing unit through the approval and action of higher authorities. And "personnel establishment" has to do with the number of positions authorized by supervising bureaus (within the health care sector) for jobs to be carried out (Weishengbu, PRC 1985: 486).

6 Cited in the Minister Qian Xinzhong's concluding speech on January 5, 1980 (Qian, 1983c).

7 Cited in the Minister Qian Xinzhong's concluding speech on January 5, 1980 (Qian 1983c).

8 Since 1979, the revenue retention system has become an essential ingredient for revenue-generating activities, having first occupied a central place in reforming industrial management (Lee 1987; Shirk 1993). As being discussed here, it has subsequently become a main theme in market-oriented reform in the medical care sector throughout the economic reform period in China.

9 In terms of interpretative scheme commonly used within the health care circle, here "undertaking" (chengbao) refers to the obligation of the subordinate to the superior on the basis of a commitment pledged by the former to the latter in a command relationship. It differs from the contract (qiyue or hetong) that pertains to quid pro quo transactions between two parties on an equal economic footing. The notion of undertaking is often used in connection with "responsibility system," which also entails a command relationship. This was further articulated in the form of the "undertaking responsibility system" (chengbao zerenzhi; URS), often understood

interchangeably as "undertaking system" (chengbaozhi) or "responsibility system" (zherenzhi). It features financial accountability placing emphasis on the fulfillment of revenue targets in accordance with an "undertaking agreement" (chengbao xieyi).

10 It is claimed that the government's appropriation to the health care sector increased from 72.69 percent of the total of wage bill in 1957 to 99.88 percent in 1965 and 135 percent in 1979 (Liu 2012: 16).

11 The drastic reducing share of state appropriation in the total of health care expenditure to providing units took place in the midst of shrinking share of government revenue in the total GNP, a decrease, percentage-wise, in the central government's revenue relative to the total national revenue, and rapid inflation (Sun & Du 2006: 24).

12 This is understood in the colloquial expression as "the management of total volume, differential-quota appropriation, revenue retention, performance appraisal, and rewards schemes" (Du 2007: 32). This means that the government still has maintains its hold over entire budgetary process, but only provides partial subsidy (a portion of the total expenditure) on the basis of performance of the providing unit concerned.

13 According to the "1979 Supplementary General Circular," the method of calculating revenue/saving as well as its actual retained amount for the providing unit should follow the "planned indicators" of revenue and expenditure as having been approved by the supervising unit (Weishengbu et al. 1982; Weishengbu & Guojialaodongzongju, 1980).

14 This is loosely understood as "the relations of interests among the state, work unit, and individual workers and staffers" in policy papers and discussions of the health care circle, in conjunction with the issues of material interests, entitlements, and benefits raised in the public arena (Chen, 1990; Peng, Cai, & Zhou 1992: 76–81).

15 The result of a survey of 2,000 hospitals above the county level indicates, as of 1990, that in the total income, the breakdowns of revenue from medical care services, state appropriation (differentiated quota), and special grants are 86 percent, 10 percent, and 4 percent, respectively (Peng, Cai, & Zhou 1992: 38).

16 The "indicators" pertain to a measuring criterion (e.g., revenue, infection rates from surgery, etc.) and the "fixed norms" refer to the expected level of actual attainment (e.g., amount of revenue fulfilled, actual days of annual hospital bed utilization, etc.), given that a set of measuring criteria has already been chosen.

17 URS requires the providing units to take part and sign an undertaking agreement for a fixed term (say, three years) often through negotiations voluntarily, although the supervising bureaus can unilaterally impose a chosen, likely high, set of targets without consent of the providing units concerned.

18 During the early phases of inaugurating URS, the MOH made mention of not discouraging providing units by further reducing state appropriation to them because they already had practiced saving and created revenue (Weishengbu, PRC 1985; Weishengbu et al. 1982).

19 The title of the "1981 Provisional Measure" is: "Provisional Measure for Hospital Management" that is issued on March 18, 1981 (Weishengbu et al. 1982).

References

Cai, R. 1988. Yiyuan "liang quan fenli" lue lun (A preliminary analysis on the separation of two powers in hospitals). *Zhongguo Weisheng Jingji(China's Health Care Economics)*, 1: 5–9.

Cao, P. 1988. Lue lun heli gouzao yiyuan chengbao jingyiing jizhi (A preliminary discussion on the re-structuring of the managerial mechanisms in the hospital chengbao system). *Zhongguo Weisheng Jingji(China's Health Care Economics)*, 12: 4–7.

Carter, N., Klein, R., & Day, P. 1992. *How Organizations Measure Success: The Use of Performance Indicators in Government*. London: Routledge.

Chang, T., Zhou, H., & Wang, X. 1990. Yiyuan chengbao jingying zerenzhi de xian-chuangyu shenhua gaige de shexiang (The current state of the hospital chengbao managment system and considerations on its further reform). *Zhongguo Weisheng Jingji(China's Health Care Economics)*, 6: 38–40.

Chen, L. 1990. Shilun yiyuan liyi daoxiang jizhi (A preliminary discussion on interest-oriented mechanisms in hospitals). *Zhongguo Weisheng Jingji(China's Health Care Economics)*, 5: 34–35, 37.

Chen, M. 1992. Chen Mingzhang buchang zai 1990 nian quanquo weisheng ting-juchang huiyi shang de baogao (The report of Minister Chen Mingzhang at the 1990 national conference of chiefs of bureau/office of health care). In R. Peng, R. Cai, & C. Zhou (Eds.), *Zhonggou gaige quanshu (Encyclopedia of China's Reform)*, 191–200. Dalian: Dalian chubanshe.

Chen, Z. 1990. Yao yiyuan chengbao zerenzhi ji qi juxianxing yinqi de sikao (Obser-vations arising from the hospital chengbao responsibility system and its limitations). *Zhongguo Weisheng Jingji(China's Health Care Economics)*, 4:12–14, 34.

Cui, Y. 1992. Cui Yueli tongchi zai yijiu basan nian quanguo weisheng tingjuchang huiyi pimushi de jianghua (Comrade Cui Yueli's speech at the conclusion of the 1983 national conference of chiefs of bureaus/offices of health care). In R. Peng, R. Cai, & C. Zhou (Eds.), *Zhongguo gaige quanshu (Encyclopedia of China's Reform)*, 119–122. Dalian: Dalian chubanshe.

Downs, A. 1967. *Inside Bureaucracy*. Boston: Little, Brown and Company.

Du, L. 2007. Hongguan jingji he weisheng fazhan de liangxing xunhuan ho exing xunhuan—ershihnian weisheng zhengce yanjiu huigu (Positive and vicious cycles of macro economy and health care development). In L. Du, & W. Zhang (Eds.), Zhongguo Weisheng Chanye Zazhishe (Ed.), *Zhongguo wesheng yiliao fazhan baogao, No. 3* (The Report of Development of Health and Medical Care in China, No. 3), 25–40. Beijing: Shehui kexue wenxian chubanshe.

Du, L., Zhang, W., & Zhongguo Weisheng Chanye Zazhishe (Eds.) *Zhongguo yiliao weisheng fazhang baogao No. 5* (The Report of Development of Health and Medical Care in China, No. 5), Beijing: Zhonguo weisheng canye zaizhishe.

Ferlie, E., Ashburner, Fitzgerald, L., & Pettigrew A. 1997. *The New Public Management in Action*. Oxford andNew York: Oxford University Press.

Ge, Y., & Gong, S. 2007. *Zhongguo yiliao gaige: Wenti, genyuan, chulu* (China's Health Care Reform: Problems, Roots and Solutions). Beijing: Zhongguo fazhen chubanshe.

Gortner, H. F., Mahler, J., & Nicholson, J. B. 1997. *Organization Theory: A Public Perspective* (2nd ed.). New York: Harcourt Brace.

Graham, C. B., Jr. and Hays, S. W. 1991. Management functions and public admin-istration—POSDCIRB revisited. In J. Ott, J. Steven, A. C. Hyde, M. Jay & J. M. Shafritz (Eds.), *Public Management: The Essential Readings*, 10–27. Chicago: Lyceum Books/Nelson-Hall Publishers.

Gu, X. 2008. *Zouxiang quanmin yibao: Zhongguo xingyigai de zhanlue yu zhanshu* (Toward Comprehensive Medical Insurance: Strategy and Tactic of China's New Medical Care Reform). Beijing: Zhongguo laodong chubanshe.

Hughes, O. E. 1988. *Public Management and Administration: An Introduction* (2nd ed.). Houndmills and New York: Palgrave.

Lee, P. 1987. *Industrial Management and Economic Reform in China, 1949–1984.* Hong Kong, Oxford and New York: Oxford University Press.

Li, J. 1999. Gaige suoyouzhi wanshang chengbaozhi (Improve ownership sysem and perfect chengbao system). *Zhongguo Weisheng Jingji(China's Health Care Economics),* 4: 9–11, 20.

Li, X., Zeng Q. & He, M. 1988. Qianyi yiyuan chengbaozhi de yanze (Preliminary discussion on the principle of the hospital chengbaozhi). *Zhongguo Weisheng Jingji (China's Health Care Economics),* 11: 13–15.

Lindblom, C. E. 1977. *Politics and Markets, The World's Political-economic Systems.* New York: Basic Books.

Liu, J. 2012. *Zhongguo yigai xiangguan zhengce yanji* (Study on Policies related to China's Medical Care Reform). Beijing: Jingji kexue chubanshe.

Luo, Y. 1990. Woguo weisheng gaige ruogan tezheng de yanjiu yu sikao (Study and thoughts on some salient characteristics of health care reform in China). *Zhongguo Weisheng Jingji(China's Health Care Economics),* 3: 4–8.

Massey, A. 1993. *Managing the Public Sector: A Comparative Analysis of the United Kingdom and the United States.* Aldershot and Brookfield, VT: Ashgate.

Mintzberg, H. 1983. *Structure in Fives: Designing Effective Organizations.* Englewood Cliffs, NJ: Prentice-Hall.

Peng, R., Cai, R. & Zhou, C. (Ed.). 1992. *Zhongguo gaige quanshu* (Encyclopedia of China's Reform). Dalian: Dalian chubanshe.

Pollit, C. 1993. *Managerialism and the Public Services: The Anglo-American Experience* Oxford: Basil Blackwell.

Pollit, C., & Bouchaert, G. 2004. *Public Management Reform: A Comparative Analysis* (2nd ed.). Oxford, New York: Oxford University Press.

Qian, M. 1990. Yiliao weisheng danwei shixing chengbao zherenzhi de jige wenti (Several problems regard the trial implementation of contractual responsibility system in medical and health care units). *Zhongguo Weisheng Jingji(China's Health Care Economics),* 2: 40–41.

Qian, X. 1983a. Ba weisheng bumen gongzuo zhuozhongdian zhuanyidao yiyao weisheng xiandaihua jianshe shanglai (Shift the central gravity of the task of health care sector to the modernization of medical and health care). In Zhongguo weisheng nianjian bianji weiyuanhui (Ed.), *Zhongguo weisheng nianjian 1983* (China's Yearbook on Health Care, 1983), 22–26. Beijing: Zhongguo weisheng chubanshe.

Qian, X. 1983b. Zai quanquo weisheng juchang huiyi shang de xiaojie (A summary at the national conference of bureau chiefs of health care). In Zhongguo weisheng nianjian bianji weiyuanhui (Ed.), *Zhongguo weisheng nianjian 1983* (China's Yearbook of Health Care 1983), 27–30. Beijing: Zhongguo weisheng chubanshe.

Qian, X. 1983c. Zai quanquo weisheng juchang huiyi shang de zongjie jianghuig (The concluding speech at the national conference of bureau chiefs of health care). In Zhongguo weisheng nianjian bianji weiyuanhui (Ed.), *Zhongguo weisheng nianjian 1983* (China's Year Health Care 1983), 36–40. Beijing: Zhongguo weisheng chubanshe.

Rainey, H. G. 1991. *Understanding and Managing Public Organizations.* San Francisco: Jossey-Bass.

Ren, H. 1988. Chengshi yiyuan chengbao jingyin erti (Two issues concerning hospital chengbao management in urban area). *Zhongguo Weisheng Jingji* (China's Health Care Economics), 11: 10–13.

Shirk, S. L. 1993, *The Political Logic of Economic Reform in China*. Berkeley: University of California Press.

Schurmann, F. 1968. *Ideology and Organization in Communist China*. Berkeley and Los Angeles: University of California Press.

Song, W. 1990. Jiaqiang hongguan tiaokong wanshang yiyuan chengbaozhi (Strengthen macro management and perfect hospital chengbao system). *Zhongguo Weisheng Jingji(China's Health Care Economics)*, 3: 24–27.

Sun, N., & Du, L. 2006. Gongli yiyuan yunxin jizhi gaige (The reform of operating mechanisms of public hospitals). In L. Du (Ed.), *Zhongguo yiliao weisheng fazhan baogao No.2* (The Report of Development of China's Medical and Health care, No. 2), 119–179. Beijing: Shehui kexue wenxian chubanshe.

Wang, W. 1992. Wang Wei tongchi zai yijiu basan nian quanguo weisheng tingjuchang huiyi shang de jianghua (Comrade Wang Wei's speech at the 1983 national conference of chiefs of bureaus/offices of health care). In R. Peng, R. Cai, & C. Zhou (Eds.), *Zhongguo gaige quanshu, yiliao weisheng tizhi gaige juan (Encyclopedia of China's Reform)*, 117–118. Dalian: Dalian chubanshe.

Weishengbu. 1982. Guanyu jiaqiang zhishu ji shuangchong lingdao shiye danwei caiwu guanli gongzuo de shixing banfa (The provisional measure of the task of financial management regarding the service units of directly affiliation and under dual command). In Zhonghua Renmin Gongheguo Weishengbu Bangongting (Ed.), *Zhonghua renmin gongheguo weisheng fagui huibian 1978–1980* (The Collection of Laws and Regulations of Health Care of the People's Republic of China 1978–1980), 630–634. Beijing: Falu chubanshe.

Weishangbu. 1985. Yiyuan jingji guanli zanxing banfa, xiugaigao (The provisional measure of hospital economic management, revised draft). In Weishengbu Bangongting (Ed.), *Zhonghua renmin gongheguo weisheng fagui huibian, 1981–1983* (The Collection of Laws and Regulations of Health Care 1981–1983), 485–492. Beijing: Falu chubanshe.

Weishengbu, PRC. 1985. Yiyuan jingji guanli zanxing banfa (The provisional measure of economic management). In Weishengbu Bangongti (Ed.), *Zhonghua renmin gongheguo weisheng fagui huibian* (The Collection of Laws and Regulations of Health Care of the People's Republic of China), 485–492. Beijing: Falu chubanshe.

Weishengbu *et al.*1982. Weishengbu, caizhengbu guojialaodongzongju guanyu yiyuan jingji guanli shidian gongzuo de buchong tongzi (The supplementary general circular of the Ministry of Health Care, Ministry of Finance and State General Bureau of Labor concerning the pilot task of hospital economic management). In Weishengbu Bangongting (PRC) (Ed.), *Zhonghua renmin gongheguo weisheng fagui huibian* (The Collection of Law and Regulations of Health Care of the PRC), 627–629. Beijing: Falu chubanshe, Xinhua shudian.

Weishengbu & Guojialaodongzhongchu. 1979. Guanyu jiaqiang yiyuan jingji guanli shihdian gongtso di yijian (Opinion concerning the strengthening of pilot work of hospital economic management). *Laodong zhengce fagui huibian* (The Collection of Policies and Laws of Labor). Beijing: [n.p].

Weishengbu & Guojialaodongzongju. 1980. Guanyu yiyuan jingji guanli shidian gongzuo de bucong tongzhi (The supplementary general circular concerning economic management of hospitals). *Laodong zhengce fagui huibian* (The Collection of Policies and Regulations of Labor), 563–566.

Wu, Q. 1992. Shenhua yiyuan gaige, chuangjian biaozhuenhua guanli xinmoshi (Further reform in medical care, build a new model of standardization management). In

R. Peng, R. Cai, & C. Zhou (Eds.), *Zhongguo gaige quanshu* (Encyclopedia of China's Reform), 448–450. Dalian: Dalian chubanshe.

Xie, Hong, & Li, X. 1988. Zouchu kunjing zhenqiang huoli (Step out of the difficult situation, revive vitality). *Zhongguo Weisheng Jingji(China's Health Care Economics)*, 7: 14–17.

Yang, H. & Sun, N. 2006. Weisheng gaige yu fazhan de pingjia yu jianyan (The evaluation and examination of health care reform and development). In L. Du (Ed.), *Zhongguo yiliao weisheng fazhan baogao No. 2* (The Report of Reform and Development of Medical and Health Care in China No. 2), 47–85. Beijing: Shehui kexue wenxian chubanshe.

Zhang, J., & Lin, M. 1988. Yiyuan chengbao jinying xiaoguo de pingjia (An evaluation of the results of hospital chengbao management). *Zhongguo Weisheng Jingji (China's Health Care Economics)*, 11: 16–19.

Zhang, S. 1990. Yiyuan chengbaozhi ying buduan wanshang (Continuously perfect the hospital chengbao system). *Zhongguo Weisheng Jingji(China's Health Care Economics)*, 4:15–16.

Zhang, X., & Cui, X. 1990. Qianyi yiyuan chengbao chenggonglu de tigao (Preliminary discussion on how to improve the success rates of hospital chengbao management). *Zhongguo Weisheng Jingji(China's Health Care Economics)*, 3: 28–29.

8   Franchising of medical care services and unintended policy consequences

Further to introduction of ESM, this chapter is devoted to an analysis of the second installment of reform focusing on the rebuilding of a franchise system for medical care services. To trace the roots of franchising in policy history, the early version of a franchise system remained dormant in the health care sector prior to 1979.[1] It has been, since 1979, resurrected and developed into the principal funding source at the providing unit level. One may treat franchising as one kind of market-oriented tool employed by the state. It pertains to the rights of market entry, and it constitutes one of the most important components in financial management at the providing unit level.

Franchising is an integral part of funding package for health care, combining with the other two—government subsidies and public insurances. Contrary to the characterization of the "state's retreat" (Duckett 2013), the study argues that the state still actively intervened in health care by making use of franchising creatively to allow the providing unit to generate revenue to render medical care services and propel the rapid growth of health care sector. In colloquial expression within the policy circle, franchising is taken as "lending policy, but not necessarily money" (geizhengce, bugeiqian). This chapter deals mainly with the franchise of curative care services (focusing on special care services) and medical devices, whereas the next chapter covers the franchise for prescription drugs. The chapter will also assess various theoretical alternatives regarding two forms of non-compliances, one focusing on the providing unit as an enforcing subordinate unit in the Party-state hierarchy, and the other treating the providing unit as a franchise-holder in the market place.

Commercialization of curative care services

As the study has just examined the articulation of a new classification of various types of health care services in light of the changing roles of the state and markets in Chapter 2, it is warranted here to have a close look at how the government started to guide the providing unit to establish an entirely new charges system centering on the curative care services as well as considerations behind this policy episode. From a comparative perspective, franchising is often used as a powerful revenue tool to substitute for a taxation system, ensuring a revenue stream for rapid growth in the industrial sector in socialist countries in the past (Naughton 1996: 25–56; Lee 1987; Peng, Cai, & Zhou 1992: 28). Learning from the industrial sector of the CPE in China after 1949, policymakers have promoted the use of franchising in the health care sector in order to generate revenue and finance medical care services with user charges during the reform era (Guan & Dong 2007: 44; Zhou 2008; 52–80, 125).

Franchise refers to rights given to a certain category of economic unit (e.g., industrial enterprises and service work units alike) to enter into market transactions for a variety of services and products. Here the term "franchise" is used interchangeably with "monopoly" depending on the number of holders of the right to market entry for providing medical care services. In a broad and systematic fashion, franchising may cover the totality of heath care resources, embracing various points of market entry, such as investment, establishment and organization, medical and health care practice, facilities, equipment and clinical technologies, pharmacy, insurance, etc. (Wang 2008: 244–7). More narrowly, "commercialization" mainly refers to transactions regarding medical care services only, for example, treatment and regular examinations, prescription drugs, advanced medical devices, and various types of insurance (Wu 2002).

As a rule, the providing unit charges the users (including both patients and insurers) a fee for the service provided on the basis of franchise, and the amount of charges depends upon which type of service. In Professor Gu Xin's view, China's health care reform is marked by the introduction and expansion of various categories of paid services in order to finance medical care provision (Gu 2008: 275–80). Public hospitals are subject to double control by the government. On the one hand, they are "service work units" that are governed as extensions of the Party-state organization, for example, by financial accountability, budgetary procedures, responsibility systems, and the system of resources management. On the other hand, they are franchise-holders subject to regulatory control in the markets. By and large they take part in market transactions and are under considerable pressure to fulfill revenue targets and to maintain budgetary balance (Zhang 1990; Lu & Yang 2005).

Ministerial policymakers began to initiate commercialization as early as 1979, focusing on embryonic forms of franchise provision.[2] Through several stages from 1979 to the late 1980s, re-engineering the franchise system involved redefining and readjusting the categories of medical care services in order to improve those services and to increase revenue flow to the providing unit level.[3] As mentioned previously, the expanded franchise system was interlocked with budgetary reform centering on the current expenditure accounts and revenue retention schemes (Sun & Du 2006: 124; Du 2007: 32: Liu 2012: 15–18). And the system was subsequently fused with the "undertaking responsibility system" (URS) (Gu 2008: 276).

There is no mistake that policymakers stressed narrow revenue concerns when they first introduced URS during the early phase of economic reform, albeit they later shifted to other policy priorities. In the early 1980s, ministerial leadership tried to convince provincial and inter-ministerial audiences that franchise provision was an effective revenue tool. For example, Cui Yueli, a ministerial ranking official, observed that from the total of annual expenditure for providing units in 1984, the state appropriation amounted only to 30,700 million RMB out of a national total of 145,700 million RMB, while the providing units contributed the remaining 115,000 million RMB (about three-quarters of the national total) (Cui 1992). In the same vein, Chen Mingzhang, another ministerial ranking leader, stressed that the franchise-based responsibility systems furnished substantial funding for badly needed development projects. For instance, local government and providing units contributed 500 million out of an estimated total of 800 million RMB for capital investment (Chen 1992c). It became obvious by the mid-1980s that not only did providing units have to generate sufficient revenue to maintain daily operation and delivery of medical care services, but they also needed to finance investment projects at the providing unit level.

It does not appear that sovereign planners were in full unison or maintained consistency over time from 1979 to the 1990s with regard to policy priorities in adopting a franchise system for providing medical care services (Du 2006a: 125). However, it is apparent that, as a salient feature of commercialization, the franchise system was introduced mainly as a financial tool. After Deng Xiaoping's tour to the southern part of the country on June 6, 1992, the Central Committee, CCP, and State Council jointly promulgated the policy paper known as the "1992 Decision," proposing to a majority of those tertiary units of welfare, charity, and services to shift into a business-oriented mode and adopt the model of enterprise management. The policy paper further urged service work units to transform themselves into entirely autonomous entities and to become fully accountable for earning and loss.[4] Some authors interpret the 1992 Decision as a call for all health care providing units to take further steps toward commercialization (Chang 1993).

Repackaging and managing franchise provision

The whole process of commercialization took place in an incremental fashion in the sense that the policymakers depended upon the policy precedents of the past and navigated forward in bringing in new ideas of financial management. In record, an entirely new category of special care services had been introduced on an experimental basis in the first stage during 1979–1983 but was expanded further in the second stage from 1985 onward (Weishengbu 1985; Song 1990). On April 25, 1985, the MOH took the first step to propose a major repackaging of the franchise provision in the "1985 Report."[5] Making the second installment of commercialization, the "1985 Report" proposed an expanded franchise for health care services with two tiers: the primary tier of basic (or essential) curative care services to be provided to all patients at regulated, and in fact, low prices in full congruence with the affordable care policy; and in addition, a secondary tier that was taken as special care service going beyond essential care to be charged at flexible rates, as previously mentioned. At this juncture of policy history, it was evident that the policy-makers tried to find an appropriate policy mix to accommodate both the basic medical care and non-basic types. This policy package of commercialization accompanying the idea of affordable care was further elaborated and confirmed in the "1988 Opinion."[6]

Furthermore, the "1985 Report" and the "1988 Opinion" proposed policy measures to deal with the meager pay of medical personnel (Weishengbu et al. 1993b; Weishengbu 1985; Fu 1989). It also encouraged medical staff to render additional and overtime services including outside practices, concurrent appointments in the non-state sector such as COEs, and outside-office-hour medical care services in non-state sectors. In addition, providing units as well as medical personnel were advised to take part in "collaborative projects" with collectively owned facilities and clinics. (Luo 1990; Weishengbu, PRC 1992b; Weishengbu et al. 1993a). This means that doctors and other medical personnel were allowed to earn additional income through overtime and/or extra work while their pay schedule remained unchanged.

Policymakers further proposed looking into new ways of financial management between the core and periphery of medical care services in accordance with tertiary industry managerial principles in order to enhance financial accountability and to expand the scale of production/services and increase savings (Ma 2006). According to Luo Yiqin, a research officer at the MOH, the repackaged hospital franchise could embrace three portions (depending how closely related a portion was to core medical care technology) as follows: the main portion, auxiliary portion and affiliated portion (Luo 1985; Luo 1990). As early as 1984, it was proposed to mark charges up for peripheral services such as logistic services in order to shift costs from core services (i.e., curative care services) that were lowly priced. Being subsequently incorporated into the "1985 Report," providing units were encouraged to earn revenue not only from main services but also from auxiliary services and affiliated enterprises (Weishengbu 1988).

The degree of commercialization can be measured by the amount of user charges for health care services and this amount's proportion of the total payment. Due to commercialization since 1979, the patients' share of the financial burden has been on the increase as the state appropriation and public insurances have been drastically curtailed.[7]

The repackaging of franchises has irreversibly created a new mix of services, representing not only new sources of revenue for providing units, but also a new pattern and higher level of consumption among users. Some authors characterize non-basic curative care services (including special care services) as "consuming beyond one's means" (chaoqian xiaofei), and of course, these services are charged at a high price (Du 2006b: 20–8). At the providing unit level, a patient would normally have the choice of a new mix of services (including both basic and non-basic care categories), often consulting doctors and being given advice by doctors. In light of the asymmetry of information and the uncertainty in a decision-making situation as noted in Chapter 1, doctors are in a better position to advise and recommend options at the higher end of the price range and thus ensure better financial returns to the providing unit (Du 2006b: 20–8). As a financial strategy, medical doctors could advise and/or induce patients to move from the choice of basic medical care types to that of non-basic ones for revenue consideration, given other things equal. Most likely the new mix of services catering to the demands of users with greater purchasing power represents an upgraded category of services and often commands a higher value than the pre-reform package does. (Zhou, Qu, & Li 2003: 144–5).

Moreover, the practice of drug franchise was an established practice in financial management in the health care sector during the pre-reform period, and it has grown into a principal funding source and become an effective and reliable vehicle for cost shifting from lowly priced curative care services to drugs in order to maintain financial balance at the providing unit level since 1979. In an investigation of one provincial jurisdiction, for example, authors have suggested that "yiyao yangyi" (to foster curative services by [revenue from] pharmaceuticals) has been part of the deliberative health care policy in China ever since the 1950s, and therefore it is controversial but not entirely "unintended" (Zhou, Qu, & Li 2003:137–67). In addition to drug franchise, advanced medical devices constitute an integral part of policy of franchising at the providing unit level, marking an entirely new policy feature during the reform era. The study will dwell on franchising of advanced medical devices briefly in following passages in next section, and leave the issue of drug franchise to Chapter 9 and 10 in view of complexity and profound policy implications.

According to Bai Zhipeng, Secretary of the China Medical Device Association, China has been keeping pace with Western countries in the acquisition and installation of large and expensive medical devices. For instance, China imported the first set of CT (computerized tomography) scanners in 1978, building up to 170 scanners by 1987, 1,300 (including ECT: electro-convulsive therapy) by 1993, and reaching an estimate of 4,258 by 2000. Moreover, China started using MRI (magnetic resonance imaging) scanners in 1985, the figure reaching 200 in 1993 and 950 in 2000 (Sun & Du 2006: 164). A similar trend of growth has been observed in some selected jurisdictions, such as Fujian Province and Bejing Municipality.[8]

As China began to accelerate the importation of advanced medical devices in 1985, the government promulgated the first set of regulations governing the coordination of imports between the central ministries and provincial/local jurisdictions. In 1995, the MOH issued the 1995 Provisional Measures, stipulating duties, responsibility, and functional areas at the central provincial and municipal levels. Meanwhile, the 1995 Provisional Measures established, for the first time, regulatory control over the acquisition, installation, and use of large medical devices, including a licensing system.[9] From a broad policy perspective, sovereign planners faced several concrete issues: lack of planning, coordination, and regulatory control in the midst of rapid expansion; low utilization rates on the whole; and regional imbalance in deployment with an over-concentration on metropolitan area (Zhu & Wang 2010). Other policy analysts stressed that the unreasonable increase in expenditure for medical care services was attributable to the sub-optimal allocation of health care resources, especially advanced medical devices and lack of regulatory control (Liu, 2012: 92–5).

In 2004 the MOH, the State Development and Reform Commission (SDRC), and the Ministry of Finance jointly promulgated the 2004 Measures, strengthening the licensing system and tightening control over market entry.[10] According to the 2004 Measures, medical devices were classified into two categories: Category A and Category B. While the central ministries took charge of the former, the provincial jurisdictions the latter. In 2005, sovereign planners started addressing uncoordinated importation, excessive charges, and the financial burden for the patient regarding advanced medical devices (Duan & Huang 2011). Subsequently the central ministries promulgated a set of policy papers as follows: the first trying to strengthen managerial power over planning for and installation of advanced medical devices at the provincial level in 2005, the second regarding a policy for procurement in 2007, and the third detailing the approval procedures of Category A medical devices at the ministerial level in 2008 (Sun & Du 2006: 164–5; Zhu & Wang 2010: 33).

At the policymaking level, sovereign planners expressed concern that the expensive advanced devices might go uncontrolled and that this would undermine the low-price policy for medical care services. In September, 2005, for example, the SDRC and the MOH promulgated the 2005 Advisory Opinion, announcing for the first time the principle of "non-profit orientation and compensation for reasonable costs" in the adjustment of prices for examinations and curative care services with large medical devices.[11]

In fact, there have been pros and cons regarding the use of advanced medical devices. In allegations by Sun Huizhu and Yu Runji, doctors who were often driven by personal interests chose to use large and advanced medical devices at much higher charges and fees than those normally used for ordinary medical examinations. Being against the excessive use of devices, they claimed that it was medically unnecessary for doctors to stick to the standard operational procedure of advising/inducing each inpatient to go through at least one or more examination (s) with advanced devices under the pretext of upgrading the level of diagnosis in a given case. On the basis of a study of five selected medical devices, Sun and Yu asserted that the hospitals recovered their investment in such devices within one year and get a revenue return of 300 percent of the investment within the devices' standard life span in accordance with relevant regulations. According to Sun and Yu, for instance, some hospitals made use of the revenue from investment in advanced medical devices in unreasonable ways—thus putting an unwarranted burden on patients—to compensate for the loss of medical care services (Sun & Yu 2010: 10).

On the contrary, some other policy analysts have maintained that advanced devices did not actually guarantee success in revenue-raising in all cases, even though in some cases revenue from advanced devices often played a role in cross-subsidizing the loss from low-priced curative care services. To deflect blame on medical personnel and hospitals, besides, some authors pointed to the fact that the patients themselves show a clear preference for the application of advanced medical devices (Mao & Lei 2009: 90).

Pro-device policy analysts argue, moreover, that it is a matter of an overall trend in the increase of health care costs amidst the evolution of medical devices and technology, albeit accompanied in some cases by low utilization rates as well as an overheated pursuit of economic utility. Overall, some policy analysts question the proposition that the employment of advanced devices is driven solely by revenue-maximizing motives and cast doubt on the assertion that their use has guaranteed excessive revenue return in all cases. As noted by Bai Zhipeng, the utilization rates of large medical devices have been less than optimal, never reaching one-third or one-half of capacity. An investigation in the Xian area suggests that in eight hospitals with a total of ten CT scanners and three MRI scanners, the utilization rate of CT was able to reach only 39.2 percent and that of MRI, only 46.8 percent, respectively. As Bai adds, it is not unusual that those hospitals that have installed large medical devices have suffered considerable loss due to low utilization rates (Sun & Du 2006: 164–5).

Some hospitals registered complaints from time to time about the broad tendency of price cuts that decreased revenue from advanced medical devices (Zeng 2006). To implement the 2005 Advisory Opinion, for instance, the price of an examination with large medical devices was cut by 60 percent in the Jiangsu Province starting September 1, 2005. Director Guo Xinghua of the Heath Care Office of Jiangsu Province commented in an interview that the rate of said reduction was too large to maintain a surplus of revenue from examinations using large medical devices (Zeng 2006: 41). In the case of Nanjing, the revenue from examinations using medical devices, which consisted of 30 percent of the total expenditure of municipal hospitals, was reduced considerably after September 2005, resulting in the loss of about 10 to 15 percent of total revenue (Zeng 2006: 41).

In fact, it was by no means easy for the government to enforce price cuts for the use of advanced devices, as many public hospitals took counter-measures to resist government pressure. In cases surveyed in Fujian Province from 2001 to 2007, for example, the providing units involved tried to cope with the financial pressure generated by price cuts by changing the schedule of charges for medical devices, coupled with increasing the numbers of patients examined.[12] In fact, price control on advanced devices stalled in the case of Fujian (Feng 2009: 9).

Unanticipated policy outcomes at the providing unit level

It is noteworthy that a pattern of unintended and undesirable policy consequences began to take hold at the providing unit level in conjunction with commercialization of health care services in the early 1980s.[13] As previously mentioned, the public providing unit enjoys an amphibious existence as a subordinate, enforcing unit at the bottom of the Party-state hierarchy, and as a franchise holder in market transactions. To examine unintended policy consequences, one may deal with two analytical dimensions: one concerning command-oriented management, that is, authority relations of bureau to the providing unit, and other pertaining to transaction-oriented management, namely, the issues of regulatory control over the providing unit (as a franchise holder) in medical care markets.

Focusing on the authority relations of bureaus to the providing unit, analysts and policymakers have articulated the following interpretative categories regarding abuses and irregularities at the providing unit level: first, irregular practices in the collection and schedules of fees and charges, for example, unnecessary treatments, laboratory tests, and prescription drugs; second, violations of accounting rules pertaining to management, maintenance, procurement, and patient debt; third, irregularities of collaborative ventures between publicly owned units; fourth, irregularities in the remuneration, bonus and wages of medical personnel; and fifth, illicit income of medical personnel from the practice of referrals, part-time and concurrent services, outside practices and commissions, bribery and extortion involving medical care services, and drug sales (Chen 1992b). Most of these activities/behaviors are concerned supervision and control by the bureaus over the providing units in the arena of financial management.

To account for unanticipated policy outcomes at the bureaucratic level, one has to go beyond the bureau level and examine the choice of policy goals in policymaking process above the bureau level. As gaps always exist between policy and performance, one needs to examine both policy implementation and results, intended or unintended, desirable or undesirable.[14] Theoretically speaking, one may assume that multiple policy goals are an important cause leading to unanticipated policy outcomes. In other words, the fulfillment of either one policy goal or a set of policy goals is not equivalent to the successful implementation of the others. Moreover, one policy might be in contradiction with the other. In addition, as policymakers often change their policy priority from time to time, policy results must be evaluated from a changing policy perspective. Besides, one cannot simply assume that policy actors are always capable of choosing right policy goals, and thus any undesirable policy outcomes must be "unintended." In fact, health care reform was and still is considered successful if one merely addresses the narrow issue of revenue target, a policy priority endorsed and adopted by top policymakers for the first decade of the reform and beyond as noted above (Sun and Du 2006: 124). It was entirely appropriate for policymakers to restore the balance between economic utility and social utility when the urgency of funding receded in the late 1980s, but this poses as a main cause of non-compliances, irregularities and even abuses at the providing unit level.

Unanticipated policy outcomes take place in market transactions as well, since the providing unit started to rely upon user charges as major funding source. Seen from the angle of health care policy, commercialization may be appraised in a balanced and positive light. For instance, it has created some new modes of services representing an improvement in both quantity and quality, and it has satisfied the demands for new types and a high quality of service as the purchasing power of the people visibly improved during the economic reform. Although the fulfillment of revenue-generating targets ought to be treated as a favorable policy outcome, meeting targets often produced undesirable results at the expense of medical-professional standards. For examples, the revenue-maximizing pressure often impaired the normal operation of some large, advanced hospital units when they deferred or assigned low priority to the tasks of training, teaching, and research, to say the least (Weishengbu 1985).

In commercialization on the basis of franchising, government policy often put providing units in an untenable position by subjecting them to a "double squeeze" ("liangtou kesi" in colloquial Chinese): dwindling of government subsidies on the one hand and ever-tightening price control over curative care services on the other (Peng, Cai, & Zhou 1992: 36). Thus, providing units were left with an untenable position: generating revenue through user charges in market transactions, as they were confronted with financial burdens of various kinds, for instance, the costs of curative care services, drugs, medical materials, wages and subsidies to medical personnel, loans for medical devices, and new construction of hospitals (Gao 2006: 51). Such financial pressure put hospital units and medical personnel in a dilemma of choosing between maintaining budgetary balance and risking irregularities and abuses. And this prepared the soil for the growth of over-provision and over-prescription (Weishengbu 1988: 1–6).

The tensions between the government and providing units were not limited to the issue of economic concerns versus social utility. Even if one focuses on the purely economic dimension, the commercialization policy could be taken as undesirable, for instance, in that it created the unintended propensity of hoarding the largest possible portion of retained revenue for the providing unit and share of income for managerial and medical personnel while ignoring the value of the providing unit's property and assets (Liang & Huang 1990). In the case of the URS, for example, neither did the undertaking agreement lend much priority to the financial accountability of the providing units over capital investments, nor did it provide effective legal or economic levers to enhance the value of fixed assets and equipment. This often results in many cases of irregularities in accounting and asset management. For example, the providing unit often endeavored, under pressure to maximize its revenue, either to postpone or skip regular maintenance jobs, since it understood that it would not be held accountable for the value of assets and property (Xie 1990).

Franchises are definitely a focal area leading to unintended policy consequences. Franchise here means a share of health care market, but not necessarily total control of it as in the case of monopoly.[15] Franchise refers to the rights of market entry, entailing double advantage to its holder: on the one hand, it denies competitors an opportunity, real or potential, from taking part in transactions; on the other hand, it gains better bargaining position through dictating pricing and limiting the choices of the clients.

According to Ma, the providing unit, assuming the role of "rent-seeker" because of power [in the form of franchise], and medical personnel tended to undermine the government efforts to enforce financial and budgetary discipline that is directly relevant to affordable care policy (Ma 2006). In Wu Ming's view, rent-seeking behavior has taken place at all levels of the hierarchy of command in the health care sector, including at the public hospital level.[16] As medical personnel make decisions jointly with hospital management pertaining to the curative care services and dispensary services, they have often been in a position to "seek rent," that is, payment of some kind, whether legal, illegal, or quasi-legal. Bribery, for instance, is illegal. Quasi-legal kinds of payment include kickbacks and commissions in addition to unnecessary prescriptions or unreasonable and excessively expensive choices of drugs (Wu 2002).

Through franchise, for instance, the hospital unit tried to generate additional revenue by referring patients to its affiliated branch hospital or joint entity where regulations and accounting rules were less than rigorous. Given the considerable ambiguity of the ownership status of the providing unit, in many cases, the providing units created "little treasuries" by making use of "subsidiary collective units" for accounting purposes in order to shelter its illicit funds (Xie 1990). In some cases, franchise funding is clearly related to the issue of pricing and affordability. According to Yang Hongwei and Sun Naqiang, franchise provision is responsible for undesirable consequences such as artificially high prices of certain categories of services (Yang & Sun 2006: 71–80).

With its drug franchise, moreover, the providing unit is still a principal actor in the transactions of drugs in the sense that not only does it enjoy strong bargaining power as the buyer in relation to the drug industry, but it also assumes a dominant position as the seller in relation to the masses of patients. In Xu Bing's view of "rent-seeking" behavior, for example, the providing unit often gains the upper hand, as holder of a franchise, in drug transactions; and such advantage tends to be enhanced further because of the relative scarcity in the drug markets.[17]

Medical personnel and unanticipated policy outcomes

Medical doctors play a pivotal role in the operation and management of the franchise system in the sense that not only do they enjoy considerable discretion over diagnosis and treatment, the use of drug prescriptions and devices, but they also have a say over which option among several in a range of prices for technical-medical alternatives is to be chosen. That is to say, because of the medical personnel, the providing unit is able to make use of franchising in order to secure, or even maximize, revenue to maintain budgetary balance and to avoid sinking into a deficit. Several theoretical formulations highlight the strengths of medical personnel in playing their role in curative care with financial implications in the midst of commercialization: the equity theory on compensation, the principal-agent relationship, information asymmetry, the theory of uncertainty and limited control, and the limitation of performance appraisals.

First, some policy analysts and policymakers trace the root of undesirable policy outcomes to the compensation policy in the health care sector. Almost immediately after 1978, many ranking officials and policy analysts addressed the issue of poor pay among medical personnel, doctors and nurses alike. Efforts to improve the compensation of medical personnel were deemed jus-tifiable because they had been underpaid for decades since the 1960s and for a long period during the reform era (Cai 1993: 7–9).

According to equity theory, organizational members (e.g., medical personnel) are likely to object when they perceive that they are not compensated equally in comparison with those who work at comparable jobs within or outside the same work unit (Mowday 1996; Gortner, Mahler, & Nicholson 1997: 285–6). This dissonance tends to produce a number of behavioral responses: job dis-satisfaction, withdrawals and slowdowns, exit seeking, and a search for reme-dies and solutions (Gortner, Mahler, & Nicholson 1997: 285–6). Among these responses are revenue-maximizing behaviors manifested in kinds of financial irregularities and abuses involving medical personnel, in addition to the pro-viding unit's endeavors to find solutions through formal and legitimate channels of compensation reform that enjoyed some measure of support within the bureau in charge of medical care. In the later phase of health care reform, policymakers, officials and analysts finally reached a consensus according to which, by nature, the labor input of medical personnel carries a higher value than that of ordinary labor in the sense that they belong to the category of "labor with a high technical component" (Qing & Yu 2006: 28–9).

In fact, medical personnel's demand for better pay reflected an overall pressure for improvement in compensation, notably manifested in the con-troversy over "indiscriminate payment of bonus and wage" in the health care profession and other sectors of the CPE during the early phase of the eco-nomic reform. In connection with an effort to seek an improvement in pay for medical personnel, examples of financial irregularities and abuses are many, including soliciting bribery, unjustifiable extra charges for referrals, bribery for treatment and drug prescriptions, and cases of marketing and retailing non-medical commodities in the name of prescription drugs, just to name a few (Chen 1992a; Chen 1992b). Furthermore, it appears that the peer group interests of staff members carried weight in designing remuneration schemes, often resulting in unfair share of compensation allocated to a given office/ department (Zhang & Lo 1989; Xia 1990; Du 2006; Zheng 2006).

Second, the principal-agent theory represents a theoretical endeavor to bring the managerial experience of business firm to a generic analysis of power relations in the public organizations. According to the principal-agent theory, the user originally has a say over the issues of services (curative care and dispensary) and payment, but loses his/her power to ensure the selection of services to the best of his/her interest, owing to leakages of authority in the actual process of delegation of power to the medical personnel (Wang 2008:52–6; Zhou et al. 2003: 144–5). There is an ingredient of truth in the say theory that medical doctors enjoy double advantage in relations to their patients not only regarding asymmetric information, but also concerning asymmetric power.

However, principal-agent theory represents an analogy, failing to address explicitly the superiority of medical doctors in relations to users in an asymmetric power scenario. This study argues that the principal-agent analysis applies better to a corporate context; hence it would be overly stretched in the case of informal patient-doctor relations in the absence of required underpinnings of corporate laws. In fact, doctors wield discretional power that is endowed by the convention of medical profession, and authorized by hospital management, and legally recognized by public authorities. Doctors are never appointed formally as representatives of patients, and therefore the former assume no legal obligation to the latter in accordance with corporate laws similar to the principal-agent analogy.

Third, the uncertainty approach can better account for the medical doctor's position of advantage in the asymmetric information scenario involving not only users, but also external monitors such as government officials. The jobs of curative care and dispensary services entail considerable medical-technical uncertainties (namely, risks), requiring medical personnel to make a series of assessments, judgments, and decisions in the process of diagnosis, tests and examinations, treatments, and drug prescriptions. Zhou et al. apply this theoretical scheme regarding the professional's upper hand in the power game with laymen when the organizational members face uncertainty-bearing consequences (desirable or undesirable or both) (Zhou et al., 2003: 148–9).

To a certain extent, the uncertainty approach provides an alternative explanation to asymmetric information not only between medical personnel and patients in transactions in the medical care markets, but also between providing units and their external monitors in the bureaucratic context. In a formal sense, the external monitors do enjoy considerable advantage in relations to medical personnel in an asymmetric power situation. However, in practical terms, the former are more likely to tighten its control over the latter's violations and abuse *only* when the former are either able to exercise competent evaluation and/or to standardize the work process and skills involving uncertainty (Downs 1967: 49–81; Crozier 1971: 145–74; Mintzberg 1983: 163–87). Because of limited information and competence on the part of supervising authorities, medical personnel are able to enjoy considerable room of maneuver with respect to pricing for both curative care and dispensary services.

Neither can the clinical job be easily standardized, nor can it be readily incorporated into routine, leaving considerable room for discretion coupled with the possible abuses so entailed. Medical personnel not only enjoy using their discretion in making clinical decisions, they also dictate choices within a full range of price options from low end to high end (also see Chapter 9). It is difficult to monitor and control doctors who are motivated to choose more expensive options for material gain in the process of diagnosis and treatments (Zheng 2006). Furthermore, as Cao Beiwen suggests, it is by no means easy to employ quantitative measures to gauge contribution by medical personnel to medical care services, even though the overall results of medical services might be measurable (Cai 1993). Similarly, James Q. Wilson treats the hospital unit as a "craft organization" where its members' activities are difficult to observe but outcomes might be relatively easy to monitor (Wilson 1989: 165–8).

Fourth, some Chinese economists suggest that medical personnel are able to circumvent controls imposed from above because they enjoy a relative advantage in terms of "asymmetric information" in their interactions/transactions with patients, insurers, and/or even administrative superiors (Hu 2001: 49–59; Wu 2002: 5; Zhou et al. 2003: 144–5; Ma 2006). From the perspective of microeconomics in China's medical care sector, Professor Hu Suyun cites principal-agent theory to illustrate how asymmetric information accounts for medical staff attempting either to induce demands for or to recommend more expensive options of care and dispensary services, or both, for patients. It is argued that, by the same token, medical personnel enjoy a considerable advantage in the medical care service market because of asymmetric information (Hu 2001: 45–51). And such advantage is again reinforced by not only "technical monopoly" but also "administrative monopoly" created under specific contexts in the Chinese medical profession during the reform, e.g., by restricting market entry for new providers and/or through selection and designation of public hospitals and pharmacies (Wang 2008: 47–9). In relations with insurers, moreover, medical personnel and patients may collaborate with each other in choosing certain curative interventions and drug prescriptions in order to avoid price control, as just noted (Zhou, Qu & Li 2003: 144–6).

It is noteworthy that the original formulation of "asymmetric information" refers to two sides of a transaction in the sense that either the buyer or seller has much more information than his/her counterpart (Chapter 1). As it is borrowed from the business circle, the formulation, without taking into further theoretical considerations, has been over-stretched to analysis of authority relations between the superior and subordinates, analogy of principal-agent relations, and the relationship between external monitors over the supervised units in case of regulatory control.

Fifth, the theory of performance appraisal highlights the diminishing effectiveness of such appraisals in the area of less quantifiable and less measurable policy objectives. During the early phase of health care reform, the use of performance appraisals contributed to a remarkable success in revenue-generating together with the introduction of URS. Due to ESM for the first decade of the reform, budgetary reforms, including URS, were largely revenue-centered, and therefore performance appraisals were basically based on measurable financial indicators (or "hard indicators") as noted previously (Chapter 7). By the late 1980s, some policymakers and analysts suggested that the medical care sector differed from the industrial and agricultural sectors where some forms of URS had been successfully implemented. Thus, revenue targets were not to be taken as the sole measurement of success for medical care services. As distortions became apparent in URS, policymakers felt strongly that public hospitals should return to the ideals of the medical profession. While consensus on URS among policymakers slowly eroded, there were attempts to move away from the revenue-centered mode of performance appraisal to a multiple-goal mode, e.g., the "comprehensive undertaking responsibility system" (CURS) as previously mentioned (Chapter 7).

According to Henri Mintzberg, performance appraisals tend to be effective in the functional realm where policy purposes are definable, quantifiable, and measurable in theoretical terms (Mintzberg 1983: 73–8). As illustrated in the case of CURS, it is more difficult to define, measure, and evaluate public policy objectives, often enlarging the gap between goals and designs on the one hand and performance and results on the other hand. Owing to the limited measurability of public policy goals, thus, CURS is likely to produce unintended policy results, in turn leading to a fresh round of search for new indicators and another cycle of bureaucratic control. The restructuring of URS to CURS appears to confirm V. F. Ridgway's empirical study on the tendency for performance indicators to proliferate while these same indicators lose their effectiveness as they involve less measurable policy goals in a planned economy such as the former USSR (Ridgeway 1956).

In the foregoing analysis, the study has dealt the issue of control over medical personnel's abuses such as over-provision and over-prescription in case of public hospitals in China. Among five alternative formulations dealing with discrepancy between policy goals and outcomes, one focuses on motivation of organizational members, and the other four formulations are based on the theoretical assumption that cost of information is larger than zero in the administrative-managerial process. It appears that according to the fourth theoretical formulations, medical doctors had upper hand in dictating the price and thus the compensation of their services because of asymmetric information in transactions with the patients. Furthermore, it is evident that supervising bureaus, in spite of their dominant position in terms of asymmetric power, would often find less than effective in applying commonly used managerial tools to impose control over medical personnel, coupled with public hospitals. As just noted, neither their medical behavior could be fully standardized and routinized in light of the third theoretical alternative concerning uncertainty, nor could it be subject to performance appraisal according to the fifth alternative. To put it simply, they could be better characterized as free-range chicken than dogs as the metaphor goes (Chapter 1.) In fact, the similar phenomenon repeats in policy episode of drug franchise to be discussed in next two chapters.

Concluding remarks

China has witnessed the transformation of its mainly government-subsidized medical care system to an increasingly franchise-funded one. This transformation was accompanied by a major change in financial strategy in terms of increasing reliance on revenue generated from patients themselves through charges and fees, and a dwindling share of state financial subsidies. Also providing units start to operate as financial entities driven by revenue concerns. As for patients and the general public, they feel the pinch in paying charges and fees, and suffer in long lines in crowded hospitals. As demonstrated in the foregoing analysis, neither providing units nor markets should be held solely responsible for high fees and long lines. Minister of Health Gao Qiang takes exception to the allegation that providing units and medical personnel should shoulder the blame for the "difficulty and expense of seeking cure" (Gao 2007: 54). As it turns out, government failures to provide affordable and accessible care are intertwined with market failures, and they are not actually separable from each other.

Notes

1 Although the providing unit enjoyed franchise for all kinds of services, there was no need to charge the patient for services provided due to appropriation in full amount requested and a highly restrictive price policy as shown in three major price cuts for curative care services in 1958, 1960, and 1972 (Dangdai Zhongguo Congshu Bianjibu 1988: 464–74; Zhou 2008 120–1).
2 In his report to the first National Health Care Conference of Bureau Chiefs on March 22, 1979, Minister of Health Care Qian explained the idea of "economic management" (Qian 1983). The Ministry of Health Care, Ministry of Finance, and State General Bureau of Labor put forth on April 28, 1979, the "Opinion Concerning the Task of the Pilot Program for Strengthening Hospital Management (hereafter, "1979 Opinion") (Weishengbu & Guojialaodongzhongju, 1979).
3 For instance, through part-time services and outside practices, appointments with specialists, upgraded wards, tests with expensive equipment, affiliated services (e.g., pharmaceutical processing), and auxiliary services (e.g., canteens, guest houses, laundry, etc.) (Peng, Cai, & Zhou 1992).
4 The title of the policy paper is "Decision Concerning the Acceleration of Tertiary Industry" (hereafter, "1992 Decision") (Zhonggongzhongyang 2002).
5 The full title of the policy paper reads as follows: "Report on Several Health Care Task Policy Problems" (hereafter, "1985 Report") (Weishengbu1985); the policy paper was subsequently endorsed by the State Council (often known as "Document Guofa No. 62 1986").

6 The full title of the "1988 Opinion" is "Opinion Concerning Problems in Expanding Medical and Health Care Services" (hereafter, "1988 Opinion") filed by the Ministry of Health Care, the Ministry of Finance, the Ministry of Personnel, the State Price Bureau, and the State Taxation Bureau on November 8, 1988; it was further endorsed and circulated by the State Council on January 15, 1989, (known as "Document Guofa No. 10, 1989") (Weishengbu et al. 1993b).

7 For illustration, though maybe somewhat extreme in light of the general pattern analyzed in Chapter 4, the result of a survey of 2,000 public hospitals above the county level indicated that, as of 1990, the breakdowns of medical care services covered by (1) the patients, (2) insurers, and (3) the government subsidies (through differentiated quota subsidies and special grants) were 86 percent, 10 percent, and 4 percent of the total revenue, respectively (Peng, Cai, & Zhou 1992: 38).

8 According to Feng Dan et al., the number of CTs in Fujian Province registered a rapid growth from 4 in 1990, 33 in 1993, 113 in 2004 to 137 in 2007; MRIs increased from 0 in 1990, 2 in 1993, 22 in 2004 to 37 in 2007 (Feng 2009: 9). As cited for Beijing for the period from 1990 to 2005 in a study by Mao Ayan and Lei Haichao, the number of CTs per one million residents grew from 0 in 1990, 7.29 in 1995, 9.48 in 2000 to 13.89 in 2005, exceeding the levels of both France and Canada as of 2004; the number of MRIs per one million residents increased from 0 in 1900, 1.59 in 1995, 3.16 in 2000 to 5.50 in 2005, already surpassing the numbers in UK, France and Canada as of 2004 (Mao & Lei 2009: 89–90).

9 The title of the policy paper reads as follows: "Provisional Measures for Deployment and Management of Use of Large Medical Equipment" (hereafter, 1995 Provisional Measures) (Zhu & Wang 2010: 33).

10 The title of the policy paper is "Measures for Installation, Management and Use of Large Medical Equipment" (hereafter, "2004 Measures") (Zhu & Wang, 2010: 33).

11 The title of the policy paper reads as follows: the Advisory Opinion concerning the Making and Adjustment of Prices of Examinations and Curative Care Services of Large Medical Devices (abbreviated as the 2005 Advisory Opinion hereafter) (Zhu & Wang, 2010: 33–4).

12 Fujian offers an illustration of "counter measures" by the providing units to cope with government policy to tighten control over the use of medical devices. After the implementation of a new charge schedule in October 2004, charges for an examination were calculated according to each portion of the body examined rather than each case. Moreover, the number of patients under examination increased considerably both before and after the price adjustment, i.e., the increase in CT examinations by 148.48 percent and that of MRI examinations by 183.75 percent. Overall, average charges for each patient increased by 34.83 percent in the case of a CT examination and decreased by 3.36 percent in the case of an MRI examination (Chen, Huang, & Guo 2010).

13 Policymakers advanced conceptualizations of these unintended and undesirable policy outcomes in order to facilitate monitoring and supervisory work. Such outcomes included the incorrect and "unreasonable" approach, "undesirable tendency," "revenue maximizing behavior" (liyi zueidahua xingwei), "short-sighted behavior" (duanqi xinwei), problems of "work style" (zuofeng), and the "work ethic of medical care services" (yifeng yide), etc. (Weishengbu et al. 1982: Weishengbu 1983; Chen 1992b).

14 According to Charles Lindblom, there exist byproducts or epiphenomena in both Model I (i.e., the command-coordinated system) and Model II (i.e., the market-coordinated system) (Lindblom, 1977: 257–8).

15 "Franchise" here refers to the right of entry into the market, but does not necessarily mean "monopoly" or exclusive control over market entry. Conceptually speaking, some authors have tended to equate franchise with monopoly (Liu & Yuan 2001; Wang 2008; Zhao & Yue 2010; Yan & Chen 2011).

16 In Wu's view, this also occurred at the level of government (e.g., ministerial, provincial, and municipal authorities) that had the power of licensing of production, wholesale, and retail, as well as approval of new drugs (Wu 2002).

17 Xu further explains that rent is generated because of relative scarcity, resulting from rapidly expanding medical care demand, part of which is in turn amplified by public insurance programs (e.g., PFMC and LIMC). To alleviate such scarcity, doctors who work with hospitals could assume the position of "rent collector" by dictating the volume of supply to satisfy demand. In Xu's view, moreover, rent-seeking activities in drug markets can hardly be restrained and balanced out by upward price adjustments, an option which is ruled out because of the government's rigid price control (Xu 1988: 12).

References

Bendix, R. 1962. *Max Weber: An Intellectual Portrait*. Garden City, NY: Anchor Books.

Cai, R. 1993. Neilun yiliao fuwu yu shichang jingji (Preliminary discussion on medical care services and market economy). *Zhongguo weishengjie(China's Health Circle)*, 2: 7–9.

Chang, P. & Liang, Z. 1993. Shenhua weisheng gaigge jidian sikao (Considerations of further reform in health care). *Zhongguo weisheng jingji(China's Health Care Economics)*, 7: 36–37.

Chen, M. 1992a. Chen Mingzhang buchang zai 1990 nian quanquo weisheng tingjuchang huiyi shang de baogao (The report of Minister Chen Mingzhang at the 1990 national conference of chiefs of bureau/office of health care). In R. Peng, R. Cai, & C. Zhou (Eds.), *Zhonggou gaige quanshu (Encyclopedia of China's Reform)*. Dalian: Dalian chubanshe.

Chen, M. 1992b. Chen Mingzhang buchang zai quanquo weisheng tingjuchang huiyi shang de zongjie jianghua (Minister Chen Mingzhang's concluding speech at the national conference of chiefs of bureaus/offices of health care). In R. Peng, R. Cai, & C. Zhou (Eds.), *Zhongguo gaige quanshu (Encyclopedia of China's Reform)*, 184–190. Dalian: Dalian chubanshe.

Chen, M. 1992c. Chen Mingzhang tongzhi zai yijiu bawu nian quanguo weisheng tingjuchang huiyi shang de zongjie jianghua (Comrade Chen Mingzhang's concluding speech at the 1985 national conference of chiefs of bureaus/offices of health care). In R. Peng, R. Cai, & C. Zhou (Eds.), *Zhongguo gaige quanshu (Encyclopedia of China's Reform)*, 135–138. Dalian: Dalian chubanshe.

Chen, Y., Huang, Y., & Guo, X. 2010. Fujiansheng daxing yiyong shebei (CT, MRI) jiage tiaozheng dui yiliao jiguo shouru de yingxiang (The impact of price adjustment of large scale equipments CI, MRI on the revenue of medical care institutes in Fujian province). *Zhongguo weisheng jingji(China's Health Care Economics)*, 29(6): 47–48.

Crozier, M. 1971. *The Bureaucratic Phenomenon* (5th impression). Chicago: University of Chicago Press.

Cui, Y. 1992. Cui Yueli tongchi zai yijiu balu nian quanguo weisheng tingjuchang huiyi shang de jianghua (Comrade Cui Yueli's speech at the 1986 national conference of chiefs of bureaus/offices of health care). In R. Peng, R. Cai, & C. Zhou (Eds.), *Zhongguo gaige quanshu, yiliao weisheng tizhi gaige juan (Encyclopedia of China's Reform)*, 145–151. Dalian: Dalian chubanshe.

Dangdai Zhongguo Congshu Bianjibu. 1988. *Dangdai zhongguo de yiyao shiye* (The Pharmacy Enterprises of Contemporary China). Beijing: Zhongguo shehui kexue chubanshe.

Downs, A. 1967. *Inside Bureaucracy.* Boston: Little, Brown and Company.

Du, L. 2006a. Woguo weisheng gaige zhengce de jingjixue fenxi (An economic analysis of health care reform policy in China). *Zhongguo weisheng jingji(China's Health Care Economics)*, 2: 5–9.

Du, L. 2006b. *Zhongguo weisheng yiliao weisheng fazan baoguo, No. 2* (The Report of the Development of Medical and Health Care in China, No. 2). Beijing: Shehui kexue wenxian chubanshe.

Du, L. 2007. Hongguan jingji he weisheng fazhan de liangxing xunhuan ho exing xunhuan—ershihnian weisheng zhengce yanjiu huigu (Positive and vicious cycles of macro economy and health care development). In L. Du, W. Zhang, & Zhongguo Weisheng Chanye Zazhishe (Ed.), *Zhongguo wesheng yiliao fazhan baogao, No. 3 (The Report of the Development of Health and Medical Care in China, No. 3)*, 25–40. Beijing: Shehui kexue wenxian chubanshe.

Duckett, J. 2013. *The Chinese State's Retreat from Heath.* Abingdon and New York: Routledege.

Duan, M., & Huang, X. 2011. Guochang he jingkou daxiang yiyong shebei caigou jiage bijiao yanjiu (A comparative study of procurement prices of domestic and imported brands of large medical care equipment). *Zhongguo weisheng jingji (China's Health Care Economics)*, 30(2): 67–69.

Feng, D. 2009. Daxing yiyong shebei jiancha yiliao jiage tiaozheng de yingxian ji duice (The impacts and policies of price adjustments for the examinations by large medical equipment). *Weisheng jingji yanjiu(Research on Health Care Economics)*, 12: 9–10.

Fu, X. 1989. Danqian weisheng gaige de jige xintedian (Several new characteristics of current health care reform). *Zhongguo weisheng jingji(China's Health Care Economics)*, 6: 15–17.

Gao, Q. 2007. Dangqian kaizhan weisheng jiufeng gongzuo, jiejue kanbingnan kanbinggui wenti mianlin de xingshi he jiben silu (The current task of rectification in health care, the situation and basic consideration to solve the problems of difficulty to see doctors and expensiveness to see doctors). In Zhongguo Weisheng Nianjian Bianji Weiyuanhui *(Ed.)*, *Zhongguo weisheng nianjian 2007 (China's Yearbook of Health Care 2007)*, 61–69. Beijing: Renmin weisheng chubanshe.

Gao, Q. 2006. Fazhan yiliao weisheng shiye, weigoujian shehui zhuyi hexie shehui zuogongxian (Develop further the enterprises of medical and health care, contribute to building a harmonious socialist society). In Zhongguo weisheng nianjian bianji weiyuanhui *(Ed.)*, *Zhongguo weisheng nianjian 2006 (China's Yearbook of Health Care 2006)*, 48–56. Beijing: Renmin weisheng chubanshe.

Gao, Q. 2007. Zai 2006 nian jixushenru kaizhan 'yibienren wei zhongxin, yitigao fuwu zhilian wei zhuti" yiyuan guanlinian gongzuo huiyi shan de jianghua (Speech at the work conference of continuing and launching 'the theme of patient-centered and quality service' in the year of hospital management in *2006*). In Zhongguo weisheng nianjian bianji weiyuanhui *(Ed.)*, *Zhongguo weisheng nianjian 2007 (The 2007 Yearbook of China's Health Care)*, 52–57. Beijing: Renmin weisheng chubanshe.

Gortner, H. F., Mahler, J., & Nicholson, J. B. 1997. *Organization Theory: A Public Perspective* (2nd ed.). New York: Harcourt Brace.

Gu, X. 2008. *Zouxiang quanmin yibao: Zhongguo xingyigai de zhanlue yu zhanshu (Toward Comprehensive Medical Insurance: Strategy and Tactic of China's New Medical Care Reform)*. Beijing: Zhongguo laodong chubanshe.

Gu, X. 2010. *Quanmin yibao de xintansuo (The New Exploration of National Health Insurance)*. Beijing: Shehui kexue wenxian chubanshe.

Guan, Z., Chui, B., & Dong, C. 2007. Chengzhen zhigong jiben yiliao baoxian zhidu de fazhan (The developlement of basic medical care insurance system of staff and workers in cities and towns). In J. Chen & Y. Wang (*Eds.*), *Zhongguo shehui baozhang zhidu fazhan baogao, 2007 (The 2007 Report of the Development of China's Social Insurance System)*, 37–63. Beijing: Shehui kexue wenxian chubanshe.

Guowuyuan. 1993. Guowuyuan pizhuan guojiajiaowei de bumen guanyu shenhua gaige guli jiaoyu keyan weisheng danwei zengjia shehui funwu yijian de tongzhi (The circular of the state council on the opinion of the state education commission and other units regarding the further reform of and encouragement to the increase of social services of educational, scientific research and health care units). In Weishengbu zhengce faguisi (*Ed.*), *Zhonghua renmin gongheguo weisheng fagui huibian, 1989–1991 (The Collection of Laws and Regulations of the Ministry of Health of the PRC, 1989–1991)*, 1–2. Beijing: Falu chubanshe.

Henderson, A. M., & Parsons, T. 1967. *Max Weber: The Theory of Social and Economic Organization*. New York and London: The Free Press.

Hu, S. 2007. Jianli guojia jiben yaobing zhidu de zhengce (To establish the national policy of basic medicine system). In L. Du, W. Zhang, & Zhongguo Weisheng Canye Zachishe (*Ed.*), *Zhonguo yiliao weisheng fazhan baogao, No. 3 (The Report on the Development of Medical and Health Care in China, No. 3)*, 340–352. Beijing: Shehui kexue wenxian chubanshe.

Hu, S. 2001. *Yiliao baoxian he fuwu zhidu (Medical Care Insurance and System of Services)*. Chengdu: Sichuan renmin chubanshe.

Lee, P. N. 1987. *Industrial Management and Economic Reform in China, 1949–1984*. Hong Kong, Oxford and New York: Oxford University Press.

Liang, Jiguang & Huang, Bisheng. 1990. Yiliao weisheng danwei de duanqi xingwei ji duce yanjiu (A study on shortsighted behavior of medical and health care units as well as counter-measures). *Zhongguo weisheng jingji(China's Health Care Economics)*, 2: 33–36.

Lindblom, C. E. 1977. *Politics and Markets, the World's Political-economic Systems*. New York: Basic Books.

Liu, J. 2012. *Zhongguo yigai xiangguan zhengce yanji* (Study on Policies related to China's Medical Care Reform). Beijing: Jingji kexue chubanshe.

Lu, F., & Yang, B. 2005. Yiliao jiage zhengce yu hangye zunru (The policy of pricing and entry to trade in health care). *Shehui baozhang zhidu(Social Security System)*, 1: 32–35.

Luo, Y. 1985. Weisheng shiye de chulu zaiyu gaige (Reform is the only way out for health care enterprises). *Jiankong bao(Health Bulletin)*, 1: 8.

Luo, Y. 1990. Woguo weisheng gaige ruogan tezheng de yanjiu yu shkao (Study and thoughts on some salient characteristics of health care reform in China). *Zhongguo weisheng jingji(China's Health Care Economics)*, 3: 4–8.

Ma, A. 2006. Weisheng gaige guilu lun (Theory on the law of health care reform). *Zhongguo weisheng jingji(China's Health Care Economics)*, 9: 13.

Ma, L. & Wu, Q. 2006. Gongli yiyuan gaige moshi de huigu yu fansi (Retrospect and reflection on the reform model of public hopitals). *Zhongguo weisheng jingji (China's Health Care Economics)*, 2:16–19.

Ma, W. 2006. Yiliao gaige de hexin wenti he wailai chulu (The core problems of medical care reforms and solutions for the future). *Zhongguo weisheng jingji (China's Health Care Economics)*, 9: 52–59.

Mao, A., & Lei, H. 2009. Beijingshi yiliao fuwu shichang yiliao zhuangbei jingsai xianxiang yanzheng (The phenomenon of arm race of medical care equipment as attested in the market of medical care services in Beijing municipality). *Zhongguo weisheng jingji (China's Health Care Economics)*, 28(11): 88–90.

Mintzberg, H. 1983. *Structure of Fives: Designing Effective Organizations*. London and Englewood Cliffs, NJ: Prentice-Hall.

Mowday, R. T. 1996. Equity Theory Predictions of Behavior in Organization. In J. S. Ott (*Ed.*), *Classic Readings in Organizational Behavior* (2nd ed.), 94–102. New York: Harcourt Brace.

Naughton, B. 1996. *Growing out of the Plan*. Cambrige: Cambridge University Press.

Peng, R., Cai, R., & Zhou, C. (Ed.). 1992. *Zhongguo gaige quanshu (Encyclopedia of China's Reform)*. Dalian: Dalian chubanshe.

Qian, X. 1983. Ba weisheng bumen gongzuo zhuozhongdian zhuanyidao yiyao weisheng xiandaihua jianshe shanglai (Shift the central gravity of the task of health care sector to the modernization of medical and health care). In Zhongguo Weisheng Nianjian Bianji Weiyuanhui (Ed.), *Zhongguo weisheng nianjian 1983 (China's Yarbook on Health Care, 1983)*, 22–26. Beijing: Zhongguo weisheng chubanshe.

Qing, G., & Yu, R. 2006. Yiyao weisheng lingyu shangye huilou wenti touxi (Analysis on bribery in the arena of medical care and medicine). *Zhongguo weisheng jingji (China's Health Care Economics)*, 11: 28–29.

Ridgway, V. F. 1956. Dysfunctional consequences of performance measurements. *Administrative Science Quarterly*, 1(2): 240–247.

Song, W. 1990. Jiaqiang hongguan tiaokong wanshang yiyuan chengbaozhi (Strengthen macro manaement and perfert hospital chengbao system). *Zhongguo weisheng jingji(China's Health Care Economics)*, 3: 24–27.

Sun, H. & Yu, R. 2010. Yiyao yangyi he yixie yangyi yingxian yiji yangyi zhuanbien (Transform from 'finance medical care through pharmacy' and 'finance medical care through equipment' to finance medical care through skill). *Zhongguo weisheng jingj (China's Health Care Economics)*, 29(3): 9–10.

Sun, N. & Du, L. 2006. Gongli yiyuan yunxin jizhi gaige (The reform of operating mechanisms of public hospitals). In L. Du (*Ed.*), *Zhongguo yiliao weisheng fazhan baogao No.2 (The Report of Development of Medical and Health Care in China, No. 2)*, 119–179. Beijing: Shehui kexue wenxian chubanshe.

Sun, N. & Du, L. 2006. Jiankang yu yiyao baojiian de fazhan (The development of health and drug services). In Du Lexun et al. (Ed.), *Zhongguo yiliao weisheng fazhan baogao, No. 2* (The Report of Development of Medical and Health Care in China, no 2), 145–179. Beijing: Shehui kexue wenxian chubanshe.

Wang, B. 2008. *Zhengfu yiliao guamzhi moshi ghonggou yanjiu (Research on the Restructuring of Mode of Governmental Control)*. Beijing: Renmin chubanshe.

Wang, Y. 2008. *Zhongguo weisheng gaige yu fazhan shizheng yanjiu (An Empirical Research on the Reform and Development of Health Care)*. Beijing: Zhonguo lao-dong shehui baozhang chubanshe.

Wang, Y. & Wang, W. 2007. Kuaisu shangzhang de yiliao feiyong yu kanbingnan, kanbinggui wenti (The issue of the rapid increase of medical care expences and the difficulty to seek cure and expensiveness to seek cure). In J. Chen, & Y. Wang (*Eds.*), *Zhongguo shehui baozhang fazhan baogao 2007 (The 2007 Report of the*

Development of China's Social Insurance), 18–36. Beijing: Shehui kexue wenxian chubanshe.

Weber, M. 1987. Bureaucracy. In J. M. Shafritz & A. C. Hyde (*Eds.*), *Classics of Public Administration* (2nd. ed.), 50–55. Chicago: The Dorsey Press.

Weishengbu. 1983. Weishengbu guanyu zhuyi zhizhi yiliao jigou lankai da chufeng buliang qingxiang de tongzhi (The circular of the Ministry of Health Care concerning the prohibition of the undesirable tendency of excessive drug prescriptions by medical care institutes). *Guowuyuan gongbao(Bulletin of the State Council)*, 22: 798–799.

Weishengbu. 1985. Guanyu weisheng gongzuo gaige ruogan zhengce wenti baogao (The report concerning several policy problems in the reform of health care work). In R. Peng, R. Cai, & C. Zhou (Eds.), *Zhongguo gaige quanshu (Encyclopedia of China's Reform)*, 139–142. Dalian: Dalian chubanshe.

Weishengbu. 1988. Weishengbu guanyu weisheng gongzuo gaige ruogan zhengce wenti de baogao (The report of the Ministry of Health concerning several policy problems in the reform of health care tasks). In Weishengbu Bangongting (*Ed.*), *Zhonghua renmin gongheguo weisheng fagui huibian, 1984–1885 (The Collection of Laws and Regulations of Health Care of the PRC, 1984–1985)*, 1–6. Beijing: Falu chubanshe, Xinhua shudian.

Weishengbu, PRC. 1990. Yufang baojian sihixing youshang fuwu de huigu yu sikao (A review and observations on the implementation of paid services in preventive care). *Zhongguo weisheng jingji(China's Health Care Economics)*, 6: 26–28.

Weishengbu, PRC. 1992a. Guanyu weisheng gongzuo gaige ruogan zhengce wenti baogao (The report concerning the policy problems of reform of health tasks). In R. Peng, R. Cai, & C. Zhou (Eds.), *Zhongguo gaige quanshu (Encyclopedia of China's Reform)*, 139–142. Dalian: Dalian chubanshe.

Weishengbu, PRC. 1992b. Qiwu shiqi weisheng gaige tiyao (Outline for health care reform of the seventh five year plan period). In R. Peng, R. Cai, & C. Zhou (Eds.), *Zhongguo gaige quanshu (Encyclopedia of China's Reform)*, 157–161. Dalian: Dalian chubanshe.

Weishengbu *et al.*1982. Weishengbu, caizhengbu guojialaodongzongju guanyu yiyuan jingji guanli shidian gongzuo de buchong tongzi (The supplementary general circular of the Ministry of Health, Ministry of Finance and State General Bureau of Labor concerning the pilot task of hospital economic management). In Weishengbu Bangongting (PRC) (*Ed.*), *Zhonghua renmin gongheguo weisheng fagui huibian (The Collection of Laws and Regulations of Health Care of the PRC)*, 627–629. Beijing: Falu chubanshe, Xinhua shudian.

Weishengbu *et al.*1993a. Guanyu kuoda yiliao weisheng fuwu yaoguan wenti de yijian (The opinion of problems regarding the expansion of medical and health care services). In Weishengbu Zhengce Faguisi (*Ed.*), *Zhonghua renmin gonghegui weisheng fagui huibian (The Collection of Laws and Regulations of the Ministry of Health of the PRC)*, 10–13. Beijing: Falu chubanshe.

Weishengbu *et al.*1993b. Guanyu kuoda yiliao weisheng fuwu yaoguan wenti de yijian (The opinion concerning the related problems of expansion of medical and health care services). In Weishengbu Zhengce Faguisi (*Ed.*), *Zhonghua renmin gongheguo weisheng fagui huibian, 1989–1991 (The Collection of Laws and Regulations of Heath Care of the PRC, 1989–1991)*, 10–12. Beijing: Falu chubanshe.

Weishengbu & Guojialaodongzhongchu. 1979. Guanyu jiaqiang yiyuan jingji guanli shihdian gongtso di yijian (Opinion concerning the strengthening of pilot work of hosptial economic management). *Laodong zhengce fagui huibian (Collection of Policies and Laws of Labor)*. Beijing: Falu chubanshe.

Wilson, J. Q. 1989. *Bureaucracy: What Government Agencies Do and Why They Do It*. New York: Basic Books.

Wu, R. 2002. Yi woguo weisheng fuwu shichang zhengfu quanzhi (On regulating the market of health care services by the government in China). *Zhongguo weisheng jingji(China's Health Care Economics)*, 8: 5–6.

Xia, J. 1990. Weisheng gaige de nanti yu duice (The difficulties and proposals of health care reform). *Zhongguo weisheng jingji(China's Health Care Economics)*, 1: 33–35.

Xie, H. 1990. Dangqian caiwu xianzhuang yu zhili fangfa (The current state of hospital finance and managerial measures). *Zhongguo weisheng jingji(China's Health Care Economics)*, 2: 12–14.

Yang, H., & Sun, N. 2006. Weisheng gaige yu fazhan de pingjia yu jianyan (The evaluation and examination of health care reform and development). In L. Du (*Ed.*), *Zhongguo yiliao weisheng fazhan baogao no. 2 (The Report of Development of Medical and Health Care in China no. 2)*, 47–85. Beijing: Shehui kexue wenxian chubanshe.

Zeng, C. 2006. Daxing yiyong shebei 'baoben bu yinli' qianjin (The prospect of 'making no profit but retaining the principal' in the case of large medical equipment). *Zhongguo weisheng(China's Health Care)*, 8: 40–42.

Zhang, J., & Lo, J. 1989. Dachufang wenti de diaocha yu fenxi (The investigation and analysis of the problem of unneccessary prescriptions). *Zhongguo weisheng jingji (China's Health Care Economics)*, 6: 20–21.

Zhang, S. 1990. Yiyuan chengbaozhi ying buduan wanshang (Continuously perfect the hospital chengbao system). *Zhongguo weisheng jingji(China's Health Care Economics)*, 4: 15–16.

Zhang, Y. 1990. Lun yiliao fuwu shichang de longduanxing (On the monopoly characteristics of medical care markets). *Zhongguo weisheng jingji(China's Health Care Economics)*, 11: 11–13.

Zheng, D. 2006. Shichang jizhi he zhengfu tiaojie zai weisheng fuwu lingyu de gongneng yu jiaose dingwei (Defining the role and functions of market mechanisms and governmental adjustment in the realm of health care services). *Zhongguo weisheng jingji(China's Health Care Economics)*, 1:18–21.

Zhonggongzhongyang. 2002. Guanyu jiakuai fazhan disan chanye de juedin (The decision concerning the acceleration of development of the tertiary industry). In Laodong he Shehui Baozhang Bu, Zhonggong Zhongyang Wenxian Yanjiusi (*Ed.*), *Xinshiqi laodong he shehui baozhang zhongyao wenxian xuanbian (Selection of Important Documents of Labor and Insurance of the New Era)*, 109–115. Beijing: Zhongguo laodong shehui baozhang chubanshe, Zhonggong wenxian chubanshe.

Zhou, L., Qu, Q. & Li, G. 2003. *Jujiao weisheng gaige (The focus of health care reform)*. Beijing: Zhonggui shehui kexue chubanshe.

Zhou, X. 2008. *Zhongguo yiliao jiage de zhengfu guanzhi yanjiu (A study on the Government Control of Medical Care Pricing in China)*. Beijing: Zhongguo shehui kexue chubanshe.

Zhu, P., & Wang, Q. 2010. Daxing yiyong shebei peizhi yu guanli yanjiu jinzhan (The progress of research on the deployment and management of large medical equipment. *Zhongguo weisheng jingji (China's Health Care Economics)*, 29(4): 33–36.

9 Drug franchising and financial management

Along with franchises in other types of curative care services, franchise in dispensary services represents another market-oriented approach that sovereign planners have adopted in order to finance affordable care during the economic reform. It remained in embryonic form during the pre-reform period (Dangdai Zhongguo Congshu Bianjibu 1988: 471–6). However, since the beginning of economic reform, it has grown into a full-fledged construct, occupying a prominent place in the financial management of medical care provision throughout all public providing units across China. And it represents one of the largest revenue sources at the providing unit level during the era of economic reform. Some analysts indicate, for example, that in 2005 the sales of medicine through all kinds of providing units in various echelons across all jurisdictions in China were equal to an estimated sum of 240,000 million RMB out of a total volume of sales of 300,000 million RMB, that is, approximately 80 percent of the total expenditure for drugs by public hospitals in China in the 2000s (Yu 2008:15).

Within the circle of policymakers and analysts, there have been pros and cons with reference to revenue sources from drug franchising at the providing unit level. Those who argue against it often point not only to its abuses and excesses but also to adverse results in undermining low-priced, affordable care policy. And some of them specifically hold the wholesale-and-retail differentials (or W/R differentials) scheme in drug sales responsible for abuses and distortions in financial management at the providing unit level. The supporters of the existing policy of drug revenue often highlight its pivotal role in funding public hospital medical care services and in cross-subsidizing various essential links that are priced artificially low within the delivery of medical care services in order to maintain affordable care.

The role of revenue from drugs is essential to maintain budgetary balance at the providing unit level. It is argued in this chapter that any policy alternative that undermines the stability of revenue flow from drugs is not viable unless a new revenue source can be found to substitute for drug revenue. The study here deals with the following issues, one by one: the tension between drug franchising and price control, cost-shifting at the providing unit level, price control, rent-seeking behaviors, and experiments in the restructuring and abolition of W/R differentials.

Drug franchising versus price control

With regard to the tension between drug franchising and price control, the providing unit is financially driven to seek higher charges to maintain a reasonable revenue flow leading to budgetary balance through a franchise funding mode on the one hand; and on the other hand, the government is committed to an affordable care policy, meaning to tighten up price control over curative care in general and dispensary services in particular. That is to say, in the case of drugs, the actual amount of revenue from a franchise source hinges upon price control, meaning that the more or less tight the price control, the less or more the revenue to the hospital unit. As noted by former Minister of Health Gao, providing units often exhibited their concern about revenue and budgetary deficits when they faced the pressure of price control for drug sales (Gao 2007: 64).

As prices of prescription drugs, often considered "exorbitant" to use a subjective, if not emotionally charged, term, have developed into a focal point of complaints from patients, they have also increasingly become a serious concern of policymakers at all levels. Policy analyst Wang offers his diagnosis of the problem: the "artificially" high prices of drugs are inseparable from drug franchises, which fortify a zone of discretion for hospitals and doctors in the use and procurement of medicine for curative care services (Wang 2008: 47–9). As a result, it is difficult to monitor whether the revenue-maximizing orientation of doctors and hospitals prevails over their concern for safety, quality, effective and affordable dispensary services for their patients. With such discretion medical personnel would put at risk their own morality by giving priority to revenue over quality, effective and safe curative care for patients.

Theoretically speaking, the pharmacist is supposed to be in charge of dispensary services. How does one explain the ascendancy of the doctor in the matter of prescription drugs? In the Chinese context, the hand of the doctor was strengthened owing to the absorption of dispensary services by curative care services through the so-called "collaborative practice between medical care and pharmacy" (yiyao heye) (Zhou 2008: 113–4; 120–1). Moreover, the role of the pharmacist was further eroded with the incorporation of dispensary services into hospital management (Si, He & Song, 1999; Zhou, Qu & Li 2003:118–35; Zhang, 2009a; Zhang, 2009b; Li 2011).

Some policy analysts argue that as the pharmacist plays the role of counterweight to the doctor in financial management, any move by hospital management to undercut the former's professional and accounting autonomy tends to bring about excessive and often uncontrollable spending on drugs (Si et al. 1999; Zhang 2009a; Zhou et al. 2003). Li Daping, a health care economist, argues, furthermore, that in actual practice in China, not only does the doctor's expanding power over drug prescriptions often weaken the pharmacist's professional autonomy (e.g., in terms of dispensing, checks and audits, advice and consultations, collection of information, evaluation and monitoring of unexpected side-effects), but also undermines the latter's role as guardian of the principle of "value for money," that is, value in terms of quality, effectiveness, safety and affordability in dispensary services (Li 2011). According to Li, moreover, a pharmacist's accounting integrity was likely to be compromised under the total control of hospital management, as the drug franchise was often employed as a revenue-maximizing tool. Li emphasizes that hospitals' exclusive control over the financial side of pharmacy tended to forfeit market alternatives, limit competition, and thus cause the tendency of an uncontrolled upward increase of prices and costs (Li 2011).

In fact, drug franchising does produce policy consequences, the evaluation of which depends on which policy stand is chosen to examine it. While drug franchising is taken as undesirable with reference to the tendency to push prices of prescription drugs upward and thus less affordable from the advocates of the patient's welfare, it is considered desirable from the perspective of financial management in terms of cost-shifting from artificially low-priced items of medical care services to higher ones, a topic to be examined next.

Drug franchising and cost-shifting

As just mentioned, revenue from drug franchising is the largest revenue source at the providing unit level, and it is often used for cost-shifting from curative care services. Cost-shifting is also taken as a form of financial cross-subsidizing that is termed colloquially in the policy circle in China as the policy design of "fostering medical care through [revenue of] drugs sales" (yiyao yangyi) (Chen, 2008: 8; Wang 2008: 47–51; Zhang, 2009a: 19).

In financial and accounting terms, cost-shifting from curative care services (i.e. diagnosis and treatment) to drugs may be analyzed in two ways. First, as a rule, dispensary services earn an exceedingly large portion of total revenue relative to curative care, devices, and other items for the hospital units in question (Peng, Cai, & Zhou 1992: 36–40). As cited by Chen and Wang, revenue from drugs consisted of more than 60 percent of the total revenue of the providing units on average; and in most small and medium hospitals in the early 2000s, it could even have reached 70 percent (Chen & Wang 2007: 27). Second, it was not unusual for all parties concerned to argue that dispensary services commanded "artificially" higher value in contrast to curative care services whose real value was underestimated for a considerable period of time. Because of the low-price policy, which brought about several major reductions of drugs prices from the 1950s to 1980, the hospital unit received revenue for curative care services which was much less than their real value, and the pay to medical care personnel grew only slowly and lagged behind that of employees from other sectors, both preceding and succeeding the economic reform as previously mentioned (Peng, Cai, & Zhou 1992: 23).

From the viewpoint of the health care circle, some flexible applications of drug franchising were justifiable in the sense that they could alleviate stringent financial conditions when the pricing of curative care services was distorted continuously and the true value of the contribution of medical personnel was not rightfully reflected in the pricing system. During the transition from CPE, the medical care circle complained constantly about the policy and practice of pricing, saying that curative care services involving less tangible input (such as human labor, often of a high skill and with risk taking) were consistently undervalued, and that tangible inputs such as drugs and devices were often priced measurably higher.[1] In financial and accounting terms, revenue derived from cost-shifting, that is to say, from low-price curative care services to high-price drugs. Also, non-basic medical care services (including special care services) were marked up higher than basic care categories, and hence it was expected that the former could "subsidize" the latter. Working with the franchise system, the hospital unit collaborated with doctors who enjoyed drug prescription power and thus had considerable say over choice of drugs and volume of sales, ensuring a desirable amount of revenue flow at the hospital level.

Sovereign planners tackled the issue of drug franchising as an integral part of their pricing exercise for medical care services. They then found it necessary to scale down the "excessive" proportion of drug revenue after the mid-1990s, entailing some noticeable adjustments among several revenue sources. Given that the government's financial subsidies remained relatively small percentage-wise, it appears that, theoretically speaking, the reduction in drug revenue needed to be offset proportionally by increasing revenue from curative care services. From the vantage point of hospital management and medical personnel, it was reasonable for them to claim a rightful share of revenue from drug franchising for two reasons: the need to fill the gap created by the cuts in the share government's subsidies and a rightful compensation for the skilled labor contribution by medical personnel in both curative care and dispensary services.

The issue of cost-shifting was often politicized. Some policy analysts argued against "excessively" large revenue from drugs saying that, for example, hospital units and doctors were politically motivated and they were acting as an "interest group" (liyi jituan) in order to secure revenue and fill the shortfall in government funding by making use of franchises for medical care services (including drug retail with the W/R differential) (Chen 2008: 8–9). In such a view, an "interest group" driven by a rent-seeking tendency would find any feasible means to reach its revenue/income goals, e.g., over-provision in drug prescriptions and overuse of advanced devices (Hu 2001: 283–7; Chen 2008: 8). Condemning irregularities and abuses in drug franchising at the hospital level, for example, a research report put together by a research project in the Research Office of the State Council states in a critical light:

> In view of the existence of the mechanisms of "fostering medical care through drug sales" (yiyao yangyi), the income from drug expenses derived through doctors' prescriptions was linked to revenue of departments/offices as well as to the productivity of the hospital. The larger the expenditure on drugs, the more revenue was derived from the price markup ratios, which made doctors, hospitals, and drug industries all

happy and hence created the "alliance of common interests." When the price of a given kind of drug was [ordered by authorities] to be reduced, the doctor would accordingly practice substituting one kind of drug [often of a higher price] for the other; thus, irregularities in unnecessary and expensive prescriptions couldn't be stopped. Drug dealers had their own counter-measures by practicing either changing the brand name of a drug or swapping between types of drug. If all these counter-measures did not work, they simply stopped production and/or sale of a given drug, resulting in the distortion of procurement through collective bidding (Zhang, 2009a:19). (Translation provided.)

The issue of "fostering medical care through drug sales" is concerned with three interrelated conceptual dimensions which need further articulation. The first pertains a political dimension, namely, what ought to be a fair allocation of material interests among various sectors through the mandatory power. In light of anti-intellectual legacy of Maoism, some policymakers treated compensation for medical care as a low priority in public finance for a considerably long period (Peng, Cai, & Zhou 1992: 23; 36–40). In a sarcastic expression, it is circulated among the people that "surgeon's knife is not worthy of barber's shaving knife," meaning that surgeon's earning is not better than a barber's. From a corporatist perspective, it is put in general terms that the interests of the medical care circle were continually thought of as subsidiary to the interests of the general populace, but comparing with other profession, medical personnel are not paid commensurate with the contributions which they are entitled to. The second dimension has to do with a managerial consideration. At the level of resource management, the question is raised with regard to appropriate pricing to ensure adequate revenue for the providing unit to maintain its regular and continuous services and reasonable compensation for medical personnel, lending due recognition to their special skill, long and hard training, and the risks and responsibility under for the job. On the third dimension, there is an issue of the government's new policy strategy in promoting the use of franchising as an alternative funding source.

Beginning in 1996, sovereign planners appeared to reach a consensus on the need to address the issue of the undervalued, skilled labor contribution by medical personnel, coupled with revenue consideration for the providing unit, and to make upward adjustments in prices by increasing fees for curative care services and decreasing charges for prescription drugs (Wang, 2001: 3–4). The State Planning Commission and the other ministerial units promulgated the 1996 Circular trying to assume a balanced position in the handling of price adjustments for medical care services, that is, to ensure proper compensation for costs to the providing units on the one hand and to defend the interests of the patient and prohibit "indiscriminate" fee-collection by medical care institutes on the other hand.[2] Nonetheless, the interests of the health care profession were still expected to defer to that of the general populace, meaning a low priority to upward adjustment of pay to medical personnel (Gao

2007:17). Thus, the issue of reasonable compensation for medical personnel still remained entangled with franchising mode of funding source.

The issues of price control over drugs

Further to the discussion on the overall patterns of price control, it is germane here to examine some thorny issues relating to pricing on a case-by-case basis. Two salient issues deserve analysis in depth: the policy of W/R differentials and the use/abuse of doctors' prescription power. First of all, there was a controversy over whether revenue from drug franchising with the policy of so-called "wholesale/retail differentials" (piling chajia; W/R differentials) is appropriate (Zhou 2008: 91). According to Tian's historical account, the policy of W/R differentials was adopted first in 1954, stipulating that W/R differentials were to be fixed at no more than 15 percent of wholesale price for Western medicine, for manufactured herbal medicine at no more than 16 percent, and for folk herbal medicine at no more than 29 percent. The same policy was re-adopted in 1978, but each jurisdiction enjoyed considerable latitude in adopting methods of calculation, and there was no strict control over marking up prices either. The providing unit was often given room to take part in the pricing exercises by adding a few percentage points here and there to each phase from production to wholesale and finally to retail at the pharmacy. This relaxation of control, which was held responsible for soaring drug prices, became a focal point for complaints from the public and criticism by the media throughout the economic reform (Tian 2010).

For example, public hospitals were liberally allowed to retain a revenue through W/R differentials roughly at 13–14 percent (estimated wastage rate of an additional 1–2 percent), coupled with a 5 percent discount allowed by the policy, and a legitimate commission of 7–13 percent to the hospital concerned (Wu, 2002: 4). The above figures could easily add up to more than 30 percent of earning in the name of W/R differentials. Nonetheless, there was considerable variation in the enforcement of W/R differentials.[3] Moreover, in the 2000s greater relaxation of W/R differentials was considered (e.g., 30–40 percent) (Zhou 2003:139). As demonstrated in research by Hu Shanlian, Gong Xianguang, and Xu Ke in the late 1990s, it was assumed that there existed a range of variations for W/R differentials in clinical services and hospital care across provincial jurisdictions (Hu, Gong, & Xu 2000). This meant that the provincial and municipal/local jurisdictions had considerable leverage over how large the W/R differentials were, depending on the amount of revenue flow allowed to the providing unit in the light of alternative mixes of funding to the basic medical care service.

From the early 1990s onward, it was evident that price control through W/R differentials was no longer effective. Accordingly, the government began to experiment shifting from controlling W/R differentials to controlling the ceiling of retail prices. In some cases that were even more generous than before, sellers and buyers were allowed to fix the ceiling of retail prices, at 35–40 percent higher than the wholesale price and even as high as 66 percent, which was openly and legally allowed to enter into the accounting book (Zhou 2003: 139). In Zhou Liangrong's estimate, the actual rate of earning for retail sales was as high as an average of 26.7 percent of total sales (averaging 28.4 percent for urban hospitals, 22.4 percent for county hospitals, 39.7 percent for hospital pharmacies, and 21.6 percent for retail drug stores) (Zhou 2003: 139).

Circulated in the mass media and among the general public, allegations of doctors' abuse of prescription power often focused on the lack of price control over drugs in the midst of the growth of regulated drug markets. Nonetheless some evidence indicates that, for reasons other than price control, a pro-doctor viewpoint enjoyed firm support within the top policymaking circle, as the safety of drugs assumed importance by the mid-2000s (Sun & Du 2006:147). Accordingly, on March 4, 2004, the MOH and the State Food and Drugs Management Bureau (or SFDMB) filed the 2004 Report to lend weight to the role of medical doctors in control over drugs.[4] Overall, this provided rationale for medical doctors to retain a say over drug prescriptions (implicitly including pricing), adding complications for price control simply in the name of affordable care.

From January 1, 2005, onward, the MOH issued a series of directives requiring a doctor's prescription for the sale of anti-cancer drugs, hormones, and neurological drugs. By December 31, 2005, the sale of all kinds of drug required a doctor's prescription and instructions from a pharmacist, virtually ending the "double-track system" that had previously made a doctor's pre-scription optional in drug sales (Sun & Du 2006:147). As a consequence, the prescription power of doctors was further strengthened due to the concern for drug safety and quality; and with this expansion of doctors' say over the use and procurement of drugs, the government's price control over drugs was eroded further. As the government faced the dilemma of choice between the concern of drug safety and quality on the one hand and price control on the other, it had to yield to medical personnel on the issue of price control.

While the pro-doctor viewpoint still enjoyed the upper hand, a series of assaults was launched, suggesting that hospitals and medical personnel alike might compromise their professional and medical concerns in order to engage in revenue-maximizing endeavors. According to Yu Tezhi et al., the medical profession, under the policy of drug franchising, might become oriented purely toward the "commercial value" of prescription drugs, together with medical devices, often allowing exorbitant billing charges, kickbacks, and commissions (Yu 2008:14–15). In Yu's view, furthermore, the policy of drug franchising produced numerous cases of prescription irregularities that increased the financial burden of the patient; it also tended to encourage choices for high-priced drugs, but neglect the safety, quality, and effectiveness of drugs.[5] More seriously, the policy of drug franchising often led to the pre-scription of expensive but high-risk drugs. Contrary to the positive image of doctors in terms of drug safety, a set of statistical data noted by Wei Jigang indicates that in 2003, the use of antibiotic drugs reached 30 percent of the total expenditure on drugs in China, in contrast with an amount of less than 10 percent of expenditure on antibiotic drugs in the world markets in the same year. It was also found, on the basis of an analysis of inpatient cases in 2005, that an estimated 19.6 to 20 percent of illnesses was due to misuse and/ or abuse of drugs (largely antibiotics) (Wei 2009: 206–7).

In the worst-case scenario, prescriptions for and sales of "unnecessary" drugs are, allegedly, motivated by the interests of stakeholders (i.e., hospitals, medical personnel, drug manufacturers, and distributors) at the expense of patients. This kind of "unnecessary" use of medicine includes expensive drugs and new brands of drugs (to be discussed further in Chapter 10).[6] In the view of Chen Xinzhong, moreover, hospital management and medical personnel often collaborated with each other to ensure the flow of a desirable amount of revenue from the drug franchise (Chen 2008). According to Zhou, Liangrong et al., moreover, public hospitals often adopted various charging strategies in order to earn a larger share of revenue (see Chapter 10).[7]

With regard to the hard issue of price control, however, policy analysts and policymakers have to consider that doctors are not easily amenable to regulatory control. According to Zhou et al., the medical care profession is characterized as "high input, high technology, extensive coordination, and high risks," requiring expensive training and long experience to enhance the ability to cope with medical risks (Zhou 2003:148–9). In actual practice, however, it is not easy to standardize the work procedures and skills adopted in the case of uncertainty in the process of diagnosis, examination, and treatment, including prescriptions for drugs (see also Chapter 1 and Chapter 8).

Former Minister of Health Gao Qiang put forth proposals to prevent medical personnel from opting for "artificially" high-priced drugs in prescribing practices during his term in office, as illustrated by the following examples: endeavors to establish specialist panels/teams and to keep and computerize records of prescriptions in order to limit doctors' (possibly abusive) discretion; efforts to standardize the issuing of doctors' prescriptions to eliminate cases of over-provision; and the establishment of operational and financial transparency and thus better scrutiny of the delivery of curative and dispensary care services (Gao 2007). Nonetheless, Gao did not address the shortage of knowledge and technical competence on the part of relevant bureaus for the implementation of his recommendations. Furthermore, even if Gao's ideas had been technically enforceable, he would have yet to find solutions to curtail the existing deficit and maintain budgetary balance caused by the loss of revenue from drugs at the providing unit level.

Remaking drug franchises

For about two decades since 1996, the relevant ministries, provincial and municipal jurisdictions have worked with a variety of policy themes and conducted pilot programs in order to remake the drug franchise system, lower the "exorbitant" prices of drugs, and lessen the patients' burden of expenditure on drugs.[8] Accordingly, policymakers experimented with three approaches: first, centralizing management of revenue from drugs at the bureau level, and working out a proper division of drug revenue and reasonable return rate to providing units; second, scaling down the actual percentage of W/R differentials by about one-half or more (say, from roughly 30 percent to 15 percent); and third, abolishing the policy of W/R differentials totally. Thus in 2009, sovereign planners prioritized the restructuring of drug franchising, and price management was put formally on policy agenda.[9]

Sovereign planners formally commenced the policy experiment with the centralization of drug revenue at the bureau level in 1997 (Zhonggong zhongyang & Guowuyuan 1999). Through installing so-called "two-line management," the government took charge of one line by exerting direct control over distributing drug revenue, while the providing unit was held responsible for the other line by maintaining autonomy to manage the drug franchise, e.g. the sale of and charges for prescription drugs to patients (namely, inpatients) with the same W/R differential ratio remaining intact.[10] For instance, on July 8, 2000, relevant ministerial authorities promulgated a policy paper authorizing the supervisory bureau to collect all "pure revenue" (excluding all dispensing-related costs which had remained undifferentiated and unaccounted for in the past) directly and put it into an account for special funds which were to be returned to the hospitals on the basis of a performance appraisal and overall balancing on a seasonal basis.[11]

The original intent of two-line management was to prevent medical personnel from involving themselves in how revenue was to be divided and shared within the providing unit. It was only meant to take direct control over drug revenue at the bureau level and return an appropriate, if not full, amount of revenue back to the providing unit. Neither did it intend to make any overall restructuring of dispensary services, nor did it mean for the bureau to replace the providing unit in terms of the jobs needed to manage the drug franchise system. According to Wang Baozhen, two-line management did not intend to sever dispensary services from curative care services in any professional sense, nor did it mean to undermine the close working relationship between doctor and pharmacist (Wang 1999). In Zhang Anfa's view, through two-line management, in practice, the bureau was to take over only parts of the financial management of drug franchising.[12] Moreover, the providing unit's responsibility for drug franchising was not totally removed.

It still had to take charge of managing the drug franchise and of engaging in prescription drug transactions with inpatients and outpatients as well as take charge of implementing established formulae and calculating W/R differentials (Wang, 1999). As claimed by Gu in his critical note, for sure, two-line management entailed reversing the policy of delegating financial and managerial autonomy to the providing unit, and represented a tendency to retreat back to excessive bureaucratization under the CPE (Gu, 2008: 285–92).

In some jurisdictions, two-line management explicitly targeted hospital units at the county level or above and those hospitals whose revenue from drugs exceeded 30 percent of the total of revenue, while excluding most of the community clinics dealing with common and frequent illnesses (Weishengbu & Caizhengbu 2001). For example, the Shanghai municipal government started a pilot program of two-line management for drug revenue on July 1, 2000. The pilot program was introduced to all public hospitals affiliated with all kinds of establishments and government departments at the municipal level and urban district/ rural county level in Shanghai. The Municipal Health Care Bureau announced the rates of drug revenue remittance for the current year according to the average saving in drug revenue in the preceding year; then the bureau worked out the drug revenue return rates on the basis of the workload of each hospital unit, the percentage of drug revenue within the total revenue, average expenditure for each clinical visit, and average expenditure for hospital care per day, in addition to other quality indicators. Upon concluding the pilot program in Shanghai, however, it was not considered feasible to extend it further to all hospitals citywide in view of limitations in the methods and criteria for allocating returned revenue because municipal policymakers were not able to account fully for the differences in economic conditions, characteristics of services, specializations of the hospitals, nature of the clients, and various combinations of medical cases (Chen 2002).

Meanwhile, the introduction of two-line management for drug revenue created more problems than the government was able to solve for its full implementation. First, it entailed an additional workload for both the local government and the hospital unit, requiring not only the bureau level to undertake the extra workload of auditing, accounting, and preparing statistics, information, and relevant data regarding drug revenue but also requiring hospital management to devote additional effort to the financial exercises of separation and remittance of drug revenue. Secondly, two-line management ran risks of undermining the accountability systems at the government and providing unit levels. To prevent the government from evading its financial responsibility for hospital management, for example, the 2000 Provisional Measures made sure that neither would the collected drug fund be diverted, nor would the returned portion of revenue be counted as part of the government's budgetary appropriation to the providing unit (Weishengbu & Caizhengbu 2001). In addition, this often-undermined accountability as the providing unit was given an excuse to attribute a deficit to the portion taken away through the two-line management, potentially creating disputes among bureaus as well as between echelons of the government. Thirdly, the two-line management system often resulted in dispute over the deficiency of the accounting procedures that had left the under-defined and undifferentiated portion of revenue accrued through medical-technical labor by medical personnel unaccounted for, and pointed to a larger overhaul of pricing and accounting in drugs than what had been originally prepared for. Accordingly, the government took a preliminary step by adding new items of accounting like "prescription fees" and "pharmaceutical services charges" to recognize the said portion of medical-technical labor at the stage of policy experiment.[13]

Alternatives to the policy of W/R differentials

To bring down the "exorbitant" charges of prescription drugs, the second approach intended to cut the percentage of W/R differentials and therefore reduce charges to the patient for drugs. No solid evidence was made available to shed light on the extent the financial conditions would be affected if the said revenue were either reduced or totally eliminated amid the debates and complaints on "exorbitant" charges of drugs during the early and mid-2000s. Accordingly, policymakers sponsored a series of pilot programs on the issue of W/R differentials and tried to answer how they impacted financial conditions at the providing unit level.

Illustrated in an investigative report on 13 hospitals undergoing a pilot program in Shangdong Province from 2003 to 2007, the reform attempt to bring down the percentage of W/R differentials was proven a difficult task due to the pressure on these providing units to maintain budgetary balance and financial viability. All of these hospitals belonged to the modern, top tier hospitals (namely Tier 3, Grade A) that were specialized for rare and difficult illnesses. The report shows that while the percentage of W/R differentials was officially fixed at 15 percent, the average of the actual percentage in hospitals stood around 30 percent, which was considered undesirably high from the government's official position (Tian 2010:11–12). Through the pilot program, the percentage of W/R differentials was required to be reduced to around 20 percent in 2004 and further to about 13 percent in 2006, in accordance with relevant policies. On the whole, the average percentage was on the decline steadily from 29.06 percent in 2003 to 30.54 percent in 2004, 27.35 percent in 2005, 20.18 percent in 2006, and 13.42 percent in 2007 (Tian 2010:12).

How did the shrinking ratio of W/R differentials impact the financial well-being of these hospitals? Given the government's financial subsidies remained low, in the range of 2.89 percent of the total expenditure in 2005 to 2.77 percent in 2007, the overall financial position of these 13 hospitals deteriorated somewhat from 2005 to 2007 with regard to their capacity to repay short-term and long-term loans. Meanwhile, the financial loss remained at an average of 4,135 million RMB for the 13 hospitals as of 2007, along with a general decrease in net revenue from drug sales, from about 30 percent to 21.12 percent in 2005, and 22.56 in 2006 (Tian 2010: 13).

The investigative report of these 13 hospitals further demonstrates that the policy objective to control the "exorbitant" prices of drugs did not produce expected policy outcomes. To begin with, there was actually no significant reduction in charges for drugs to patients when the pilot program was carried out from 2005 to 2007.[14] Instead, considerable, unintended, and undesirable consequences were produced from distortions in financial management at the providing unit level. First, the providing units appeared to have lost sensitivity toward price differences in the sense that higher prices for drugs, rather than low prices, were chosen in the procurement exercises. Secondly, in actual cases of prescriptions, expensive—though substitutable—drugs were chosen in order to ensure better revenue flow. Thirdly, the hospitals and medical personnel tended to maximize revenue through the choice of the "optimal combination" of services, e.g., more of the high-priced devices versus less of low-priced labor services and treatment. Fourthly, they exhibited "expansionist" tendencies by generating more revenue through the increase of quantity of services rather than improvement in quality of medical care (Tian 2010: 15–16).

With comparable research results, Yu Fenghua et al. conducted an investigation on a Tier 3 hospital unit with 1,813 hospital beds in Shangdong Province during the period from 2005 to 2008, shedding light on the role of W/R differentials in financial management at the providing unit level. In fact, the hospital unit was not considered successful in curtailing expenditure on drugs, this being attributed to the revenue motivation of the hospital management as well as the distortion created by medical personnel through prescribing expensive—though substitutable—drugs to bolster drug revenue.[15]

To deal with the soaring charges for drugs, top policymakers implemented an even more drastic reform initiative by adopting the third approach, that is, to abolish the policy of W/R differentials in the sale of prescription drugs altogether, not only for hospital care but also for clinical services. In a pilot program conducted in a hospital in a municipal jurisdiction in Hebei Province from 2006 to 2008, for example, the municipal government claimed to adopt a "zero ratio of W/R differentials" in order to abolish once and for all cost-shifting, namely "cross-subsidization" (or "subsidizing curative care through drug sales"), to eliminate the over-provision of drug prescriptions, and, hence, to lessen the financial burden on patients (Li, Zhang, & Liu 2010). As the franchising of drugs was not formally abolished, the hospital management was only allowed to charge patients an amount according to the zero ratio of W/R differentials, so patients could pay for medication an amount less than retailers' mark-up prices. In the year 2008, the number of outpatients was 704,000 and the number of inpatients was 38,000. However, there was no substantial reduction in charges for prescription drugs. Owing to the zero ratio of W/R differentials, for example, each outpatient was charged 8.63 RMB less for prescription drugs while each inpatient was charged 160.68 RMB less for the same (Li et al., 2010: 75). For the three years of 2006, 2007, and 2008, moreover, the percentage of revenue from prescription drugs was controlled at the tolerable levels of 38.07 percent, 40.00 percent, and 42.46 percent of the total expenditure for medical care services, respectively (Li et al. 2010: 75). As recorded, however, the hospital unit registered red on the balance sheets for revenue and expenditure in those three consecutive years, which resulted in a shortage of funding for new investment projects (Li et al. 2010: 75).

In another pilot program conducted in Hebei, drug franchising was not set aside albeit the W/R differentials scheme was terminated. In implementation, policy issues were raised with reference to the deficiency of accounting procedure once again: the existing W/R differential scheme did not recognize some unaccounted portion of contribution from medical personnel for costs, for instance, the costs of various dispensary services provided by hospitals, doctors, and pharmacists, respectively. Accordingly, new charge schemes were recommended, such as a 10 percent drug service charge to recognize the doctor's contribution in prescription and the handling charges for the pharmacy as well as 30 percent more in charges for the doctors' work in diagnosis, examination, treatment, etc. As reported, furthermore, the experiment of abolishing the W/R differential scheme in Hebei led to exposure of shortfall in the government's subsidies to public, non-profit hospitals—the government's subsidies to the hospital merely consisted of 2.74 percent in 2008 (Li et al., 2010: 76).

A survey reviewing the program piloting a zero ratio for W/R differentials for 1,812 hospital units in Jiangxi Province from 2003 to 2008 shows that, to varying degrees, there was a decrease in the charges on medical bills for both outpatients and inpatients.[16] Nonetheless, the providing units at all levels invariably suffered steadily from increasing loss from 2003 to 2008. For instance, the year 2008 showed an average loss of 14.997 million RMB for each hospital unit at the provincial level, 8.4450 million RMB at the municipal level, 3.1447 million at the county level, and almost half a million RMB at the township level. It is observed in the same case that the financial deficit of providing units at the county and township levels increased from 58.25 percent in 2003 to 71.12 percent in 2008, while the deficits of providing units at the provincial and municipal levels remained stable from 2003 to 2008. In this pilot program, however, no policy directly addressed financial deficit at the providing unit level (Li et al. 2010: 24–5).

Concluding remarks

The foregoing narrative shows how the government granted providing units drug franchise-right of entry into transactions for drugs in the market place, and the ability to fix W/R differential ratios to allow providing units a share of revenue from drugs, marking the adoption of a new funding strategy to provide affordable care to the populace during economic reform. Accordingly, the providing unit was expected to shoulder a large portion of the financial burden of health care, and, theoretically speaking, assume an intermediary role by passing some earnings from drugs franchising to users (i.e., patients). It was apparent that no workable mechanisms had ever been in place to ensure that the providing unit could play the intermediary role effectively without addressing the budgetary balance.

On the basis of the policy experiments on restructuring drug franchise and control of W/R differentials cited above, it is evident, however, that considerable strain developed between the government and the providing unit due to contradictions inherent in the drug franchise policy throughout the era of economic reform. On the one hand, the government needed to ensure some "rate of self-sufficiency" and budgetary balance in a providing unit's revenue generating effort. On the other hand, the government adopted measures undermining such a policy by reducing revenue to the providing unit, for instance by curtailing subsidies to the providing unit and by maintaining low charges for users.

Besides, it remained a challenging task to implement the W/R differentials policy intended to create a franchise funding source throughout the reform era for a couple of reasons, including variations among jurisdictions with reference to W/R differentials ratios and difficulties for supervising bureaus and providing units to reach agreement on such ratios. As noted previously, moreover, policymakers introduced a series of pilot programs either to control or reduce the revenue volume from drug franchise through lower or even zero ratios of W/R differentials; these pilot programs invariably produced adverse financial results for providing units, proving that new and workable proposals for restructuring the drug franchise system were very much in need.

Notes

1 For illustration, an estimate regarding the breakdowns of the total revenue of hospitals in the 1990s are as follows: 1.6 percent from registration fees, 4.9 percent from hospitalization, 25.1 percent from diagnosis and medical tests, and 61.6 percent from drugs (Peng, Cai, & Zhou 1992: 36).
2 The full title of the policy paper is the "Circular Concerning the Strengthening and Improvement of Management of Fee Collection in Medical" (abbreviated as "1996 Circular)," promulgated by the State Planning Commission, Ministry of Health, and Ministry of Finance. Wang Yang tried his best to argue that, after all, the increase in prices for curative care services had already been put on the policy agenda nationwide, requiring provincial and municipal jurisdictions to draft plans for price adjustments and to carry them out in due course from 1996 to 2000. According to Wang, this resulted in overall price rises of an estimated 6,500 million RMB, representing the first step toward improving the low-price medical care services that had existed for decades since the 1950s (Wang 2001).
3 It is estimated, according to Wu, that state-owned pharmaceutical enterprises could give a total of 25–35 percent of the price of drugs as commission to a hospital; the representatives of manufacturers could offer the hospital at least 10–20 percent of the drug price as commission (Wu 2002: 4).
4 The title of the report is "Report on the Adverse Effects of Drugs, and Management Measure for Monitory" (abbreviated as 2004 Report). Starting in July of the same year, the Ministry of Health Care began to enforce restrictions over the sale of antibiotic drugs at the level of retail drug stores, resulting in a drastic 20 percent reduction of antibiotic drugs in these stores (Sun & Du 2006: 147).
5 Yu Tezhi et al. argue additionally that doctors are blameworthy for the violation of the principle "administer cure according to illness; reasonably prescribe medicine" in the case of drug franchise abuses (Yu 2008:14–5).
6 In the case of "expensive drugs," for example, doctors who were motivated for a better income could choose the option of drugs at the higher end of the price range (cf. Liu & Yuan, 2001; Y. Wang, 2008, p. 49). The case of so-called "new brands" often involved the repackaging of old drugs which were approved by respective authorities under less rigorous law enforcing circumstances, a case to be examined further in the next chapter (Zhou et al., 2003: 137; Wang, 2008: 49).
7 These charging strategies include: (1) the increase of the total volume of expenditure on prescription drugs, (2) the expansion of the portion of high-priced drugs in

the total expenditure on prescription drugs, and (3) the pursuit of net profit in drug sales and high rates of kickbacks in the total volume of expenditure on drugs (Zhou 2003: 140).

8 Policy themes of price control, including W/R differentials, were first articulated in the "Provisional Measures of Price Management of Drugs in 1996" (hereafter, "1996 Provisional Measures") (Wang 2001: 2–3). Furthermore, the government explored a variety of policies and measures regarding pricing of drugs and the problems associated with W/R differentials. Beginning in 2000, for example, the government adopted a policy experiment to fix the price ceilings of selected drugs directly. In 2006 the Development and Reform Commission promulgated a policy paper requiring hospital units to return to the original limits—around 15 percent of W/R differentials. The policy paper is entitled the "Opinion on Further Rectification of the Pricing Regime in the Drugs and Dispensary Services Market" (hereafter, "2006 Opinion") (Tian 2010:11).

9 For example, on November 9, 2009, the State Development and Reform Commission, Ministry of Health, and Ministry of Human Resources and Social Security promulgated the "Opinion concerning the Reform of Pricing Mechanisms for Drug and Medical Care Services" (hereafter, "2009 Opinion"). It proposed to restructure the mechanisms of compensation to the providing units in line with the separation of accounting and management between curative care and dispensary services. The "2009 Opinion" even went further by proposing to take steps to phase out the W/R differential policy for drug sales gradually (Zhao & Xue 2010: 48).

10 This policy position was repeatedly affirmed in a series of policy papers later, notably, the "Opinion regarding Further Institutional Reform of Medical Care, Drugs, and Health Care" promulgated by the Central Committee, CCP, and State Council in April 2009, among other policy papers. On July 1, 2000, the Ministry of Health and Ministry of Finance lent considerable weight to the two-line management pilot programs in accordance with the "Provisional Measures for Two-line Management of Revenue and Expenditure on Drugs in Hospitals" (Chen, 2002: 12).

11 The Ministry of Health and Ministry of Finance were able to draft and promulgate a policy paper for implementation of the "Provisional Measures for Two-line Management of Revenue and Expenditure on Drugs in Hospitals" (hereafter, 2000 Provisional Measures) on July 8, 2000 (Weishengbu & Caizhengbu 2001: Article 3).

12 As suggested, for instance, the bureau could take part in the tasks of accounting for revenue and expenditure, as well as could be held accountable for gain and loss (Zhang 2000).

13 "Pharmaceutical service charges" were first articulated and formally proposed in the "Opinion Concerning the Reform of Pricing Mechanisms of Drug and Medical Care Services" (henceforth, "2009 Opinion") promulgated by the State Development and Reform Commission, Ministry of Health, and Ministry of Human Resources and Social Security on November 9, 2009 (Zhao & Xue 2010; Li & Yong, 2010).

14 In the case of clinical visits, the average charge for drugs stood at 84.37 RMB, 81.43 RMB, and 84.43 RMB in 2005, 2006, and 2007, respectively; and for inpatients, the average charge for drugs was 288.4 RMB, 261.61 RMB, and 291.72 RMB in 2005, 2006, and 2007, respectively (Tian 2010: 14).

15 It took three years for the hospital unit to scale down the percentage of its ratio of W/R differential from 38.31 percent in 2005 to 13.66 in 2008. Meanwhile, unexpectedly, the revenue from drugs increased from 37,090,000 RMB in 2005 to 73,680,000 RMB in 2008—a nearly 98 percent increase. The revenue rate from drug retail decreased from 32.7 percent in 2005 to 6.91 percent in 2008 in the wake

of the expansion of medical care services to 857,447 clinical visits in 2008 (a 94 percent increase from 2005) and 51,481 cases of inpatients (upon checkout) in 2008–a 105 percent increase from 2005 (Yu 2010).

16 It is estimated that in 2008 each outpatient paid 9.87 RMB less for medication and each inpatient paid 248.13 RMB less (Ao, Wang, & Xiong, 2011).

References

Ao, J., Wang, Y., & Xiong, W. 2011. Gongli yiliao jigou yaopin lingjiacheng hou de yinxian ji duice fenxi (An analysis of the impact and policy of zero marking-up of drugs in public medical care institutes). *Zhongguo weisheng jingji (China's Health Care Economics)*, 30(9): 24–26.

Chen, J., & Wang, Y. (Ed.). 2007. *Zhongguo shehui baozhang fazhan baoguo, 2007 No. 3* (The Report of China's Social Insurance Development, 2007, No. 3). Beijing: Shehui kexue wenxian chubanshe.

Chen, W. 2002. Yaopin shouzhi liantiaoxian guanli chaozuo xingshi yu kexingxin yanjiu (A study concerning the operational pattern and, feasibility of the two-line management of revenue and expenditure of pharmaceutical products). *Weisheng jingji yanjiu(Research on Health Care Economics)*, 5: 12–15.

Chen, X. 2008. Guanyu "yiyao buyi" wenti de shanque (Discussion on the issue of subsidizing medical through pharmacy). *Zhongguo weisheng jingji(China's Health Care Economics)*, 9: 8–9.

Crozier, M. 1971. *The Bureaucratic Phenomenon* (5th impression). Boston: Little Brown & Co.

Dangdai Zhongguo Congshu Bianjibu. 1988. *Dangdai zhongguo de yiyao shiye* (The Pharmacy Enterprises of Contemporary China). Beijing: Zhongguo shehui kexue chubanshe.

Downs, A. 1967. *Inside Bureaucracy.* Boston: Little Brown & Co.

Gao, Q. 2007. Dangqian kaizhan weisheng jiufeng gongzuo, jiejue kanbingnan kanbinggui wenti mianlin de xingshi he jiben silu (The current task of rectification in health care, the situation and basic considerations for solving the problems of the difficulty to see doctors and the high expensive of seeing doctors). In Zhongguo Weisheng Nianjian Bianji Weiyuanhui (Ed.), *Zhongguo weisheng nianjian 2007 (China's Yearbook of Health Care 2007)*, 61–69. Beijing: Renmin weisheng chubanshe.

Gao, Q. 2007. Quannian guanche luoshi wuzhongquanhui jingshen,zuo weihu renmin jiankang de zhongcheng zhanshi (To implement thoroughly the spirit of the fifth plenum of Central Committee, CCP, to serve as loyal fighter to defend the health of the people). In Zhongguo weisheng nianjian bianji weiyuanhui (Ed.), *Zhongguo weisheng nianjian 2007 (China's Yearbook of Health Care 2007)*, 13–22. Beijing: Renmin weisheng chubanshe.

Gao, Q. 2006. Fazhan yiliao weisheng shiye, weigoujian shehui zhuyi hexie shehui zuogongxian (Develop further medical and health care enterprises and contribute to building a harmonious socialist society). In Zhongguo weisheng nianjian bianji weiyuanhui (Ed.), *Zhongguo Weisheng Nianjian 2006* (China's Yearbook of Health Care 2006), 48–56. Beijing: Renmin weisheng chubanshe.

Gu, X. 2008. *Zouxiang quanmin yibao: Zhongguo xingyigai de zhanlue yu zhanshu* (Toward Comprehensive Medical Insurance: Strategy and Tactic of China's New Medical Care Reform). Beijing: Zhongguo laodong chubanshe.

Gu, X. 2008. "Shouzhi liantiaoxian": Gongli yiliao jigou de xingzhenghua zhilu (The two lines of revenue and expenditure: The road to bureaucratizing public medical care institutes). *Zhongguo weisheng jingji (China's Health Care Economics)*, 27(1):14–16.

Hu, S. 2001. *Yiliao baoxian he fuwu zhidu* (Medical Care Insurance and its System of Services). Chengdu: Sichuan renmin chubanshe.

Hu, S., Gong, X., & Xu, Ke. 2000. Quanguo yiliao jigou yaopin piling chajia shouru yanjiu (Research on the revenue of price differentials between wholesale and retail pharmaceutical products in health care institutes throughout the country). *Zhnogguo weisheng jingji (China's Health Care Economics)*, 19(6): 5–7.

Li, D. 2011. Yaojia xugao de chengyin fenxi yu zhili duice (An analysis of causes as well as policy in dealing with the artificially high prices of drugs). *Weisheng jingji yanjiu(Research on Health Care Economics)*, (286):7–8.

Li, W., Zhang, S., & Liu, Y. 2010. Shixin jiben yaopin lingchalu dui yiyuan de yingxian ji duice (The impact on and policy toward hospitals in the implementation of zero marking up of basic drugs). *Zhongguo weisheng jingji (China's Health Care Economics)*, 29(2): 75–76.

Li, W. & Yong, Y. 2010. Woguo shishi yaoshi fuwufei de kexingxin fenxi ji shiishi celue (A feasibility analysis and strategy for the implementation of dispensary services charges' in China). *Weisheng jingji yanjiu(Research on Health Care Economics)*, 5: 18–19.

Liu, H., & Yuan, J. 2001. Dui yiyuan yaopin jingying zhong fanchang xianxian de fenxi (An analysis of irregular phenomena in the hospital medicine business). *Weisheng jingji yanjiu(Research on Health Care Economics)*, 3: 6–8.

Mintzberg, H. 1983. *Structure in Fives: Designing Effective Organizations.* Englewood Cliffs, NJ: Prentice-Hall.

Peng, R., Cai, R., & Zhou, C. (Eds.). 1992. *Zhongguo gaige quanshu* (Encyclopedia of China's Reform). Dalian: Dalian chubanshe.

Si, G., He, H., & Song, L. 1999. Guanyu yaopin jingying guanli tizhi wenti de tiaocha (An investigation into the problems of operational and managerial systems in pharmacies). *Zhongguo weisheng jingji(China's Health Care Economics)*, 3: 15–18.

Sun, N., & Du, L. 2006. Jiankang yu yiyao baojiian de fazhan (The development of health and drug services). In Du Lexun et al. (Eds.), *Zhongguo yiliao weisheng fazhan baogao, No. 2* (The Report on the Development of Medical and Health Care in China, No. 2), 145–179. Beijing: Shehui kexue wenxian chubanshe.

Tian, L. 2010. Yaopin chajialu bienhua dui yiyuan jingji yunxing he yiyao feiyong de yingxian (The influence in the variation of drug price differential rates on economic operation and medical care expenditure). *Weisheng jingji yanjiu(Research on Health Care Economics)*, 1: 11–17.

Wang, B. 1999. Zaitan yiyao fenkai hesuan, fenbie guanli (Revisiting separate accounting and management of medical care and medicine). *Zhongguo weisheng jingji(China's Health Care Economics)*, 10: 8–9.

Wang, Y. 2008. *Zhongguo weisheng gaige yu fazhan shizheng yanjiu* (Empirical Research on the Reform and Development of Health Care). Beijing: Zhonguo laodong shehui baozhang chubanshe.

Wang, Y. 2001. Yinru jinzheng jizhi jinyibu shenhua yaopin he yiliao fuwu jiage gaige (Introduce a mechanism for competition, go further in the price reform of medicine and medical care services). In Guojia Fazhan Jihua Weiyuanhui Jiagesi (Ed.), *Yiyao jiage zhengce zinan* (The Guide for Price Policy in Medicine), 1–15. Beijing: Zhongguo wujia chubanshe.

Wei, J. 2009. *Zhongguo yiyao tizhi gaige yu fazhan* (The Reform and Development of the Medicine System in China). Beijing: Shanwu yinshuguan.

Weishengbu, & Caizhengbu. 2001. Yiyuan yaopin shouzhi liangtiaoxian guanli zanxing banfa (A provisional measure for two separate channels between revenue and expenditure for medicine in hospitals). In Guojiafazhan, Jihuaweiyuanhui, Jiagesi (Ed.), *Yiyao jiage zhengce zhinan* (The Guide for Price Policy in Medicine), 138–143. Beijing: Zhongguo wujia chubanshe.

Wu, M. 2002. Yaopin fuwu tigong gecheng zhong xunzu xingwei chansheng yuanyin fenxi (An analysis on the cause of rent-seeking behavior in the provision of dispensary services). *Zhnogguo weisheng jingji (China's Health Care Economics)*, 21 (11): 4–6.

Xu, B. 1998. Cong yiyaoye de xunzu xingwei kan zhidu chuangxin de biyaoxing (Examining the necessity of institutional innovation in light of rent-seeking behavior in the medical and pharmaceutical sectors). *Zhongguo ruanexue* (China's Soft Science), 10: 22–25.

Yan, S., & Chen, W. 2011. Woguo gongli yiliao jigou yaopin jiage xugao ji tizhi yuanyi fenxi (An analysis of artificially high prices for drugs and structural factors in public medical care institutes in China). *Zhongguo weisheng jingji (China's Health Care Economics)*, 30(7): 33–35.

Yu, D. 2008. Quexiao "yiyi buyi" qieduan yiyao jingji liyi lianxi jianli fangkong yiyao gouxiao lingyu shangye huilou de changxiao jizhi (Abolishing "fostering medical care through drugs" to sever the connection to pharmacy's economic interests and establishing long-lasting mechanisms to curtail commercial bribery in the sphere of drug sales and procurement). *Zhongguo weisheng jingji (China's Health Care Economics)*, 27(2): 14–16.

Yu, F. 2010. Gongli yiyuan yaopin jiacheng zhengce shishi xiaoguo de yanjiu (A study on the effect of implementing the policy of marking up drugs prices in public hospitals). *Zhongguo weisheng jingji (China's Health Care Economics)*, 29(5): 14–16.

Zhang, A. 2000. Qiantan yiyao fenkai hesuan, fenbieguanli de zuofa (A preliminary discussion on the approach separating curative care from dispensary services in accounting and management). *Zhongguo weisheng jingji(China's Health Care Economics)*, 6: 13–15.

Zhang, C. 2009a. Mingque yiyuan dingwei, shixing yiyao he guanban fenkai (Clearly positioning hospitals and implementing the separation between control and management in medical care and dispensary services). In Guowuyuan Yanjiushi Ketizu (Ed.) *Shenhua yiyao weisheng tizhi gaige yanjiu* (Research on the Further Reform of Medical and Health care), 53–73. Beijing: Guowuyuan yanjiushi ketizu.

Zhang, C. 2009b. Wangshan yiliao baoxian zhidu, gaige yiyao liutong tizhi (Perfecting the medical care insurance system, and reforming the system of transactions for drugs). *Shenhua yiyao weisheng tizhi gaige yanjiu* (Research on the Further Reform of Medical and Health Care), 65–73. Beijing: Guowuyuan yanjiushi ketizu.

Zhang, C. 2001. Yiyao fenkai,yaopin shouzhi liangtiaoxian guanli banfa yu feiyingli xing yiyuan de fazhan daolu (The managerial measure of the separation of curative care and dispensary services, the two separate channels of revenue from and expenditure for medicine as well as the developmental paths of non-profit-oriented hospitals). *Zhongguo weisheng jingji(China's Health Care Economics)*, 4: 32–33.

Zhao, L., & Xue, B. 2010. Qianghua disanfan zeren, dapo yiyuan shuanxian longduan: Gaibian 'yiyao yangyi' dizhi de lujin (Strengthening the third party's responsibility and breaking the hospital's bilateral monopoly: The chosen path to transform the structure of financing medical care through pharmacy). *Zhongguo weisheng jingji* (China's Health Care Economics), 29(7): 47–50.

Zhonggong Zhongyang & Guowuyuan. 1999. Guanyu weisheng gaige yu fazhan de jueding (The decision concerning the reform and development of health care). In D. Zheng, D. Liu & B. Zhang (Eds.), *Shehui baozhang zhidu gaige* (The reform of social security system), 43–51. Beijing: Gaige chubanshe.

Zhou, L., Qu, Q., & Li, G. 2003. *Jujiao weisheng gaige* (Focusing on health care reform). Beijing: Zhongguo Shehue Chubanshe.

Zhou, X. 2008. *Zhongguo yiliao jiage de zhengfu guanzhi yanjiu* (A study on government control of medical care pricing in China). Beijing: Zhongguo shehui kexue Chubanshe.

10 Regulatory control in expanding drug markets

The role of the state in drug markets is exceedingly large and complex in China's health care reform. Not only does the state take a very active part in building drug markets, but also it heavily intervenes, through regulatory control, in the market transactions of drugs. Throughout the reform era, sovereign planners have encountered considerable challenges to shape drug markets and install some forms of regulatory control in order to fulfill the policy purposes, namely meeting medical and professional criteria (e.g. quality, safety and effectiveness of medicine) on the one hand and ensuring affordability and accessibility of health care to users on the other hand.

In fact, one can find that the state and markets are intertwined in the realm of medicine in the era of economic reform in China. The state acts as both a builder and regulator of drug markets. Its role is pivotal in unleashing the energy for the growth of free markets in drug during early decades of the reform, subsequently converting the free markets into regulated markets, and build quasi-markets amidst the introduction of the basic medical care insurance programs across municipal jurisdictions. The state is often fused with the markets. For example, not only is it an integral part of institutional infrastructure and legal foundation for regulated markets, but also it represents the mechanisms of regulatory control that are necessary conditions without which regulated markets cannot operate. The study will demonstrate the role that the state assumes in developing and licensing of new drugs, in upholding of standards of safety, quality and effective use of drugs, in enforcing drug pricing policy, in devising and applying drug pricing mechanisms, in monitoring and controlling irregular market behaviors, and in ensuring affordability and accessibility of medicine to all users (Guojia Yaopin Jiandu Guanliju 2003).

Endeavors to build drug markets and the drug industry have produced unanticipated and uncontrollable outcomes often contrary to the intent of policymakers. To be discussed in the ensuing pages, this study focuses on some main policy episodes relevant to the success and failures in enforcing regulatory control, especially price control, for drugs in the providing units. The study also addresses broad theoretical issues regarding policymaking in the case of developing and building the mechanisms of regulatory control in the rise of drug markets. Is it appropriate to characterize it in terms of

government politics model? To what extent has bureaucratic politics penetrated into the policymaking arena? How does the state differ from the model
of business/industrial management in policymaking in these policy episodes?
A close survey of the rise of regulatory control intends to answer the above
questions and to shed light the distinctive role of the state versus the markets
in handling policymaking.

Discovery of regulatory control

As soon as the economic reform started in the post-Mao period, sovereign
planners took the initiative to build up the drug industry and rebuild drug
markets in the midst of decentralizing power and liberalizing regulatory control throughout China. It is unmistakable a significant development here that
free markets on medicine arrived, and were in full operation, albeit for a short
time span during the early phase of economic reform. Starting from 1979 to
the late 1980s, sovereign planners built up the drug industry in light of an
overall policy strategy to promote economic growth and to fulfill revenue
goals. The local government units made attempts to break away from the
SOEs' predominant position over investment, production, and distribution of
drugs, by allowing entry of a variety of enterprises into the drug market and
by accommodating a greater diversity of ownership systems and many different types of enterprises. The number of enterprises of the "three types of
investments" (foreign-owned type, Hong Kong and Taiwan types) increased
drastically within three years from 412 in 1992 to 612 in 1993, 1,000 in 1994,
and 1,500 in 1995 (Wei, 2009: 147; 220–1).

With the relaxation of control by the central government, many small drug-
manufacturing enterprises emerged at the local level, operating with poor
equipment and facilities, and producing drugs of dubious quality and safety.
The number of drug-manufacturing enterprises experienced an enormous
increase: the number of licensed manufacturers was first counted at 800 in the
late 1970s, and it grew to 5,655 in 2001 (Liu & Yuan, 2001: 6). Taken as a
"pillar industry," the drug industry was quickly built up in two-thirds of the
provinces, and 80 or so prefectural jurisdictions in the midst of the inauguration of fresh development plans and policies of support and subsidy (Wei
2009: 220–1). The number of these enterprises, including both SOEs and
enterprises of other ownership types, increased about fourteenfold, exploding
from 2,253 in 1980 to an estimated total of 33,857 (including 22,003 units of
COEs and private-owned types) in 1990 (Wei 2009: 150).

As much as a vigorous effort in meeting increasing health care demands
among the populace, the rapid rise of local drug industry was indicative of
the transformation of the CPE to a mixed economy. Meanwhile, sovereign
planners introduced decentralization with respect to planning, revenue, wages
and bonuses from central ministries to municipal/local governments while
allowing the latter to gain a considerable share of the revenue generated by
the drug industry at the local level (Ge & Gong 2007: 28–32). In addition,

local governments were able to secure more revenue sources by acquiring franchises for producing and marketing drugs on behalf of the local drug industry. For instance, 130,000 drugs of international brands were registered with local governments, representing nearly 78 percent of the total of 180,000 items registered concurrently with the central government (Wei 2009: 220–1). Consequently, the revenue-maximizing propensity of local governments and the drug industry has reinforced the providing units' pursuit of revenue, creating challenges to the exercise of regulatory control in drug markets.

In conjunction with the policy of expanding managerial autonomy, the SOEs for drugs were allowed considerable room to broaden the scope of their commercial activities and to choose more channels of procurement and sale through direct transactions with manufacturing entities at different places of production. Also, in the procurement and supply of drugs, all wholesale stations were to be decentralized to the municipal level (with prefectural status), and new wholesale corporations were to be reorganized accordingly. Meanwhile ministerial authorities encouraged various jurisdictions to organize trade centers for drugs, form joint ventures among SOEs at the local level, and promote direct transactions among bureaus and/or agencies and wholesale and retail outlets. As the regulatory restrictions on wholesale franchises were lifted at various hierarchical levels and in a fixed territorial domain, wholesale enterprises were given freedom to make optimal choices in transactions in the market place (Wei 2009: 148–51).

While municipal/local governments started to encounter issues of regulatory control in the midst of the developing drug industry and promoting the trade of drugs around the mid-1980s. Accordingly, relevant ministerial units swung back, starting to convert free markets of drugs into regulated markets. First of all, it endeavored to tighten the control and licensing of the drug industry in order to cope with the unintended and undesirable results of free drug markets, albeit in their early stage of development. For instance, 23 percent or 7,658 units (out of a total of 33,857) operated without having both a license for enterprise status and a license for commercial undertaking; and 32 percent or 10, 946 units lacked either one of the two licenses. The problem of fake drugs, as well as the problem of irregular and illegal commercial transactions, was then prevalent, posing safety and quality issues to the patients and public (Wei 2009: 150). As early as July 1989, for example, the State General Bureau of Drug Management (hereafter, SGBDM) promulgated the 1989 Circular, stipulating that only licensed, qualified, and franchised state-owned wholesalers were allowed to engage in the wholesale business of drugs.[1] The State Council issued more circulars, directives, and policies from 1992 to 1996 in order to cope with the many cases of such abuses, irregularities, and violations that took place in drug markets. (Wei 2009: 151).

A fresh round of regulatory control was introduced in 1997 when the Central Committee, CCP, and State Council put constructing of the regulated drug markets on the policy agenda in the midst of promoting the "three reforms" in medical care, medical insurance and drug policy. As a reversal from the policies implemented in the early decades of regulatory controls in the midst of the growth of regulated drug markets, 1997 was marked by an endeavor to return to centralized control through building a "unified market for drugs," coupled with establishing nation-wide agencies for wholesale and a system of chain stores for retail throughout the country (Wei 2009: 150–2). Entering into the 2000s, the SGBDM confronted the chaos created during the early years of reform by continuing its fight to restore order to drug markets, to eliminate fake and poor-quality drugs, to prohibit illegal markets and trade centers for drugs, and to stamp out unlicensed organizational entities in the drug trade (Guojia Yaopin Jiandu Guanliju 2003).

In the meantime, the government introduced another round of administrative interventions in order to scale down the "exorbitant" pricing of drugs and to control abuses and irregularities associated with the drug markets, as noted by Vice Premier Wang Yang in the early 2000s.[2] Also the MOH issued the 2000 General Circular concerning pilot programs for a collective bidding system in drug procurement.[3] This circular intended to promote fair competition among all departments and jurisdictions, to dismantle administrative protection imposed by each jurisdiction, and to break the confines of franchises granted on the basis of ownership systems and territorial boundaries. For more than two decades since 1979 the government had gone through a full cycle of policy experiments from relaxation to tight control in drug industry and drug markets. By the 2000s, a system of regulatory controls in regulated drug markets was then in operation.

Origins of the drug pricing policy

When coming to the operational issue of drug pricing policy, it is appropriate first to look into how the apparatus of regulatory control is built, coupled with an analysis of the considerations behind it. In the Chinese context, pricing is an integral part of regulatory control, and it is inseparable from the other jobs such as licensing, quality control and enforcement of safety standards among the others. As a rule, various bureaus act on behalf of the state to exercise regulatory control. As drug industry and drug markets were new, the government needed to construct governing and managing apparatus to enforce regulatory control.

In fact, it took two separate steps for the government to have organizational apparatuses in place for the task of drug pricing. During the decade of reform from 1979 to1989, the government took the first step to establish an apparatus for regulatory control over drug pricing. Subsequently, it took second step to rebuild the governing and managing apparatus of regulatory control over the same functional area beginning in 1996. As a result, the task of drug pricing normally has fallen under the jurisdiction of two sets of apparatus, which are functionally intertwined (Zhou 2008: 154–5). The first is the price bureau, affiliated with the State Planning Commission (hereafter,

SPC; later re-named as the State Reform and Development Commission, or SRDC). This bureau is directly in charge of fixing prices for drugs as well as supervising drug prices. The second, the State General Bureau of Pharmacy Management (hereafter, SGBPM), which works under the MOH, is responsible for the procurement and use of drugs, for the control of revenue from drugs at the providing unit level, as well as for the licensing of drugs, namely, the control of market entry for a given drug. In accordance with relevant regulations and laws, for example, the SGBPM has licensing power over not only general categories of drugs but also various types of medicine requiring special considerations, e.g., new drugs and special drugs under strict control (Guoweiyuan 1989; Quanguo renmin daibiao dahui changwu weiyuanhui 1989). As a rule, the provincial/local price bureau has to work with its local counterpart unit of the SGBPM when it comes to matters of pricing (Weishengbu 1989).

At the onset of the reform, price control was relaxed, but the government returned to some forms of macro-management later in response to chaos and disorder typically found in a free market situation. In the relaxation of price control from 1979 to 1992, the government basically ceased handling pricing on an item-by-item basis, as the enterprises gained ever greater discretion in the pricing of each drug in the majority of cases. By the early 1990s, the prices of a majority of drugs were marked up at the enterprise level in response to market circumstances. In the absence of regulatory control, however, this opened the floodgate for chaos and an uncontrollable market situation albeit providing units were able to generate revenue and improve remuneration to medical personnel because of some increase of drug prices.

As a consequence of a lack of regulatory control, the revenue-driven sale of drugs at the hospital level tended to intensify competition among manufacturers, wholesalers, and retailers through aggressive promotion sales. And sales representatives often offered large kickbacks and commissions to medical personnel and encouraged them to choose drugs at high prices. This was often coupled with irregularities in bookkeeping, false invoices and receipts, and artificial costs and charges, among other manipulations. Beginning to assume a political dimension, moreover, the price bureau acted on behalf of consumers by trying its best to put the brakes on such abuses and irregularities in the drug industry, and control revenue flow at providing unit level (Wei 2009: 164).

For more than one decade from the early 1980s to the mid-1990s, the price bureau addressed several pricing issues, including the policy experiment of double-track price schedules from 1983 to 1992 as noted (Chapter 9), the pricing of new services and advanced medical devices (not including labor costs) starting from 1985, rulings on adjusted wholesale/retail (W/R) differentials during 1984 and 1988, and the readjustment of price schedules, including 4,100 items in 1988 and 6,000 items in 1991, respectively, in order to cope with over-provision and multiple charges for a single service by the providing unit (Zhou 2008: 132–4). In addition, the government lifted rigid control over pricing on the basis of a calculation of the production/retail ratios between manufacturers and retailers in those enterprises that had suffered losses coupled with high costs of production and wastage. Also, the government simplified procedures for pricing by working on the mark-up of the price of products at a given manufacturing location and leaving prices at the location of sales to negotiations between supplier and retailer (Wei 2009: 162).

Furthermore, the government introduced a classification for three modes of price management: mandatory, advisory, and market-adjusted mode. This allowed the government to play a large and active role in the mandatory mode while the markets could find room through the market-adjusted mode. The advisory pricing mode applied to cases in between. Besides this, the government took the initiative to decentralize pricing power to the local government and enterprise level, and narrowed down the scope of unified pricing for Western medicine at the central level drastically, from 1,900 items to 250, as well as that of medical devices from 54 items to 9 (Wei 2009: 162–3). At the discretion of local governments and enterprises, all these decentralized items were allowed a mark-up according to floating rates. In addition, the liberalization of price control was part of the effort to loosen the rigid, mandatory planning of the CPE of the past and to underscore productivity and growth as the gateway for further economic reform. However, this gave unduly high priority to revenue targets for medical care services at the expense of medical and professional concerns, e.g., curative effects, safety, quality, and accessibility (Wei 2009: 162–3). The establishment of pricing system was indicative of the transition from free markets to regulated markets of medicine. And this price system was needed for the implementation of affordable care policy.

New pricing system in regulated markets

The pricing system reached a new phase in the early 1990s, years highlighted by a wide variety of policy experiments and many new policy options. This new phase is marked by an emphasis on professional medical care criteria in the pricing exercises, an increased application of the market approach, and a further exploration of indirect state interventions called the "one arm-length approach." Beginning in 1992, the State Institutional Reform Commission (hereafter, STRC) called for liberalizing price control and making price adjustments through a market approach; it further underscored in 1993 the need to establish market mechanisms for pricing. As a watershed for the arrival of the regulated markets for drugs, the SPC began to make explicit the position in December 1994 that the pricing of drugs ought to be distinguished from that of commodities of a general nature, and that regulatory control over drug markets be treated differently from that of ordinary market situations (Wei 2009: 164–5).

With the first attempts, sovereign planners shifted to a market approach to address the issue of pricing management by making systematic efforts to introduce regulatory control over entry into drug markets in such areas as investment, the establishment of hospitals, new lines of hospital business, practices of doctors, and advanced medical devices (Guojia Yaopin Jiandu Guanliju 2003). In 1992, for example, the SGDMB issued a policy paper allowing enterprises broad discretion in handling the mark-ups of all their pharmaceutical products except for those of vital importance to the state policy and people's health.[4] In order to focus on restructuring pricing mechanisms and to lend the market a large role in price formation, SGDMB stressed in another policy paper in July 1992 that in price management, the state should provide general guidelines, only handle the retail prices of a small number of representative types of manufactured drugs, and move away from micro-management of particularities of drug pricing exercise. For example, it stated that the state ought to reduce case-by-case administrative interventions and focus, instead, on policy and pricing measures (Wei 2009: 163).

Also, the government stepped up its effort to introduce restrictions and uphold standards for drug-manufacturing enterprises, not only to ensure the curative effect, quality and safety of drugs but also to give incentives in terms of better prices for better compliance. This represented another significant landmark to incorporate the considerations of professional criteria into pricing policy. For instance, the SBDSM worked hard to introduce quality criteria and control, Good Manufacturing Practices (hereafter, GMP), and Good Storage Practices (hereafter, GSP) throughout the country. In addition, the concern for pharmaceutical standards led to the adoption of a licensing and registration system. For example, drug-manufacturing enterprises underwent a process of reissuing of licenses with the result that unqualified and substandard enterprises were driven out of business through screening and delisting procedures. Moreover, both wholesalers and retailers were made subject to periodic reviews and license reissuing exercises. The government established a drug registration system, too. As imported drugs were required to meet the requirements of technical assessments and to secure approval, import agencies were subject to review in order to establish their eligibility. In addition, the government set up mechanisms for the approval of new medicine, including panels of experts, standards, and procedures for the evaluation of new drugs. Also, the government undertook, for the first time, certifying all pharmacists, requiring them to pass examinations and to register according to set standards and requirements. (Guojia Yaopin Jiandu Guanliju 2003).

Furthermore, the SPC put forth the 1996 Provisional Measures, stipulating the apparatus, the policy content, types of drugs, and subjects for price control.[5] The 1996 Provisional Measures introduced, inter alia, price control for a short list of drugs, namely, "three major categories of drugs": namely, first, drugs produced by a monopoly (i.e., franchise); second, drugs for extensive clinical use, basic curative care and preventive care; and third, drugs used in neurology, anesthesia, and birth control.(Zhou 2008: 136–7). By dint of the

1996 Provisional Measures, these three categories of drugs were subject to mandatory pricing and advisory pricing, ensuring their accessibility and minimizing abuses. Transactions involving these drugs were regulated through supply/sale rates and W/R differentials (Wei 2009: 165). In the next year, 1997, the SPC issued another policy paper known as the 1997 Supplementary Regulations, representing one further step in providing guidance for the detailed operation of price management, such as the pricing by manufacturers and wholesalers who work under the price limits of producers, as well as incidents of oversupply or scarcity.[6]

Indicative of a major breakthrough of pricing policy, on November 3, 1998, the SPC promulgated the 1998 Policy, recognizing the profit rates that the drug industry often enjoyed in the marketplace and, meanwhile, bringing in some form of regulatory control.[7] While the 1998 Policy demonstrated its intent to encourage research and the development of new drugs, it set out limits that the drug industry needed to observe in pricing exercise. For instance, the policy set an upper-ceiling for profit rates for a variety of drugs: newly approved drugs, the new drugs and special drugs within a protective period, foreign drugs not listed in China's drugs catalog, drugs certified according to the standards of GMP, and drugs produced by joint ventures within the protective periods. In addition, the policy specified the preferential pricing for quality drugs, including GMP-certified drugs and other drugs of higher quality as approved by relevant authorities. The 1998 Policy was intended to impose control over excessive sales expenses, and it also sought to establish the relative weight of costs of marketing within the limit of prices of sales, e.g., promotion expenses, expenses of the sales units, costs of product registration, costs associated with clinical experiments, and transportation costs. In favor of the providing unit and medical personnel, the 1998 Policy recommended raising W/R differentials and medical services charges for drugs. Moreover, it introduced some form of price control by enhancing the transparency of pricing exercises, including introducing a system of recording and publication of drug prices (Zhou 2008: 138–42).

In its policy paper circulated in 2000, the SPC made an attempt to create a large space for market competition and to move away from detailed, overly complicated procedures in pricing management.[8] The SPC tried to limit its intervention by allowing price control only on retail, and not on all three links of supply/sale ratios from manufacturing, wholesale, and retail, as listed in the basic medical care insurance program. Also, it experimented with lifting control over supply/sale differentials between manufacturer and wholesaler (Guojia Jiwei 2001). In 2005 the government endeavored to exercise effective price control over all prescription drugs listed in the basic curative care program catalog. As a result, 2,400 kinds of drugs were included within the scope of pricing by the government (i.e., 1,500 kinds by the central government, 900 kinds by local governments), representing approximately 20 percent of drugs or 60 percent of total expenditure in China (Wei 2009: 165). As the rise of a system of regulatory control does not ensure its optimal operation, it is not unusual that many issues, especially pricing issues, would be raised in the process of enforcement that is to be examined next.

The drug franchise and pricing issues

In addressing the root problem of the exorbitant prices of drugs, policy-makers, policy analysts, and even the general public often pointed their fingers at the drug industry. However, in the absence of well-defined criteria and standards, determining what ought to be a "reasonable" price for each drug is always controversial. In fact, it is arguable when one tries to define what is meant by "exorbitant" and "artificial" with regard to drug prices. Besides, one would find different answers depending upon whether one adopts a policy-oriented or a market-oriented approach. The former pertains to the government's pricing in the name of the "collective good," which often lacks agreed upon operational definitions in the first place. And in the latter, pricing policy centers solely on considerations of the market conditions, such as the relationship between supply and demand. By and large, the latter involves definable and measurable criteria, and thus is less controversial.

Some policy analysts attribute the "exorbitant" charges for drugs to problematic regulatory control measures, including such components as drug franchising, the formation of drug prices, and high transaction costs. Consequently, the application of regulatory control encounters multiple factors—a long procedural chain and an exceedingly complex situation next to impossible.[9] For instance, the calculation of the prices of retail drugs often involves several phases in which costs are added with each phase until the drugs finally reach the patients, "consumers" in a broad sense of the medical care markets (Zhu 2006: 16).

"Exorbitant" price is often attributed to "middlemen." According to Wang Shuming, there were an estimated 13,000 drug wholesalers who played an important role in the wholesale business in the mid-2000s, including sale representatives hired by wholesalers and agencies at the first, second, and third tiers. Drug retailers and pharmacists were able to earn a share of more than 40 percent of the total profit rate at the hospital level. In Wang's estimate, even if retailers and pharmacies had been required to reduce 45 percent of prices on average for drugs sold on the markets, they would have still enjoyed a 10 percent profit rate. Wang observed, furthermore, that through several transaction links, drug prices were pushed to an artificially high level, so much so not being based on real costs. Pricing involved more transaction links than necessary, and kickbacks and commissions were often required at multiple links in addition to costs for commercials/advisements, etc. (Wang 2006: 68–9).

According to Liu Hongning and Yuan Jie, three related ratios were found relevant for calculating the price of drugs sold to patients: W/R differentials, discount rates, and sales promotion. First, given that W/R differentials for a hospital's retail franchise (e.g., 15 percent for Western medicine and 20 percent for folk herb medicine) remained unaltered, the differentials tended to work in favor of the medical care circle when the total volume of sales increased (see chapter 9). Second, the discount rates (often called "commission" or "kickbacks") were given to a hospital or an individual, legally or illegally, starting with 5 percent in 1980 but increasing to 30 percent or even 40 percent by the 1990s. By the same token, as the total volume of sales increased, it bought larger revenue to the providing unit even if the discount rates remained at the same, high level. Third, sales promotion expenses, normally estimated at 5–10 percent of total drug expenditure, were given directly to doctors (as a rule, about 40 percent of drugs are sold under a sales promotion scheme), often providing incentives to doctors to write "big prescriptions" (Liu & Yuan 2001: 5–7). It is noteworthy, above all, that the three ratios just described work as leverages: an increase in the percentage of any of the three would be translated into a proportionally large volume of expenditure to be borne by patients. In Wei Jigang's view, a large proportion of expensive drugs in the total volume of transactions tended to boost the revenue of the hospitals as well (Wei 2009: 218). According to Liu and Yuan, however, patients would not benefit visibly from a decrease in volume of any of the said three ratios, the impact of which would be too small to be felt by patients (Liu & Ycn 2001: 7).

Moreover, price control was to be enforced in order to encourage the drug industry's compliance to pharmaceutical standards, such as curative effects, quality, safety of drugs, and accessibility, but such standards were often violated because of local protectionism as well as revenue concerns on the part of the drug industry. For instance, some drugs that did not fulfill GMP criteria were supposed to be fixed at a lower price, but in practice GMP criteria were often ignored because of leeway granted by local authorities (Yang 2009; Zhou, Qu, & Li 2003). It appears that local authorities often chose to intervene in price control in connection of enforcement of pharmaceutical standards, warranting a close look at how bureaucratic politics had a bearing on price control and which key actors are involved.

Key actors in pricing game

Price control is concerned with the issue of policy implementation that can be treated properly from the government process/organizational behavior model as proposed by Graham Allison (Chapter 1). In reality, however, it often involved a maneuver among several key actors, grappling with each other in order to assert their interests and to gain the upper hand in the pricing game (Zhou 2008: 106–13). Several actors included the providing unit, members of drug industry, hospital management, multitudes of consumers and of course regulatory agencies. Hospital management and the drug industry often played active parts in the pricing game in the sense that any pricing episode would have a direct bearing upon the revenue they earned.

In general terms, regulatory agencies here refers to a number of government units, institutionally positioned and functionally defined, each oriented toward a given set of policy goals. Taken together they all act on behalf of the state, but, as their duty requires, they each speak on behalf of the department they represent. Moreover, these regulatory agencies might act in the name of the "public interest," but they each choose to define "public interest" according to their own perception, interpretation, policy concerns and emphases (Zhou 2008: 107). For example, the SPC's priority is the plan for national economic development in order to promote economic growth, operationally in charge of macro-management of pricing from a budgetary concern. Under the SPC's command, the price bureau focuses on controlling prices for health care services with an eye for stability in commodities prices, often acting on behalf of consumers in order to maintain low, affordable prices for curative care services, especially for drugs. Nonetheless, it is expected for the price bureau to strike a balance between the fiscal survival of providing units and the burden of the consumers. Under the MOF, the finance bureau, which often takes a pro-growth stand, tends to lend support to price adjustments as long as they lessen the burden of government subsidies (Zhou 2008: 107).

In practice, provincial and municipal/local health care bureaus tended to divert financial resources to the industrial sector, and, they were normally supporters of price increases as well as increases in any funding source other than government subsidies in order to ensure the effective and proper operation of providing units. Subject to the overall leadership of the MOH, officials in the health care bureau not only participated in the making of policy affecting pricing but also oversaw policy implementation.[10] And as these officials were given ultimate responsibility over delivering health care services, they tended to become natural allies to the providing units when it came to the matter of pricing, thus siding with the providing units at the expense of consumers (Zhou 2008: 107).

At the end of day, however, pricing became a game mainly between two institutional players: hospital management and the government. As previously noted, the propensity of the hospital to seek revenue hinged, by and large, on the amount of government subsidies made available to it and how rigidly the government was going to enforce price control. While the proportion of government subsidies devoted to "current expenditure" (jingfei) registered a steady decline at the providing unit level after the mid-1980s, hospital management (led by the director) was compelled to generate revenue through the sale of drugs in order to cope with financial shortfalls resulting from the dwindling government subsidies (Zhao 1999: 13).

Given variations in actual cases in the reform process, municipal/local jurisdictions, by and large, had a substantial stake in ensuring that drug enterprises were able to make profits and generate revenue for their respective jurisdictions.[11] These jurisdictions were least willing to see revenue derived from the drug industry dwindle through the lowering of sale prices (Wang

2006: 69). Besides that, there were blind spots in the monitoring and supervising of the pharmaceutical industry's pricing behavior. For example, the bureau of drugs mainly focused on curative effects, safety and quality in order to control the market entry of drugs, while the price bureau often chose to focus one-sidedly on the issue of whether the price schedule and mark-up of a given drug were affordable and appropriate. Consequently, these two bureaus might not be able to reach an agreement easily on the issue at hand, albeit they were expected to look into each case while balancing medical/professional criteria and economic considerations (Wang 2006: 69).

To maximize revenue for all parties concerned, three kinds of drug-related irregular pricing behaviors occurred in a three-way collaboration among the drug industry, hospital management and medical personnel: the sale of so-called "new drugs," substitution of expensive drugs for less expensive ones, and over-prescription of drugs (Liu & Yuan 2001; Zhou et al. 2003: 137; Wang 2008: 49; Zhou 2008: 135–56). The first kind had to do with abusing the label of so-called "new drugs," often manifested in the change of the brand names of old drugs in order to find excuses for marking up prices and therefore maximizing profits. And a great many "new drugs" were actually repackaged types using expired patents. For instance, most of these drugs (say, 97 percent) were produced and distributed by making use of the expired patents of medicines from foreign countries (Zhou, Qu, & Li 2003: 137). Irregularities involving the introduction of "new drugs," coupled with imported drugs, high-priced drugs and joint-venture drugs, often took advantage of loose standards and lax supervision by the government (Liu & Yuan 2001: 6–7; Zhu 2006: 16–17; Wei 2009: 221). The profit motive of the drug industry often distorted the professional and medical care concern for the curative effect, quality, and safety of drugs that is ideally embodied in the role of a well-trained, devoted pharmacist at the providing unit level. This situation has left much to be desired under the present stage of medical education in China and other related institutional arrangements (Wang 2011: 16). For example, the central ministries and municipal/local governments had the power to license new medicine, but overall the procedures for assessment and approval tended to be less than stringent. Given as an illustration by policy analysts Zhao Lei and Xue Bai, some 1,113 "new drugs" passed testing criteria and gained approval in China in 2005, while, by contrast, only 81 were approved by the USA's Food and Drug Administration in the same year (Zhao & Xue 2010: 48). The drug industry did not have real R&D capacity to produce as many new drugs as it claimed. According to Zhou, a recent trend for price control showed a discrepancy between the policy to encourage R&D and the actual research capacity of the drug industry (Zhou 2008: 138–9). Citing statistics from 2003 to 2005, Wei Jigang illustrates the discrepancy: the government approved 212 brands of chemical drugs among which only 17 brands were considered genuinely domestically developed, meaning that authentic, "new drugs" consisted only of 0.8 percent in that period (Wei 2009: 221).

In principle, better drugs ought to fetch better prices, but the government did not seem to enforce rigorously enough the existing standards and procedures for licensing new drugs, meaning that many old brands of drugs were priced and charged as new drugs (Wang 2001a: 2–3). In practice, moreover, medical/professional standards and requirements for licensing new drugs could not be upheld consistently across jurisdictions. In addition, local governments were likely to be influenced by local, vested interests in a deliberate move to give a green light for relaxing standards and regulations for new drugs (Wei 2009: 220–1).

The second kind of irregular behavior in drug pricing is concerned with substitution of expensive drugs for less expensive ones, given the same standards of quality, safety and curative effectiveness. For instance, hospital management and medical personnel often worked together to expand the number of medically substitutable but expensive drugs in order to maximize revenue, resulting in the marginalization of good quality, effective, and reasonably priced brands (Wu 2002: 5; Zhou 2008: 139; Yu 2008: 14–15). According to Wei Jigang, the preference of hospital management and medical personnel for high-price drugs often conveyed a distorted message to the markets and upset the proper operation of pricing mechanisms. In collaboration with hospital management and medical personnel, for example, the drug industry sought to maximize profits by producing and selling highly priced but medically substitutable categories of drugs (Wei 2009: 214–5). Moreover, the goals of health care services were often compromised, with reference to those cases of irregular and unnecessary prescriptions, prescriptions entailing safety risks, and above all, stoppage of production and marketing of "good drugs" (meaning effective, safe, and affordably priced ones) all together (Gao 2007b: 30; Yu 2008: 14–15).

The third kind pertained to over-prescriptions, making patients to take more medicine and pay more than necessary to cure the same illness. There was a substantial number of cases of excessive and unnecessary use of drugs at the providing unit level, estimated at 20 percent according to some surveys (Yu 2008: 15). It is claimed that some of these cases were and still are motivated by concerns about income and revenue. As Zhou Liangrong et al. put it, medical care is a type of profession that entails working with high risks which could have serious consequences for the health of patients (Zhou, Qu, & Li 2003: 148–9). To cope with medical uncertainty, doctors are entrusted with considerable discretion in diagnosis, examination, treatment, and drug prescription. However, when motivated by income and revenue, doctors and hospital management often worked together to abuse the power of drug prescription. More serious problems concern improper use of drugs, for instance, antibiotics and hormones, which could lead to serious adverse side-effects (Yu 2008: 15; Zhou 2008: 138–9).

On top of the pricing game centering on "three kinds of drug" just noted, an analyst suggests that hospital management adopted the financial strategy by maximizing revenue flow from the following areas: first, the increase of the total volume of expenditure on prescription drugs; second, the expansion of the portion of high-priced drugs in the total expenditure on prescription drugs; and third, the pursuit of net revenue in drug sales and high rates of kickbacks in the total volume of expenditure on drugs (Zhou 2003: 140). The first two sources had to do with the drug prescribing power of doctors, while the third required drugs sales representative to find ways. Apparently, all three were irregular.

In a new trend emerging from the reform, consumers assume a role in the marketplace pricing game, too. Consumers are effective actors in the drug markets in the sense that their choices and preferences bear on pricing. To put it in another way, consumers have gained considerable purchasing power since 1979 in dictating how much they want to spend for medicine, albeit the government and public insurances (understood as "society") still contribute a significant share of funding.[12] From various analytical categories, the amount, income, purchasing power, preferences, spending patterns, and other characteristics of consumers reflect how much weight they carry with regard to the volume of expenditure in health care services.[13] It is apparent, nonetheless, that not all people equally benefit from economic growth and improvement of living standards, and therefore some users can better afford to enjoy rapidly expanding and improving medical care services.

Since the mid-1980s, health care reform has been targeted at the new stratum of higher income users who were willing to spend more and could sustain the demand for highly priced services and drugs (Wang & Wang 2007: 23). Throughout the economic reform, the increase in the income of employees has heightened the demands of consumers and has enabled them to climb the ladder of needs from the basic level of food and shelter to higher levels of security and comfort. This new trend in consumerism reflects the legitimate pursuit of quality medical care, better medicine, and advanced medical devices. In addition, higher income patients have been willing to pay extra for more effective drugs and for minimizing risks as long as they can afford it (Zhou, Qu, & Li 2003: 144). Moreover, through public insurances (either PFMI, LIMC, or the new basic medical care insurance introduced after 1998, and formally after 2001) not only would the mechanism of a third party's payment reduce the sensitivity of the insured about charges and fees for drugs, but it would also create room for medical personnel and patients to collaborate to opt for the high end of the price range, given the substitutability among prescribed drugs for comparable medical effects (Zhou, Qu & Li 2003: 146). According to Zhao Yuxing, those patients who are cushioned by public insurances are often more likely to spend excessively for new drugs and expensive drugs (Zhao 1999: 13).

Above all, several key actors, such as the drug industry, hospital management and even users were inclined to push up prices of drug, making affordable care less accessible to the populace as a whole, and prompting the government to consider some policy options to control exorbitant charges of drugs, a topic to be tackled in the remaining passages.

Policy options for exorbitant charges

For more than two and half decades since 1994, the government has been conducting policy experiments with new combinations of both administrative and market tools in order to enforce regulatory control in the health care sector.[14] In concrete terms, sovereign planners have utilized a series of vigorous remedial measures to address, amidst the rise of drugs markets, issues of unanticipated and undesirable policy outcomes such as the exorbitant prices of drugs, revenue-maximizing orientation and abuses, and irregularities in the drugs markets, among others.[15] Some of these tools were commonly available in the early period of CPE while others resemble designs adopted in public management in the West.[16]

To ensure that patients could obtain lower prices on drugs, for example, relevant ministerial units took the initiative to enforce a series of measures in order to reduce the "artificially" high price of drugs, cluster by cluster. However, there were varying assessments among analysts and policymakers on the economic results as well as effects on consumers. As noted by Wang Yang, for example, from 1997 to 2000 there was a reduction of 11,000 million RMB in drug prices, resulting in a slower annual growth in the retail price of drugs from more than 10 percent in 1996 to about −0.1 percent in 2000 (Wang 2001b: 2). Hu Shanlian cites an investigation, claiming that for more than one decade from 1997 to 2007 there were 22 price adjustments resulting in a reduction of an estimated total of 66,760 million RMB; and on average, each reduction in price was within an estimated range of 15–20 percent for a selected batch of drugs (Hu 2007). Furthermore, Zhou Xuerong observes that the government's adoption of price reduction through a cluster-by-cluster strategy meant to minimize the difficulty of the providing unit to maintain a budgetary balance in the face of a sudden, increased financial burden (Zhou 2008: 154–5). According to Hu, moreover, the actual amount of reduction was not significantly large for each cluster because the providing units were often able to find ways to circumvent these price cuts. For example, hospital management increased charges by enlarging W/R differentials for the same period.[17] It is further claimed that patients might not have felt much substantial relief from the expense of cuts.[18]

Furthermore, in conjunction with the introduction of basic medical care insurance programs across jurisdictions, the government adopted a combination of several spending control measures, including collective bidding system for drug procurement, a catalog of basic drugs, and the system of designated hospitals and pharmacies (Zhou 2008: 155–6). First of all, top policymakers promoted collective bidding measures for procuring drugs starting July 7, 2000 in order to control expenditure on drugs, allowing a time frame of three years for its full implementation. The bidding measures were targeted at drugs involving a relatively large volume and those commonly used in clinical care; priority was given to drugs included in the catalogs for basic medical care insurance programs (Weishengbu et al. 2003). The adoption of collective bidding was intended to eliminate middlemen and thus curtail "irregular work style"—practices of bribery, kickbacks, and commissions. Hospitals were encouraged to take the initiative to organize collective bidding by themselves or jointly among several hospitals. As an alternative, hospital units were advised to hire a company to act as an agent to organize the collective bidding (Weishengbu et al. 2003).

However, there have been counter-measures at the providing unit level that have frustrated collective bidding exercises for drug procurement. For instance, clinicians and pharmacists have systematically made use of drug franchising to find high-priced but substitutable drugs. A survey of selected jurisdictions indicates that a mere 25–30 percent of drugs chosen through collective bidding was adopted by providing units while the remaining 70–5 percent was to be obtained through negotiated procurements (Zhou 2008: 112–3). As a pattern, clinicians and pharmacists often made use of the drug franchise at hand, deliberately choosing medically substitutable but high-priced drugs to replace those drugs selected as "winners" in the procurement exercises done through collective bidding; as a result, "winners" in the collective bidding were often not prescribed by clinicians (Zhou 2008: 111–2).

Still another way to combat the soaring expenditure of medical care services has been the introduction of state mandatory catalogs/lists of basic drugs, especially those used in medical care insurance programs (Yu 2011; Fan & Ma 2011). According to Hu, basic drugs on a state mandatory catalog/list are understood as follows: "the kind of drugs that can satisfy the health care demands of the majority of people; they always are available in adequate quantity and suitable types; and their prices are affordable to the individuals and communities concerned" (Hu 2007: 342). Such catalogs/lists represent a collection of criteria for drugs professionally chosen for basic medical care services. Supposedly, such lists would record the most economic selections according to the consideration of cost containment.[19]

In fact, the government first promulgated the Catalog of State Basic Drugs as early as 1982, which was updated with six versions up to 2011 (Fan & Ma 2011). In the reform era, ministerial authorities endeavored to create catalogs/lists of basic care drugs in line with the practices of the WHO and various countries, coupled with a series of implementing measures and organization-building efforts. Parallel to the policy experiments and pilot programs of medical care insurance reform, the use of a state mandatory catalog/list of basic drugs shifted into a higher gear in the 1990s with several major updates subsequently for more than one decade, notably in 1992, 1996, and 1999.[20]

The task of establishing state mandatory catalog of basic drugs is not only limited to the construction of operational definition, and it requires to find effective ways of implementation. According to Hu Shanlian et al., the state mandatory catalog for basic drugs needs to go beyond the compiling, listing, and updating of basic drugs. In some policy analysts' view, it is equally important to establish compatible mechanisms, controls and procedures, and relevant institutions at every key link in the process of implementation, such as manufacturing, sales and marketing, use and pricing, taxation and public finance, and funding and payments in order to enforce the basic catalog (Hu, Zhang, & Ye 2007). Accordingly, ministerial authorities produced in 2009 a series of policy papers to support the follow-up work in enforcing the listing of basic category drugs, including mechanisms for evaluating and selecting (e. g., independent review institutes), procedures to ensure the priority listing of curative care services, the introduction of the client-oriented principle, assurances for funding and timely provision especially to providing units in the lower echelons, and responsiveness to the requests of clinics in community and rural areas.[21]

In fact, the relevant ministries continued to intervene in organizational issues relating to prescription drugs, lending considerable weight to pharmacists within the providing units. Not only did they endeavor to ensure the institutional status of pharmacy management to be properly recognized, but also strived to define clearly and sanction strongly its main functions and duties. For instance, professional qualifications and recruitment criteria for pharmacists were established and stipulated in relevant policy papers: pharmacists were in charge of dispensary services, standard operational procedures, and the matter of doctors' instructions; in addition, they managed, reviewed, and checked prescriptions. To obviate the possible abuses and irregularities of one-man rule under the head of a drug department, moreover, the 1999 Provisional Measures installed a collective decision-making mechanism through establishing the "Management Committee of Drug Affairs in Second and Third Tier Hospitals" (Laodong he shehui baoxianbu et al. 2003). In addition, starting in 2001, the use of the lists/catalogs for basic drugs has been incorporated into the framework of quasi-markets through systematically constructing networks of designated hospitals and designated drug retail stores in conjunction with establishing basic medical care insurance programs (Laodong he Shehui Baoxianbu, Weishengbu & Guojiazhong Yiyao Guanliju 2003).

In order to impose some measures of control over the costs of prescription drugs, moreover, the first attempt was made, targeting the outpatient. For example, relevant ministries promulgated a set of regulations to establish a system of designated retail drug stores in the midst of building the quasi-markets under the basic medical care insurance program. As an integral part of the contractual framework in allocation of insurance fund, these designated retail drug stores were, accordingly, given the franchise for prescription drugs for outpatients whose expenditure on prescription drugs consists of approximately 20 percent of the total spent on curative care services. The designated retail drug stores for outpatients were meant to dilute the over concentration of dispensary care services in the hands of hospital management and doctors in order to promote market competition within the quasi-market in drug sales, and thus bring down the price of prescription drugs. While the power of doctors for issuing drug prescriptions was still honored, the market share of retail prescription drugs was not exclusively given to hospitals, but, instead, it was granted to designated drug retailers in the marketplace (Laodong he Shehui Baoxianbu & Guojia Yaopin Jiandu Guanliju 2003).

From the above analysis, it has become apparent that the endeavors of cost containment regarding drugs have inter-phased with building the quasi-market pertaining to basic medical care insurances throughout the country since the late 1990s. With many innovative policy measures by the government, it is expected that the providing unit and drug industry are likely to produce counter-measures in a continuous wrestling centering on the hot issue of exorbitant charges to medicine in health care in China, an issue deserving further investigation in due course.

Concluding remarks

The foregoing analysis has covered the rise of free markets in medicine during the early period of the reform, its transformation into regulated markets subsequently, and the creation of quasi-markets in conjunction with the inauguration of basic medical care insurance starting in 2001. However, it is not expected that the performance of the markets was optimal. The growth in the drug markets accompanied the diversity of ownership and types, decentralization of macro-management, and, above all, revenue-maximizing tendencies. The drug industry also became entangled in local politics, in turn, erecting obstacles to adopting unified standards, criteria for the safety and quality of drugs, and an effective licensing system of new drugs. Many abuses such as over-provision and substitution of expensive drugs for less expensive and commonly used ones were prevalent. The core of the problem has to do with the substantial difficulty in curtailing the abuse of drug franchising, and the discretionary power of providing units and medical care personnel. Sovereign planners' measures have not appeared effective due to the lack of a clear, operational definition and workable criteria with reference to the abuses and irregularities in fees/charges. These have to do with the roots of issues that have continued to reinforce the revenue-maximizing orientation of providing units, coupled with inadequate government appropriation and excessive reliance upon drug franchising, and revenue targets, inter alia. (Gao 2007: 63–5).

The issue of non-compliances concerning the "three kinds of drugs" just noted is concerned with both micro-management and macro-management. From the perspective of micro-management, for instance, sub-optimal results of regulatory control appeared attributable to the shortage of needed information, a policy episode in congruence with the decision-making approach. To fend off bureaucratic control, in addition, medical personnel did enjoy advantage in resisting performance appraisal, as anticipated by the uncertainty approach (Chapter 1 & 8). Also, in the transactions of medical care between the two sides: the doctor and patient, the former was able to enjoy advantage in relations to the latter regarding the choice of options of treatments according to the asymmetric information theory (Chapter 1). In light of macro-management, sovereign planners failed to establish the central government's control, and maintain consistency of regulatory control across provincial jurisdictions with reference to the issues of safety, quality and effects of drugs in view of lack of trained personnel and expertise, overwhelming workload, and long-time lag required for full implementation. This makes learning from American experience of FDA next to the impossible in China, in spite of rising expectation associated with widespread globalization. As a result, sovereign planners have to accept less than desirable policy option—the decentralization of regulator control to the provincial level. (Yang 2009). As noted, for example, the local jurisdictions were involved politically in the three-way collaboration among the drug industry, providing units and medical personnel against regulatory agencies in abusing pricing policy of new drugs, expensive but substitutable drugs, and the practice of over-prescriptions. Last, but not least, the foregoing analysis of the policy episode pertaining to regulatory control on drugs has exhibited key characteristics of the government process/organizational behavior model, albeit the government politics model found pertinent to explain some irregularities in enforcing pricing control of drugs.

Notes

1 The full title of the policy paper reads as follows: "Circular Concerning the Strengthening of Market Management of Wholesale Drug Markets" (Wei 2009: 150).
2 Wang Yang gave a report about what was on the policy agenda for tackling price reform in drug and curative care services in 2000 (Wang, 2001a: 151–4).
3 The full title of the "2000 General Circular" reads as follows: "General Circular of the Ministry of Health Care concerning the Pilot Program for Strengthening Unified Bidding in Procurement by Medical Care and Pharmacy Institutes" (hereafter, "2000 General Circular") (Weishengbu Weisheng Fazhi Yu Jiandusi 2001).
4 The SGBPM put forth the "Opinion Regarding the Better Management of Large and Medium SOEs in the Drug Industry" in 1992 (Wei, 2009: 163).
5 The full title of the policy paper reads as follows: "Provisional Measures for Price Management of Drugs" (abbreviated as "1996 Provisional Measures") (Zhou, 2008: 136–7).
6 The title of the policy paper is the "Supplementary Regulations for the Provisional Measures of Price Management of Drugs" (hereafter, (Guile comment: please insert the abbreviation)) (2008: 136–8).
7 The full title of the policy paper is the "Policy Concerning the Perfecting of Prices of Drugs" (hereafter, "1998 Policy") (Zhou 2008: 138–42).
8 The State Planning Commission circulated the "Opinion Concerning the Reform of Price Management of Drugs in 2000" (hereafter, the 2000 Opinion) (Guojia Jiwei 2001).
9 For example, the pricing exercise needs to consider a long list of factors: costs of R&D, production costs, costs of marketing and sales, profits of pharmaceutical industries, costs and earnings of wholesale business units, commissions and kickbacks to medical personnel, commissions to the providing units, and costs added to procurement by the providing unit.

10 It appears that the health care bureau had a dual role, both as policymaker and policy enforcer, in accordance with the practice of "inseparability between the policymaking body and enterprise" (zhengqi bufen) (Zhou, 2008: 108).

11 It is difficult to maintain uniformity and coordination of price control among various governmental units and across various jurisdictions. For example, some local government units might opt for helping hospitals out, e.g., by allowing for flexible pricing or larger W/R differentials when they could not make funding available to subsidize basic medical care services, but some other governmental units or jurisdictions might not be so inclined (Wang, 2006: 69).

12 Moreover, the financial input of the government decreased from 32.16 percent in 1978 to 16.96 percent in 2003, and the input from social organizations (e.g., public insurers) declined from 47.41 percent in 1978 to 27.16 percent in 2003, while expenditure by individual users increased from 20.43 percent in 1978 to 55.87 percent in 2003, reflecting the increasing importance of the consumer's voice. The expanding share of the expenditure by individual users took place on the basis of overall increase of total expenditure at the national level, that multiplied by 67.87 for 25 years from 11,021 million RMB in 1978 to 759,029 million RMB in 2004 (Wang & Wang 2007: 17–8).

13 As an improved purchasing power among the people propels expanding the volume of expenditure in medical care services in general and drugs in particular, so the new style of medical care consumerism adds fuel to the skyrocketing of drug prices. It is well understood, moreover, an increase in population and aging, as well as the changing illness profile have started to reshape the demands for medical care services during the reform era (Wang & Wang 2007: 23).

14 Wang Bingyi provides a profile of macro-management of health care markets, highlighting price management in medical care services in general and in dispensary services in particular (Wang 2008: 228–85).

15 Wang Yang took inventory of policy issues and measures that had been put on the policy agenda from 1996 to 2000 (Wang, 2001a). Also, in 2006, Minister of Health Care Gao Qiang conducted a review of what was to be done about exorbitant drug prices (Gao 2007a).

16 Examples include tours of inspection and investigation, a "performance pledge" made by health care personnel themselves, transparency in fee schedules, computerized systems of financial and accounting procedures, computerized medical care cases, a licensing system for providing units, and permits of practices for medical personnel (Zheng 2003: Gao 2007a: 61–3).

17 According to Hu, although the W/R ratio was 15 percent, in many cases hospital units would fetch 30–40 percent revenue calculated through the W/R ratio in some jurisdictions (Hu, 2007).

18 In a rough estimate for seven years from 1997 to 2004, for example, the total reduction amounts to 30,000 RMB, approximately 10 percent of the total expenditure for medical care services. And only 2004 alone, it stands at 333,154 RMB (Hu 2007).

19 In 1999, several ministries offered an operational definition of "basic drugs" as drugs meeting "the essential needs of clinical care, safety and effectiveness, reasonable prices, convenient to use and market supply ensured." See "The Provisional Measures for Managing the Scope of Drug Use in the Basic Medical Care of Staff and Workers in Cities and Towns" (Laodong he Shehui Baozhangbu *et al.*, 2003: 74–6).

20 For example, in 1992, the Ministry of Health Care and four other ministerial units jointly produced the "State Catalog of Basic Drugs" (Hu 2007: 342). In 1999, the relevant ministries promulgated "The Provisional Measures for Managing the Scope of Drug Use in the Basic Medical Care of Staff and Workers in Cities and Towns" (hereafter, "1999 Provisional Measures"), endeavoring to streamline

managing the use of prescription drugs at the providing unit level (Laodong he Shehui Baozhangbu *et al.*, 2003: 74–6). The state mandatory catalog was updated further in 1996, including 2,398 items (with both Western and folk herbal drugs), and it was subsequently updated four times until 2004. Its final list contained 2,033 items as of 2004 (Hu 2007: 342).

21   Nine relevant ministries led by the Ministry of Health Care proceeded to beef up implementation of the catalog for basic drugs by promulgating, in September 2009, another set of policy papers called the "Measures for Managing the State Catalog for Basic Drugs" (Fan 2011).

References

Fan, L., & Ma, A. 2011. Woguo jiben yaowu mulu lingxuan xianguan wenti tantao (Discussion on several relevant issues of the selection of the basic drugs catalog in China). *Weisheng jingji yanjiu* (Research on Health Care Economics), 4: 3.

Gao, Q. 2007a. Dangqian kaizhan weisheng jiufeng gongzuo, jiejue kanbingnan kanbinggui wenti mianlin de xingshi he jiben silu (The current task of rectification in health care, the situation and basic consideration to solve the problems of difficulty to see doctors and expensiveness to see doctors). In Zhongguo Weisheng Nianjian Bianji Weiyuanhui (Ed.), *Zhongguo weisheng nianjian 2007* (China's Yearbook of Health Care 2007), 61–69. Beijing: Renmin weisheng chubanshe.

Gao, Q. 2007b. Weishengbu buzhang Gao Qiang zai quanguo chengshi shequ weisheng gongzuo huiyi shang de zongjie jianghua (Minister Gao Qiang, MOH, concluding speech at the national conference of community health care work). In Zhongguo weisheng nianjian bianji weiyuanhui (Ed.), *Zhongguo weisheng nianjian 2007* (China's Yearbook of Health Care 2007), 33–37. Beijing: Renmin chubanshe.

Ge, Y., & Gong, S. 2007. *Zhongguo yiliao gaige: Wenti, genyuan, chulu* (China's Health Care Reform: Problems, Roots and Solutions). Beijing: Zhongguo fazhen chubanshe.

Guojia Jiwei. 2001. Guojia jiwei guanyu gaige yaoping jiage guanli de yijian (The opinion of the state planning commission concerning the reform of the pharmaceutical price managment). In Weishengbu Weisheng Fazhi Yu Jiandusi (Ed.), 24–26. Beijing: Beijing falu chubanshe.

Guojia Yaopin Jiandu Guanliju. 2003. Guanyu guanche chengzhen yiyao weisheng tizhi gaige zhidao yijian de shishi yijian (The opinion for through implementation of the advisory opinion of institutional reform of medical and health care in cities and towns). In Guowuyuan Jiuzheng Henye Buzheng Zhifeng Bangongshi (Ed.), *Jiuzheng buzheng zhifeng gongzuo zhinan* (Guidlines for the Eradication of Irregular Work Style), 57–63. Beijing: Zhongguo fangzheng chubanshe.

Guowuyuan. 1989. Yaozheng guanli tiaoli (shixing) (The regulations of management of drugs policy, trial implementation). In Guojia Yiyao Guanliju (Ed.), *Yiyao gongzuo wenjian xuanbian* (The Selected Documents for the Task of Pharmacy), 12–17. Beijing: Zhongguo yiyao keji chubanshe.

Hu, S. 2007. Jianli guojia jiben yaobing zhidu de zhengce (To establish the national policy of basic medicine system). InL.Du, W.Zhang, & Zhongguo Weisheng Canye Zachishe (Eds.), *Zhonguo yiliao weisheng fazhan baogao, No. 3* (The Report on the Development of Medical and Health Care in China, No. 3), 340–352. Beijing: Shehui kexue wenxian chubanshe.

Hu, S., Zhang, Y., & Ye, L. 2007. Guojia jieben yaowu zhidu yanjiu (A study of state basic drugs system). *Weisheng jingji yanjiu* (Research on Health Care Economics), 10: 3–5.

Laodong he Shehui Baozhangbu *et al.* 2003. Chengzhen zhigong jiben yiliao baoxian yongyao fanwei guanli zanxing banfa (The provisional measures of management of the scope of drug use for basic medical care insurance of staff and workers in cities and towns). In Guowuyuan Jiuzheng Hangye Buzhengzhifeng Bangongshi (Ed.), *Jiuzheng yiyao guoxiaozhong buzheng zhifeng gongzuo zhinan* (Guiidelines for the Eradiction of Irregular Work Style in the Procurement and Sale of Drugs), 74–77. Beijing: Zhongguo fangzhen chubanshe.

Laodong he Shehui Baozhangbu, Weishengbu, & Guojia Zhongyiyao Guanliju. 2003. Chengzhen zhjigong jiben yiliao baoxian dingtian yiliao jigou guanli zanxing banfa (The provisional measures of designated medical care institutes for basic medical care insurance of staff and workers in cities and towns). In Guowuyuan Jiuzheng Hangye Buzhengzhifeng Bangongshi (Ed.), *Jiuzheng yiyao gouxiao zhong buzheng zhi feng gongzuo zhinan* (Guidelines for the Eradication of Irregular Work Style in the Procurement and Sale of Drugs), 68–72. Beijing: Zhongguo fangzheng chubanshe.

Laodong he Shehui Baozhangbu, & Guojia Yaopin Jiandu Guanliju. 2003. Chengzhen zhigong jiben yiliao baoxian dingtian lingshou yaodian guanli zanxing banfa (The provisional measures of management of designated retail stores for the basic medical care insurance of staff and workers in cities and towns). In Guowuyuan Jiuzheng Hangye Buzhengzhifeng Bangongshi (Ed.), *Jiuzhen yiyao gouxiao zhong buzheng zhi feng gongzuo zhinan* (Guidelines for the Eradication of Irregular Work Style in the Procurement and Sale of Drugs), 78–79. Beijing: Zhongguo fangzheng chubanshe.

Liu, H., & Yuan, J. 2001. Dui yiyuan yaopin jingying zhong fanchang xianxian de fenxi (An analysis of irregular phenomenon in the business of hospital medicine). *Weisheng jingji yanjiu* (Research on Health Care Economics), 3: 6–8.

Quanguo renmin daibiao dahui changwu weiyuanhui. 1989. Zhonghua renmin gongheguo yaopin guanlifa (the law of pharmacy management of the PRC). In Guojia Yiyao Guanli Ju (Ed.), *Yiyao gongzuo wenjian xuanbian* (Selected Documents for the Task of Pharmacy), 3–8. Beijing: Zhongguo yiyao guanliju.

Wang, B. 2008. *Zhengfu yiliao guamzhi moshi ghonggou yanjiu* (Research on the Restructuring of Mode of Governmental Control). Beijing: Renmin chubanshe.

Wang, L. 2011. Jiben yiliao baozhang kuangjiaxia woguo yaopin jiage helihua fenxi (An analysis of rationalization of prices of drugs under the framework of medical care insurance in China). *Weisheng jingji yanjiu* (Research on Health Care Economics), 4: 14–17.

Wang, S. 2006. Daya yaopin jiawei xugao yingchong yuantuo zhuaqi (To control the artificially high price of drugs one should start with their origin). *Zhongguo weisheng jingji* (China's Health Care Economics), 25: 68–69.

Wang, Y. 2001a. Yinru jingzheng jizhi jinyib shenhua yaopin he yiliao fuwu jiage gaige (To introduce mechanisms of competition, and to go further price reform of medicine and medical services). In Goujia Fazhan Jihua Weiyuanhui Jiagesi (Ed.), *Yiyao jiage zhengce zhinan* (Guides for Pricing Policy of Medicine), 1–16. Beijing: Zhongguo wujia chubanshe.

Wang, Y. 2001b. Yinru jinzheng jizhi jinyibu shenhua yaopin he yiliao fuwu jiage gaige (Introduce the mechanism of competition, go further with the price reform of medicine and medical care services). In Guojia Fazhan Jihua Weiyuanhui Jiagesi (Ed.), *Yiyao jiage zhengce zinan* (Guides for Pricing Policy of Medicine), 1–15. Beijing: Zhongguo wujia chubanshe.

Wang, Y., Wang, W. 2007. Kaishu shangzhang de yiliao feiyong yu kanbienlan kanbiengui wenti (The problems of raising medical care charges as well as the difficulty to seek treatment of illness and expensiveness to seek cure). In J. Chen, J. & Wang, Y. (Ed.), *Zhonggui shehui baozhang fazhan baoguo* (The Report of Development of Social Insurance in China), 17–36. Beijing: Zhongguo shehui kexue wenxian chubanshe.

Wei, J. 2009. *Zhongguo yiyao tizhi gaige yu fazhan* (The Reform and Development of the Medicine System in China). Beijing: Shanwu yinshuguan.

Weishengbu. 1989. Guanyu jianyi chengli guojia yiyao guanliju de baogao (The report concerning the establishment of the state general bureau of pharmacy management). In Guojia Yiyao Guanliju (Ed.), *Yiyao gongzuo wenjian xuanbian* (The Selected Documents for the Task of Pharmacy), 9–10. Beijing: Zhongguo yiyao keji chubanshe.

Weishengbu *et al.* 2003. Yiliao jigou yaopin jizhong zhaobiao caigou shidian gongzuo ruogan guiding (Several regulations of the pilot tasks in teh procurement through collective bidding of drugs of medical care institutes). In Guowuyuan Jiuzheng Hangye Buzhengzhifeng Bangongshi (Ed.), *Jiuzheng yiyao guoxiao zhong buzheng zhifeng gongzuo zhinan* (Guildelines for the Eradication of Irregular Work Style in Procurement and Sale of Drugs), 85–89. Beijing: Zhongguo fangzhen chubanshe.

Weishengbu Weisheng Fazhi Yu Jiandusi. 2001. Weishengbu guanyu jiaqiang yiliao jigou yaoping jizhong zhaobiao caigou shidian guanli gongzuo de tongzhi (The general circular of the Ministry of Health care concerning the pilot program of strengthening the unified bidding in procurement in medical care and pharmacy institutes). In Weishengbu Weisheng Fazhi Yu Jiandusi (Ed.), *Zhonghua remin gongheguo weisheng fagui huibian* (The Collection of Laws and Regulations of Health Care of the People's Republic of China), 885–886. Beijing: Beijing falu chubanshe.

Wu, M. 2002. Yaopin fuwu tigong gecheng zhong xunzu xingwei chansheng yuanyin fenxi (Analysis on the cause of rent-seeking behavior in the provision of dispensary services). *Zhongguo weisheng jingji* (China's Health Care Economics), 21(11): 4–6.

Yang, D. 2009. Rgulatory Learning and Its Discontent in China: Promise and Tragedy at the State Food and Drug Administration. In Gillespie, J. & R. Peerenboom (Eds.) *Regulation in Asia : Pushing Back on Globalizaton*: 115-39; 284-8. London: Routledge.

Yin, W., Zhang, Y., & Zhang, C. 2011. Shishi guojia jiben yaowu zhidu de shijian yu sikao (The practice and considerations of the introduction of the state basic drugs system). *Weisheng jingji yanjiu* (Research on Health Care Economics), 4:12–13.

Yu, D. 2008. Quexiao yiyi buyi qieduan yiyao jingji liyi lianxi jianli fangkong yiyao gouxiao lingyu shangye huilou de changxiao jizhi (To abolish financing medical care through drugs to sever the connection of economic interests of pharmacy, and to establish the long lasting mechanisms to curtail commercial bribery in the sphere of drugs sale and procurement). *Zhongguo weisheng jingji* (China's Health Care Economics), 27(2):14–16.

Yu, D. 2011. Guojia jiben yaowu zhidu shishi guochengzhong chuxian de wenti he jiejue duice (The problems and solutions in the process of establishment of the state basic drugs system). *Zhongguo weisheng jingji* (China's Health Care Economics), 30 (12): 9–10.

Zhao, L., & Xue, B. 2010. Qianghua disanfan zeren, dapo yiyuan shuanxian long-duan: Gaibien yiyao yangyi dizhi de lujin (strengthening the third party's responsi-bility and breaking the hospital's bilateral monopoly: The chosen path to transform the structure of financing medical care through pharmacy). *Zhnogguo weisheng jingji* (China's Health Care Economics), 29(7): 47–50.

Zhao, Y. 1999. Woguo yiliao yaopin feiyong fenxi (Analysis on expenses of medical care and pharmacy in China). *Zhongguo weisheng jingji* (China's Health Care Economics), 6:12–14.

Zheng, X. 2003. Guojia yaopin jiadu guanliju juzhang zheng xiaoyu zai quanguo jiuzheng yiyao gouxiao zhong buzhengzhifeng gongzuo dianshi huiyi shang de fayan. In Guowuyuan Jiuzheng Hangye Buzhengzhifeng Bangongshi (Ed.), *Jiuzheng yiyao gouxia zhong buzhengzhifeng gongzuo zhinan* (Guildelines for the Era-diction of Irregular Work Style in Procurement and Sale of Drugs), 29–31. Beijing: Zhongguo fangzheng chubanshe.

Zhou, L., Qu, Q., & Li, G. 2003. *Jujiao weisheng gaige* (Focusing on the Health Care Reform). Beijing: Zhongguo shehue chubanshe.

Zhou, X. 2008. *Zhongguo yiliao jiage de zhengfu guanzhi yanjiu* (A Study on the Government Control of Medical Care Pricing in China). Beijing: Zhongguo shehui kexue chubanshe.

Zhu, Y. 2006. Woguo yaopin jiage xugao liyi zhuti de liyi fenbu ji chengyin fenxi (Analysis on interest configuration among interest entities as well as its causes in case of artificial high prices of pharmaceutic products). *Zhongguo weisheng jingji* (China's Health Care Economics), 25(11):15–18.

Part IV

Conclusion

11 Review and assessment

The foregoing analysis examined the conventional medical care system first built as an integral part of CPE, and, tried to account for its transformation through several subsequent phases into a new system supported by two main pillars such as public hospitals and public insurances from 1979 to the present. It appears that China's health care reform represents a social engineering endeavor with considerable breadth, complexity and challenges, and it remains a gradual and on-going process. Sovereign planners have been trying to bridge the gaps between policy and performance, while adhering to the commitment of affordable care for all people in China. It is germane here to continue to monitor the overall policy trend and make a preliminary assessment of the outcome of re-engineering endeavors on the basis of available data and information in subsequent three sections.

The changing balance between the state and markets

Emerging from reform efforts over several decades, sovereign planners have been able to articulate an explicit view in order to delineate which types of health services ought to fall into the area of responsibility of the state, and the others are left to the markets (Chapter 2). According to the 2009 Opinion, the government acts on behalf of the state, treating the basic medical care as "collective goods," and reaffirming its commitment to the provision of affordable care for all at the essential level. Meanwhile, it outlines the roles of the state and markets respectively in four major tasks that the government plans to undertake: public and preventive health care, medical care delivery system, insurance programs and supply of drugs (Zhonggong zhongyang, Guowuyuan 2009).

First, the government plans to build professional networks for public and preventive health care, coupled with clearly defined priorities among public health care programs undertaken by both central and local governments. While the central government focuses on some well-chosen programs as an anchor, the provincial authorities are encouraged to top up with their own programs and funding schemes adaptable to the local needs. Also, the government is able to build mechanisms to address public health care emergencies. In the 2009 Priority Implementation Plan, policymakers set up concrete targets for public health care, for example, the annual average subsidies for minimum public health services at 15 RMB per person for 2009 and 20 RMB for 2011. It is required to include personnel costs, infrastructure investments, managerial expenditure and revenue from services into the government budget in full. So long as it is financially feasible, the state is expected to fund chosen immunization programs and shoulder the costs of those programs regarding serious illness such as tuberculosis and AIDS (Guowuyuan 2009).

Second, the government intends to re-structure the medical care delivery system, making public, non-profit-oriented providing units as the main pillar and allowing non-public, profit-oriented units to assume a supplementary role. The government has adopted a strategy to construct and consolidate the networks of medical and health care services in the low echelons of the Party-state hierarchy. For example, the government has chosen to build health care facilities in townships and heath care clinics in villages, serving as foundation of rural medical and health care networks coordinated by a cluster of county hospitals. Also, the government has been trying to strengthen the urban community health care centers that act as "gate-keepers" centering on primary care. In addition, the government has been taking initiatives to build the "integrated delivery system" by connecting the urban community health centers and rural health care facilities in townships to public hospitals through a referral system (Du, Zhang & Xu 2009: 17). Also, the emphasis on lower echelons means to correct the "reverse pyramid" of overconcentration of health care resources at the public hospital level, encouraging users to make full use of facilities at lower level to treat common and frequent illnesses, while reserving public hospitals for the treatment of complicated and difficult cases.

The government has also established the priority and targets to build and strengthen the medical and health care facilities in lower echelons in urban and rural areas. For example, it has planned to build and re-structure 3,700 community health care centers and 11,000 community health stations in cities throughout China within three years from 2009 to 2011. In addition, the central government has made a commitment to constructing 2,000 key county hospitals during the same period. Incorporated into the plan, moreover, it intends to support building 29,000 health institutes in townships in 2009, and further expand and rebuild 5,000 health institutes in townships (Guowuyuan 2009).

With regard to the public hospital reform, the government has made pledges ultimately to abolish the drug franchise funding system by reducing three funding sources (curative care fees, drug charges and government subsidies) to two sources (curative fees and government subsidies). As an interim arrangement, the government will undertake to re-structure financial management and address the issue of budgetary balance at the providing unit level. On the one hand it will seek to lend appropriate recognition to the value of the medical/technical component of curative care service, for example, making upward adjustments of curative care fees and dispensary service charges. On the other hand, it will try to fill up the gaps in government's budgetary appropriation to infrastructure investments, procurement of large and expensive equipment, as well as the spending in public health care programs at the public hospital level.

In order to set a brake on the irregular practices of upgrading treatments from the basic medical care to special care category unnecessarily, the government will try to impose a limit of up to 10 percent of the special care service in the total of medical care services in order to prevent public hospitals from diverting resources and manpower to revenue-earning activities at expenses of basic medical care (Guowuyu 2009: 43).

To help users to pay their medical bills, third, the government has pledged to fill gaps in coverage of public insurances. As soon as the basic medical care insurance packages formally inaugurated from 2001 onward, the state lost no time to start the NRCMCI in 2003, and URBMCI in 2007, trying to alleviate financial burden of users first focusing on catastrophic medical events and then moving gradually into a large number of common but less expensive types of services depending upon financial feasibility. For sure, this marks a change of funding mode from subsidies to providers to subsidies to users, notably in NRCMCI. The 2009 Opinion urged to accelerate the constructing of public insurance systems coupled with supplementary insurances and commercial health insurances. It adopted the strategy for building an insurance system with broad coverage, focusing on basic medical care, and sustainability, aiming at covering both the employed and unemployed population in urban area, rural peasantry, and the needy in urban area. It was proposed to embrace all those personnel of bankrupt enterprises, enterprises with financial difficulties, retirees, and "flexibly employed personnel" into URBMCI, while encouraging agricultural laborers to enroll in the BMCI (Zhonggong zhongyang & Guowuyuan 2009: 27–8; Guowuyuan 2009: 38).

By the late 2000s, the government was confident enough about the implementation of health insurance plans for all, pledging to increase insurance enrollment to more than 90 percent in the total population, including three major public insurances, i.e., BMCI, URBMCI, and NRCMCI. Also, it was in position to recommend an increase of subsidies to NRCMCI up to annual average 120 RMB per person, and a raise of the ceiling of payment to six times of annual average income of residents for all three public insurances. In view of a considerable saving of each insurance program, it was recommended to control saving to a reasonable level, for instance, no more than 15 percent of annual saving in the total of NRCMCI fund, and no more than 25 percent of accumulative saving in the same (Guowuyuan 2009: 38–9).

Fourth, the 2009 Opinion recommended to establish the state basic drug system, stressing drug safety, quality, curative effects and supply. On the one hand, the 2009 Opinion reiterates the principle of reasonable prices and affordability of drugs, and proposes to adopt concrete measures to ensure the low-price policy of drugs. For example, it lends priority to drafting the state basic drug catalog, establishing a collective bidding procedure in the basic drugs, compiling manuals and guides for clinical use of drugs, preparing a collection of model cases of basic prescription drugs, and building a supply network of drugs in rural area. On the other hand, it places emphasis on the issues of safety, quality and curative effects, urging to strengthen regulatory control on market entry, introduce licensing of new drugs, impose monitoring of drug safety incidents, and establish effective control measures (Guowuyuan 2009: 39–40).

Through the new health care reform of the 2009 vintage, it is apparent that sovereign planners have demonstrated a much clearer mapping of entire terrain of the health care services as well as the respective roles of the state and markets in it. This mapping is largely in congruence with the theoretical analysis of this study with regard to how to make the best out of the strengths of either the state or markets, while avoiding weaknesses of each, in the implementation of affordable care policy as noted in the preceding chapters.

The re-engagement of the state

As policymakers have made considerable effort to provide basic medical care services to the people, it is appropriate to ask: is medical care affordable for all residents in China at the end of the day? To address the question, one needs to examine how much each user has to pay for various services in the context of market transactions relative to their purchasing power. And do they find it affordable within their own means? It is germane here to dwell on the consequences of high percentages of personal expenditure, and sovereign planners' endeavors to restore the balance among three funding sources, and to reduce the share of financial burden on the user from the late 1990s to the present.

It is evident that there exist, varying from year to year, pockets of the population in China which cannot seek for a cure in illness. How large were these pockets during those years of the highest percentages of personal expenditure for health care during the late 1990s and early 2000s previously mentioned (Chapter 4)? For example, a survey indicates that for those residents who reported ill within two weeks of the onset of their illness but did not seek cure, there registered an increase visibly about ten percentage points from 38.5 percent in 1998 to 48.9 percent in 2003 (Wang 2008: 268).

Given that other things are equal, the percentages of residents seeking cure in illness are co-related to their income levels. According to the analysis of the third national investigation of national health care services, in the lowest 1/5th income (or low income) bracket in rural area, those residents (or normally taken as outpatients) who failed to seek a cure in illness consisted of 35.4 percent in 1993, 30.7 percent in 1998, and 46 percent in 2003, while in the same income bracket in urban area those residents who failed to seek cure in illness comprise 37.5 percent in 1993, 49.1 percent in 1998, and 60.2 percent in 2003. It appears that urban residents have higher percentages of lowest 1/5th income bracket residents failing to seek cure in illness than their rural counterparts. In case of seeking hospital care, the same analysis indicates that in the lowest 1/5th income bracket in rural area, residents did not seek hospital care (or normally taken as inpatients) were 44.2 percent in 1993, 51.4 percent in 1998, and 41 percent in 2003, and in urban area, residents in the same bracket did not seek hospital care are 31.7 percent in 1993, 46.8 percent in 1998, and 41.6 percent in 2003 (Wang 2008: 271). Overall, in the lowest 1/5th income bracket as just mentioned, higher percentages of rural residents failed to seek hospital care than their urban counterpart, except for 2003 with nearly the same percentage, suggesting that by and large rural residents found less affordable to pay for their hospital care.

How to eliminate the pockets of patients in urban and rural areas who cannot afford to seek a cure? It appears that sovereign planners began to move forward on many fronts trying their best to beef up health care at the macro level from the early 2000s onward, for instance, increasing the share of the government financial input, building up public insurances, and constructing a new tier of primary care facilities at the community health care centers in urban areas and health care institutes and clinical stations in rural areas. Meanwhile, they redoubled their effort to impose regulatory controls, especially price control regarding prescription drugs and medical devices, in order to enforce the low-price policy at the micro level.

Some analysts have borrowed the concept of "re-engagement of the state" to characterize the new trend of health care policy since 2000 (Gu 2010:33). To begin with, analysts take note of rapid recovery of the state's financial role from the early 2000s, as they hold a consensual view on the observable decline of public financing (e.g. the government subsidies and public insurances) prior to the 2000s, In Gu Xin's observation, for example, the phenomenon of "expensiveness to see cure" (kanbingnan) was substantially alleviated within a couple of years from 2002 onward: personal spending on health care started to decline, within several years, from 60 percent of the total of health care expenditure in 2002 to 40.4 percent in 2008, a trend continuing to the present (Gu 2010: 15–7). In statistical terms, the "basic fact" is that the government subsidies gained nearly 15 percentage points from 15.5 percent in 2000 to 30.4 percent in 2011, as the share of public insurances grew about 10 percentage points from 24.1 percent in 2001 to 34.7 percent in 2011 (Chapter 2). Gu Xin attributes the improvement of public insurances partly to the expanding coverage and the raise of premiums of three public insurances, namely, the enhanced BMCI, NRCMCI, and URBMCI (Gu 2010: 15; 61–3).

The advance of the state did not take place only in a mechanical way and quantitative terms, but, instead it accompanied with some significant policy changes, for instance, achieving some measure of "horizontal equality" by narrowing down the gap between the urban and rural sector. For the time span about eight years, the rapid growth of the government budgetary input to the rural sector narrowed down the gap between the urban and rural sector from 5 times in 2002 to 2.4 times in 2008 (Gu 2010: 24). A set of statistical data cited by Gu Xin indicates that the percentages of the government budgetary input to the rural sector climbed up noticeably for the five-year period from one of the lowest ebb, 15.8 percent in 2003 to 29.1 percent in 2008, and the share of government contribution to the funding of health care sector in rural area increased from 6.2 percent in 2001 to 31.8 percent in 2008 (Gu 2010: 25).

Furthermore, sovereign planners have begun to adopt the new ways in financial appropriation to the health care sector shifting from subsidies to the provider to those to the users, as often advocated in the public policy context in the West. As cited by Gu Xin, a set of statistical data indicates that there was an increase in the government subsidy to help rural residents directly pay for their medical insurance premiums to NRCMCI from 13 million RMB in 2003 to 639.2 million RMB in 2008. This subsidy directly to users reached 61.2 percent in 2008 from 7.4 percent in the total of the government budgetary expenditure to the rural health care in rural area, while, in comparison, the decline of subsidy to the provider from 88.7 percent in 2003 to 35.4 percent in 2008, indicative of a major change of method of financial appropriation to health care (Gu 2010: 32). Another piece of material cited by Gu Xin suggests that the government went beyond the discussion on paper by making substantial financial commitment of 850,000 million RMB to five major items of new medical reform, two third of which would be spent through "subsidies to demand side," namely users, for the three-year time span from 2009–2011 (Gu 2010: 30)

In addition, policymakers have installed some concrete budgetary and managerial mechanisms in order to ensure the consistency in the financial appropriation to the areas of priority. According to the 2009 Opinion on further reform of health care system, the government intended to adopt diversified input mechanisms and to maintain the balance among three funding sources. The new mechanisms of financial input ensure the following: the continuous increase of the government input in the total expenditure in health care, a fixed proportion of the government's financial input in health care higher than overall government expenditure, and priority given to public health care, rural health care, urban community health care and basic health care insurance (Zhonggong zhongyang & Guowuyuan 2009: 30–1).

No easy policy option

Given that the government has made considerable efforts to re-allocate health care resources to meet the urgent demands of public health care and rural health care, sovereign planners have also adopted several approaches to implement a low-price policy at the providing unit level amidst major policy changes during the economic reform. These approaches include the re-structuring of franchises, price adjustments, direct price control, and spending control mechanisms of public insurances.

This study has examined a number of attempts made by policymakers to control drug prices, including pilot programs to cut back the W/R ratio from about 30 percent to about 15 percent (for Western medicine), and even the proposals of the total abolishment of the W/R ratio. All these attempts resulted in varying degrees of deficit and financial difficulties in the participant providing units, some of which tried to find ways to circumvent the tightening regulatory control through legal or quasi-legal avenues (Chapter 9). Moreover, the government introduced a series of price cut for selected drugs on a periodical basis during the 2000s, providing some relief to the patients, but, this did not turn the tide of increase of drug prices (Chapter 10). There has been no evidence to suggest that the "two-line management" of drug revenue was able to control "exorbitant charges," but it has demonstrated that considerable administrative costs and complexity were involved (Chapter 9). In theory, the "two-line management" has raised a policy issue with regard to whether or not the supervisory bureau ought to substitute for the providing unit and to assume more workload than justifiable. It is theoretically problematic to "bureaucratize" the provision of medical care and to return to the old fashion mode of management during the CPE era.

Sovereign planners encountered a series of policy issues, as they tried to impose some forms of control on "exorbitant" charges" to drugs. In theoretical terms, "exorbitant charges" to drugs is inseparable from the question how to measure and therefore recognize the value of professional/medical discretion embedded in either command-oriented management or transaction-oriented management. First of all, policymakers cannot come to a scientific criterion to determine what is taken as right prices for drugs in the health care sector. In China over several decades, professional/medical components in prescription made by doctors and dispensary services rendered by pharmacists were not given proper weight on the pricing exercises of drugs. At the end of the day, it is found that one has to recognize the value of services provided by doctors and pharmacists in order to decide what is an appropriate cost for drug prescription and dispensary services. This was not included into the pricing exercise until the new medical care reform commencing in 2009.

The foregoing analysis suggests that public hospitals and medical personnel are often able to enjoy considerable say over pricing not only because of franchising but also owing to medical personnel's expertise in professional/medical care realm (Chapters 2, 8 and 10). In case of pricing over medical care in the Chinese context, three dimensions of decision-making structure need to consider as follows: the regulatory control of supervisory bureaus over providing units (including public and non-public hospitals); transactions between providing units and users (including the patient, insured or non-insured, and insurers), and, transactions between providing units and drug industry. The study observes that with regard to formal chain of command, hospital management is subordinate to supervisory bureaus, but on informal dimension the former often tends to enjoy considerable discretion because they control uncertainty, (i.e., risks entailed by professional/medical decisions) and lack of information to implement performance appraisal (Chapters 1, 8 and 10).

When it comes to the issues of abusing new brand names for existing drugs, substitutable but higher priced drugs, and over-prescription/provision, it is evident that supervisory bureaus could not effectively exercise regulatory control due to lack of medical expertise in handling uncertainty in curative care. Also, in midst of enforcing the standards of safety, quality and curative effects of drugs, supervisory bureaus need to lend public hospitals and medical personnel room of discretion (Chapter 10). As a result, this discretion, on top of franchise, further strengthened the position of public hospitals and medical care personnel to dictate the terms of negotiation with drug industry and the patient. It has become obvious that price control inevitably encounters diminishing effects in the realm of medical care, without addressing the issue of the proper value of professional/medical components of curative care and budgetary balance at the providing unit level (Chapter 10). Furthermore, it is evident that centralization of policymaking power at the national level is a prerequisite to effective regulatory control on drug issues. However, the attempt to push for centralization failed from the mid-1990s onwards, because of the overwhelming workload, long-time lag required, lack of trained personnel and expertise. As a result, consistency cannot be maintained across provincial jurisdictions, where politics penetrates into the enforcement process, leaving the issues of safety of drugs and foods unsolved, likely in the foreseeable future (Chapter 10).

Further to the issue of public hospitals, are public insurances a solution to the affordable care policy? So far, no conclusive evidence has been available for an affirmative answer. The study has argued that, in design, the enhanced BMCI package operates as a quasi-market in the sense that the insurer interacts with the providing unit through negotiation and makes a contractual arrangement. In managerial terms, a non-governmental public body, called "executive agency" (jinban jigou), acts on behalf of the insurance fund and represents the interest of enrollees to negotiate with the providing unit. With the status of the insurer, the executive agency makes payment to the providing unit on behalf of enrollees according to signed contracts, while overseeing the enforcement of the contract (Chapter 5). It is supposed that the insurer works with strengths of professional competence, taking advantage of market competition and compensating the disadvantage of the user by addressing the issue of asymmetric information between the provider and user (Gu, Gao & Yao 2006: 19). In general terms, advocates who treat insurer as a counterweight to the provider have yet to demonstrate their propositions at empirical level. Therefore, it appears that in case of enhanced BMCI, a providing unit has hardly ever negotiated through market transactions with an insurer, as the public hospitals and pharmacies have normally "designated," that is, mandated to do so by local authorities. Evidence is required to confirm that an insurer does exercise its discretion of choosing among competing providers, either among public providing units or between public and non-public units. For the time being, public hospitals are well supported by the local governments in respective jurisdictions through policy, subsidies, and investment funding. For example, most of non-public, profit-oriented providing units are restricted to access to public insurances. It is not expected that public hospitals would face real competition from their non-public, profit-oriented counterparts. Another issue about the limitation of insurance system in spending control has to do with the possible collaboration between a medical doctor and a patient. For example, a medical doctor could induce a patient to accept more expensive treatments, drugs and examination that are normally covered by an insurer, the third party, while a patient has only to assume relatively little financial burden.

Both NRCMCI and URBCMI differ from the enhanced BMCI, for the former two insurance schemes have started with a narrow focus only on catastrophic medical events, and therefore both are more affordable than the latter in terms of low premiums. From the consideration of management, the enhanced BMCI package is normally under the guidance and supervision of the bureau of labor and social security, while the providing unit is under the command of the bureau of health care. Theoretically speaking, the enhanced BMCI can act on behalf of enrollees better in the sense that it can avoid interference from the bureau of health care, conventionally the protector of the providing unit. As it is, NRCMCI and its counterpart providing units operate under the same supervisory system, namely, from the health care bureau in respective jurisdictions at the local level. There has been the question raised on whether NRCMCI should be put under command of a supervisor other than the health care bureau. As an insurer, the institutional integrity and managerial independence of NRCMCI might be in jeopardy as it has to operate under the shadow of the health care bureau—"protector" of the providing unit. So constituted, NRCMCI can hardly act as a counterweight to the providing unit in market transactions to bring down the high prices.

The re-engineering of affordable care policy began with marketization about four decades ago as early as 1979, and, since then, public hospitals and public insurances have been occupying the central stage of health care reform. Both have experienced substantial transformation, with some distinctive achievements as well as gaps of performance falling short of the ideal of affordable care. In terms of such complex and large-scale changes, time is insufficient to do justice to a comprehensive and in-depth analysis of all issues in hand. Much more assessment needs to wait until settling of dust when fresh sets of research material become available.

References

Du, L., Zhang, W., & Xu, Bo. 2009. Zongjie jingyan, jiefang sixiang, xinyigai chuixian jinjunhao (To sum up experience, liberate thought, herald the start of new health care reform). In L. Du, W. Zhang, & Zhongguo Weisheng Chanye Zazhishe (Eds.), *Zhongguo yiliao weisheng fazhan baogao, No. 5* (The Report of Development of

Medical and Health Care in China, No. 5), 1–22. Beijing: Shehui kexue wenxian chubanshe.

Gu, X., Gao, M.,& Yao, Y. 2006. *Zhenduan yu chufang, zhimian zhongguo yiliao tizhi gaige* (Diagnosis and Treatment, Facing China's Reform of Medical Care System). Beijing: Shehui kexue wenxian chubanshe.

Gu, X. 2010. *Quanmin yibao de xintansuo* (New Exploration of National Medical Insurance). Beijing: Shehui kexue wenxian chubanshe.

Guowuyuan. 2009. Yiliao weisheng tizhi gaige jinqi zhongdian shishi fangan (The priority implementation plan of the reform of medical and health care system). In L. Du, W. Zhang, & Zhongguo Weisheng Chanye Zazhishe (Eds.), *Zhongguo yiliao weisheng fazhan baogao, No. 3* (The Report of Development of Medical and Health Care in China, No. 5), 36–44. Beijing: Shehui kexue wenxian chubanshe.

Wang, B. 2008. *Zhengfu yiliao guamzhi moshi ghonggou yanjiu* (Research on the Restructuring of Mode of Governmental Control). Beijing: Renmin chubanshe.

Zhonggong Zhongyang, Guowuyuan. 2009. Guanyu shenhua yiliao weisheng tizhi gaige de yijian (Opinion concerning the further reform of medical and health care system). In L. Du, W. Zhang, & Zhongguo Weisheng Chanye Zazhishe (Eds.), *Zhongguo yiliao weisheng fazhan baogao, No. 3* (The Report of Development of Medical and Health Care in China, No. 5), 22–36. Beijing: Shehui kexue wenxian chubanshe.

Index

1951 Regulations 99
1979 Opinion 69n1, 149, 157–8, 159
1979 Supplementary General Circular
  54, 69n3, 162n13
1980 Circular 43n10
1981 Provisional Measures 69n5, 159–60
1984 National Conference of Office/
  Bureau Chiefs 31
1985 Report 30–1, 39, 128, 129, 132, 133,
  137n9, 137n14, 169–70, 181n5
1988 Opinion 39, 128, 132–3, 137n9,
  181n6
1989 Circular 210, 226n1
1989 Opinion 170, 181n6
1992 Circular 129, 137n11
1992 Decision 129, 137n10, 169
1994 Opinion 104, 105, 107
1994 Regulations 60, 70n12
1995 Provisional Measures 171
1996 Circular 135–6, 193, 202n2
1996 Opinion 70n18
1996 Provisional Measures 203n8,
  214–15, 226n5
1997 Decision 69n5, 70n13, 124
1997 Several Opinions 70n19
1997 Supplementary Regulations 215,
  226n6
1998 Decision 62, 63, 70n16, 106, 108
1998 Policy 215, 226n7
1999 Advisory Opinion 65, 66–7
1999 Decision 59, 70n11
1999 Provisional Measures 224, 227n20
1999 Several Options 61, 70n14
2000 Advisory Opinion 39, 40, 43n11, 67
2000 General Circular 211
2000 Opinion 108, 122–3, 137n4
2000 Outline 70n19
2000 Provisional Measures 198, 203n11
2004 Advisory Opinion 110

2004 Report 195, 202n4
2005 Advisory Opinion 172, 173, 182n11
2005 DRC Report 30
2005 Report 82, 90, 91, 92
2006 Opinion 203n8
2007 Advisory Opinion 112
2007 Circular 138n17
2009 Opinion 203n9, 203n13, 235, 237–8,
  240
2009 Priority Implementation Plan 236
2012 Advisory Opinion 110, 117n11,
  117n12

accountability 58, 154, 169, 170, 175;
  and incentives 152; resource
  management 150; and retained revenue schemes 152–4
adaptive behavior 19
administrative modes *36*
administrative structure, re-engineering
  59–61
advisory pricing mode of price
  management 213
affordability 26, 104, 237–8
Allison, Graham T. ix, 10–11, 12, 217
asset management 175
asset privatization 38, 43n7, 43n8
asymmetric information theory 21
Australia 88

Bai Zhipeng 171, 173
bandwagon phenomenon 8, 11–12,
  86, 113
basic control cycle within bureaucracy
  19, 24n4
Basic Medical Care Insurance (BMCI)
  ix, 34, 62, 66, 68, 84, 98, 101, 122,
  237, 239; defining "essential" 104,
  116n8; enrollees 63; evolution of

101–3; executive agency 63–4, 68–9; expectation and performance 114; five merits of 105–6; four major policy goals 104, 116n7; funding sources 105; hierarchy 62; non-planned sector 109–12; origin of 103; PA-USFA 105–6, 109, 116n10; planned sector 103–6; role of state 103–4; *see also* enhanced Basic Medical Care Insurance (BMCI)
basic medical care insurance systems 61–4, 222, 224–5
basic medical care services, policy definition 33–4, 42n2, 42n3
basic types of medical care services 31–4
Beijing 62, 93n2, 102
Blau, P. M. 19
bounded rationality 13
Brazil 79
budgetary undertaking system (BUS) 30, 152, 153
bureaucratic pathology 19

Cao Beiwen 179
catastrophic medical events 109–10
Category I, pure-public health care 28, 29, 30, 31, 42, 77, 88, 89, 90, 128, 130, 137n13
Category II, quasi-public health care 28–9, 29, 30, 31, 42, 77–8, 88, 89, 90, 128, 130, 137n13
Category III, basic medical care services 29, 42, 77–8, 128, 130, 137n13
Category IV, non-basic medical care services 29, 42, 128
Central Committee 69n6, 210–11
centrally planned economy (CPE) x, 3, 8, 13, 18, 27, 29–30, 39, 41, 42, 57, 59, 68–9, 69 n.10, 76, 84, 98, 99, 108, 124, 148, 154, 155, 168, 177, 192, 222, 235; bureaucratic framework 37; introduced 121–2; legacy of 115; low-pay policy 114–15; model of macro-rationality 13; restructuring 86–7
Certificate of Eligibility of Medical Doctors 40
Certificate of Practice of Medical Doctors 40
Chang, T. 43n4
Chang, Y. 43n4
Chen Chunhui 88, 91
Chen Jijiang 137n13, 191
Chen Jinfu 62, 104, 116n9

Chen Mingzhang 55, 137n14, 156, 169
Chen Xinzhong 196
China Medical Device Association 171
Chinese Communist Party 69n6, 137n2, 169, 210–11; 3rd Plenum of 11th National Congress of 148, 161n1; Party Center 59, 61, 137n2; Party Commission 55; Party Committee 56
Chou Yulin 113
Chu Jinhua 122
city hospitals, allocation of resources 86
classification : hospitals 5l; medical devices 172
classification management 39
clientelism 35
coalition formation 12
Cohen, Myron S. 69n7
collaborative practice between medical care and pharmacy 190
collective-bidding procurement programs 222–3
collective goods 28, 29, 30, 104, 216, 235
collective-owned enterprises (COEs) 99–100, 113, 170
collective units 176
collective welfare 60
command-oriented management 16–18, 17, 23, 53–6
commercialization 5, 38–41, 75, 82, 92; and curative care services 35–6, 43n5; curative care services 167–9; debates over 35, 147; degree of 170, 182n7; and failures of health care reform 93n1; issue of 147; objects of transactions 36, 43n5; and revenue-generation 35–6; unanticipated policy outcomes at providing unit level 174–6, 182n13; use of term 43n6, 168
compensation 91, 101, 177
compliance 11–12
comprehensive trade-wide oriented residential management (CTORM) 65–6, 69, 70n19
comprehensive undertaking responsibility system (CURS) 156–7, 180
conflict resolution 12
Congress of Representatives of Staff and Workers (CRSW) 56, 160
consumers, as actors in drug markets 221, 227n12, 227n13
contractualism 35

coordination: modes of/classification scheme 36–8; non-command centered 35
corporate governance 18
cost-based price 124
cost containment 34
cost fees 31
cost-shifting 200; and drug franchising 191–4; and price control 130–3, 136
county hospitals 65, 86
cross-subsidization 200
CT (computerized tomography) scanners 171, 173
Cuban missile crisis, case study 10–11
Cui Bin 103
Cui Yueli 55, 56, 161n9, 169
curative care services 27–8, 29, 30–1, 61; and commercialization 35–6, 43n5; commercialization of 167–9; contribution percentage 116n9; types 31–4
Cyert, R. M. 12
Cyert, Richard M. 20

decision-making approach 19, 24n4
demand, control of 101
Deng Xiaoping 169
Development and Reform Commission 203n8
Development Research Center 30
deviant behavior 19
differential-quota appropriation 154, 155, 162n11
differentiated quota subsidy 77
direct subsidies 77
directors' responsibility system (DRS) 54–6
disparity 61, 78, 84–6, 89
divergent policy views 20–1
doctors *see* medical personnel
Document Guofa No. 10 *see* 1988 Opinion
Document Guofa No. 62 *see* 1985 Report
Document Zhongyang No. 1 (1983) 153
Don Chaohui 103
double-track pricing system 130–1, 195, 212
Downs, Anthony 24n4
Dror, Yehezkel 10
drug franchising 131, 171, 225; alternatives to W/R differentials 199–201; and cost-shifting 191–4; drugs/pharmaceuticals 131, 171,176,

216–17; medical personnel 176–81, 223, 241–2; policy themes 196–7, 203n8; and price control over drugs 194–6; remaking 196–8; two-line management 197–8, 203n10, 241; wholesale-and-retail (W/R) differential scheme 192, 194, 197, 201, 202, 202n3
drug markets: calculation of prices 216; collective bidding measures 222–3; consumers as actors in 221, 227n12, 227n13; discovery of regulatory control 209–11; drug pricing 220; exorbitant charges for drugs 216, 222–5; and franchise system 131, 171,176, 216–17; government as actor in 221, 227n12, 227n13; illegal 211; key actors in pricing game 217–21; monitoring and supervising pricing, pharmaceutical industry 219; municipal/local jurisdictions 218–19, 227n11; new pricing system in regulated markets 213–16; origins of drug pricing policy 211–13; over-prescriptions 220; as pillar industry 209; profit motive 219; and public insurance schemes 221, 227n12, 227n13; reasonable price for drugs 216; regulatory control 208–28; remedial measures 222, 227n15, 227n16, 227n18; society as actor in 221, 227n12, 227n13; standards of drugs 220; three major categories of drugs 214–15, 220–1, 225–6; three modes of price management 213; versus price control 190–1; wholesale-and-retail (W/R) differential scheme 215, 216–17, 222, 227n17, 227n18
drug wholesalers 216
drugs/pharmaceuticals 212; affordability 237–8; branding/labeling 202n6, 219–20, 242; calculation of prices 216; changing status of 196, 292n7; charges for 199–200, 203n14; collective-bidding procurement programs 135, 138n17; commercial value of 195; doctors' power over 190–1, 195; double-track pricing system 130–1, 195, 212; expensive 195–6, 202n6, 216, 222–5, 241; fake 210, 211; and franchise system 176; franchising 171; high risk 195–6; illegal markets for 211; over-prescriptions 220; pharmaceutical service charges 198, 203n13; poor quality 211; prescription

fees 198, 203n13; prescription irregularities 195; pricing policy 211–13, 220, 237–8; provision of 64; rebranding 202n6, 219–20, 242; registered brands 210; research and development 219; revenue from 78; sales 189; service charges 198, 203n13; standards of 220; state mandatory catalogs/lists of basic drugs 223–4, 227n20; state-owned enterprises (SOEs) 209, 210; supply of 237–8; three major categories of 214–15, 220–1; unnecessary 196; wholesale-and-retail (W/R) differential scheme 189, 203n8, 212
Du Lexun 69 n.9, 85–6, 90, 128, 155
dual command 57, 69n8
Duckett, Jane 81–2

economic leverages 13
economic management (EM) 5, 54–6, 148–9, 151, 154, 159, 161n3, 181n2
ECT (electro-convulsive therapy) 171
enhanced Basic Medical Care Insurance (BMCI) 103, 109, 110, 112, 115, 242–3; accumulated deposit 113–14, 117n14; and catastrophic events 106–9; ceiling 114; disparities with other insurance schemes 114–15; implementation 113; and spending control 111; *see also* Basic Medical Care Insurance (BMCI)
enterprise insurance 99
Enterprise Rectification Team 55, 69n4
enterprise style of management (ESM) 7–8, 18, 147, 148–52, 158
entitlement for the citizen 42n2
equity theory 177
executive agency 242
externality 16

Fend Dan 182 n 8
Ferlie, Ewan 16
Finance Office 137n11
financial capacity of China 104
financial management, classics of 138n19
financial reform, and funding of health care services 86–9
financial stringency in lower echelons 89–92
financial undertaking system (FUS) 87, 93n3
five fixes 151–2
Five Year Plan (12th) 110

fixed norms 157, 158, 162n16
fixed-quota appropriation 154
Food and Drug Administration (USA) 219, 226
fragmented structure of authority 10
franchise system x, 4, 21–2, 60, 76, 78, 83, 92, 136, 148, 154; commercialization of curative care services 167–9; defined 167; drugs/pharmaceuticals 131, 171,176, 216–17; medical devices 167, 168, 171–3, 175/medical personnel and unanticipated policy outcomes 176–81; origins of 167; and pricing 176; re-engineering 168, 181n3; re-packaging and expansion of 131; repackaging and managing franchise provision 169–73; as revenue tool 41, 169; unanticipated policy outcomes at providing unit level 174–6, 182n13; and URS 168–9; use of term 168, 176, 182n15; *see also* drug franchising
free markets 15
Fujian 93n4
Fujian Province 173, 182n12
full-quota budget, subsidy by special funding, and savings to be remitted to the upper echelon 154
funding: health care services, and financial reform 86–9; public health approaches 93n4; public health care arena 89; severe shortage of 88

Gao Qiang 61, 70n15, 90, 93n5, 181, 190, 292n7
gatekeeper primary care 65
GDP 82, 87
Ge, Y. 93n4
General Office of the State Council 110
Geng Ying 84
Germany 16
Goldstein, Avery 11, 86
Gong, S. 93n4
Gong Xianguang 194
Good Manufacturing Practices (GMP) 214, 215, 217
Good Storage Practices (GSP) 214
Gouldner, A. 19
government politics paradigm 11
government process/organizational behavior model 11, 82, 217, 226
government subsidy 82
government(s): as actor in drug markets 221, 227n12, 227n13; addressing gap

in urban and rural sectors
239–40; as financial resource 76,
77–8, 79–82, *80*, 83; professional
networks, public and private health
care 235; re-structuring medical
care delivery system 236–7;
support for public hospitals 243;
weakened role of 88–9
Gu Xin 64, 103, 113, 114, 117n14, 124,
153, 168, 197, 239, 240
Guan Zhiqiang 103
Guangdong Province 93n4, 129,
137n11
Guangxi 93n4
Gui, J. 62–3, 117n14
Guinzhou 93n4
Guo Xinghua 173

Hainan Province 104
health care benefits and entitlements,
classification of 77
health care bureau 218, 227n10
Health Care Economics Research
Institute (MOH) 91
health care expenditure *79*; growth of
78–9; public hospitals 85–6
Health Care Office 137n11
health care reform: alternative paths to
34–8; failures of 75; 93n1
health care resources: allocation of
78–84; managing 65–8
health care services: classification
scheme 27–9, *29*; demand, and income
level 238–9; financial reform and
funding of 86–9; re-packaging, and
pricing issues 128–30; repackaging
27–31
Hebei Province 200–1
Henderson, G. 69n7
hidden subsidy 130–1
HIV immunization program 29
horizontal combination 37
horizontal equality 239–40
hospitals: classification of 5; discretion
over medical devices 154; disparity of
services 61, 70n15; enterprise managed
59–61; number of beds 161n5; revenue
of 192, 202n1
Hu Qiaomu 13
Hu Shanlian 194, 222, 223–4, 227n17
Hu Yaobang 55–6
Huang Guowu 113
Huang Xiaoping 85
Huang Yanzhong 10, 11, 54, 81, 86, 113

incentives 152, 157–60
income levels, and percentages of
residents seeking cure in illness 238–9
incrementalism 13
independent interests 92
indicators 157, 162n16
indirect subsidies 77
individual, as financial resource 77,
79–82, *80*
information, cost of 19, 20
Inner Mongolia 93n4
Institutional Reform Commission of the
State Council 43n11

Jiang Zemin 156
Jiangsu Province 40–1, 173
Jiangxi Province 201
Jingxi, Liaoning Province 102, 116n5
Jiujiang municipality 62, 105
jointly managed health care institutes 37

Korea 81

labor, division of 11
Labor Insurance Medical Care (LIMC)
viii, 31, 64, 69 n.9, 76, 77, 83, 84,
98, 99, 100, 100–1, 104, 106, 109,
112, 115, 126, 183n17, 221; control
measures 102; expectation and
performance 114; and financial
hardship 126, 137n7; revenue
growth 126
Lampton, David 12
large medical care expenditure study 107
Lee, Peter NS 13
Li Daping 190–1
Li Huaiyong 129
Li, N. 39–40
Li Pang 156
Li Shuwen 82
Li Shuxia 82
Li Xiennian 152
Li Xinmin 55
Liang, H. 33, 34, 42n3
licensing 60
Lieberthal, K. 10, 11, 12
Lindblom, C. E. 8, 23n2, 35; Model I
(preceptoral model) 23n2, 182n14;
Model II (strategic model) 13, 23 n2
182n14
line organization 57; use of term
"line" 69n8
Liu Hongning 216–17
Liu, Junmin 153

living standards ix, 27, 101, 127, 128, 129, 221
load shedding 86–9, 155
low pay 114–15
low-price policy ix, 4, 21, 121, 125, 136
Luo Yiqin 170

Ma Anning 62–3, 65
Ma, L. 43n9, 117n14
Ma, W. 176
Ma Weiwei 82
macro-rationality model 13
major illnesses 111; conceptualizing and defining 102; social unified funding 102–3; social unified funding for 116n6; *see also* SARS (Severe Acute Respiratory Syndrome)
managed competition 35, 151, 161n4
management: business/industrial 5–6, 8–9; command-oriented management 16–18, *17*, 23; economic management (EM) 7–8; enterprise style of management (ESM) 7–8, 18; by multiple bureaus 56–9; public 6–7; transaction-oriented management 16–18, *17*, 23
Management Committee of Drug Affairs in Second and Third Tier Hospitals 224
mandatory mode of price management 213
Mao Zedong 13, 53
March, James G. 12, 20, 23n2
market, definition of 35
market-adjusted mode of price management 213
market behavior 35
market de-regulation 36, *36*
market entry system 40
market-oriented approach to price regulation 5, 12, 14, 35, 41, 122, 124–8, 216
markets/marketization viii–ix, 5, 6, 26–7, 32, 34, 41–2, 109, 151, 154; caution about 27; classifications scheme 15; debate over 35; definition of market 15; effectiveness of 35; free markets 15; internal markets 16; irregularities arising from 21; partial marketization 54; path toward 15–16; pressures facing 101, 115n2; pricing policy 122; quasi-markets 15–16, 68; reach 27–8; regulated markets 15; reliance on command 8; versus state 12–13,

235–8; towards full-fledged mode 38–41; use of term 8, 43n4; utility 35
Measures of Management of Hospitals by Echelons 58
mechanisms of competition 39
medical and Health Care Fund (MHCF) 99
medical care *see* curative care systems
medical care benefits 99
Medical Care Office, State Council 110
medical care subsidies to public personnel (MCSPP) 108–9
medical devices 40, 91, 133, 136n1, 195, 213; advanced ix, 3, 5, 8, 15, 16, 33, 61, 70n15, 76, 78, 131, 135, 168, 171, 172, 173, 212, 214, 221; classification of 172; commercial value of 195; costs of 77, 132, 133, 135–6, 173; dependency upon 32; fees for 135; and franchise system 167, 168, 171–3, 175; hospital discretion over 154; market for 78, 133, 135; medical personnel discretion over 22; policymaking and 172; price cuts, and decreased revenue from 173, 182n12; standards of 63; use of 36, 76, 78, 108–9, 131–2, 172–3, 182n12, 239; user charges 147; utilization rates 173
medical personnel: asymmetric information 179, 180; cost contribution from 200–1; discretion of 33; discretion over drug pricing 16, 21–2, 23, 33, 124, 125, 126, 131–2, 135, 136, 154, 156, 176–81, 190, 220, 225, 241–2; discretion over medical devices 22; and drug franchising 176–81, 223, 241–2; incentive packages 157–60; pay 132, 170, 177, 193–4; performance appraisal 18, 35, 55, 152, 154, 156–60, 179–81; and price control 195, 196, 202n5; power over prescription drugs 190–1, 195; pricing discretion 132; special nature of job 178–9, 180–1
medical-technical services; labor input 132, 133, 135–6, 138n18; standards 32, 34, 42n3
Meng Qingyao 125
merit goods 29
Mexico 81
Ministry of Finance 31, 43n7, 59, 69n1, 69n3, 70n18, 70n19, 153, 161n1, 172, 181n2, 181n6, 202n2, 203n11, 218

Ministry of Health 40, 43n10, 54, 57, 59, 60, 61, 69 nl, 69n3, 70n18, 70n19, 91, 110, 114, 122–3, 126, 132, 137n4, 137n14, 138n17, 148, 153, 159, 161n1, 162n18, 169, 170, 171, 172, 181n2, 181n6, 195, 202n2, 202n4, 203n9, 203n11, 203n13, 211, 212, 227n20, 227n22, 228n21
Ministry of Human Resources and Social Security 203n9, 203n13
Ministry of Labor and Social Security 62, 63, 70n18, 102, 104, 116n5, 116n6
Ministry of Personnel 181n6
Mintzberg, Henri 180
mixed economy 8, 27, 29–30, 98, 102
Maoist period 98, 99; anti-intellectual legacy of 193
Mode A, administrative/managerial reform *36*, 37, 59, 68
Mode B, property rights reform; corporatization and privatization *36*, 38, 42, 43n7
Mode C, commercialization of service provision *36*, 41, 42, 54, 155
Mode D, full-fledged marketization *36*
Mode One, budgetary mode 129–30
Mode Two, budgetary mode 129–30
Model I (preceptoral model) 23n2, 182n14
Model II (strategic model) 13, 23 n2 182n14
monopoly: administrative 179; technical 179; use of term 168, 176, 182n15
MRI (magnetic resonance imaging) scanners 171, 173
Municipal Health Care Bureau, Shanghai 198
Mushi, Shantong Province 102

Nanjing 173
Naughton, B. 13
New Public Management (NPM) x, 6, 17, 148, 149
New Rural Cooperative Medical Care Insurance (NRCMCI) ix, 34, 84, 85, 98, 109–10, 113, 115, 117n11, 237, 239, 240, 243; accumulated deposit 113–14, 117n14; ceiling 114; disparities with other insurance schemes 114–15; implementation 113; spending control 111; three-tier health care system 65
NHS (National Health Service, UK) 15–16

Ningxia 93n4
non-basic curative care services 16, 28, 125, 128, 131, 170–1
non-basic medical care services, policy definition 33–4, 42n2, 42n3
non-basic types of medical care services 31–4
non-compliance 11–12, 20–2
non-profit-oriented hospitals 5, 30–41, 39, 123, 236, 243
non-public hospitals 5, 15, 39–40, 41, 123, 135, 236, 241, 243
non-public sector 3, 23, 38, 87, 104

OECD Health Care Data 81
Office of State Council 108
Oksenberg, M. 10, 11, 12
one-man management 55
organization behavior model *see* government process/organizational behavior model
organizational behavior paradigm 11
out-of-pocket payment (OPP) 32, 77, 79, *80*, 82, 85, 92
outpatients, retail drug stores for 224–5
output linkages 7

passing the buck 11–12, 86, 88–9
People's Communes 110
performance appraisal 18, 35, 55, 152, 154, 156–7, 179–81; and incentive packages 157–60
personal account (PA) 105, 106, 116n10
personnel establishment 161n5
pharmacists: professional autonomy 190–1; regulations 224
pharmacy/ies, designated 64
pilot programs 12, 13
policy, post-Weberian analysis 18, 19, 20, 21, 23, 24n4
policy actors 9–10; multiple 10–11, 20–1, 82; orientation 11; plurality of 10
policy experiments 13
policy goals 174–5, 180, 182n14
policy instruments, and changing task environment 121, 136n1
policy-oriented approach to price regulation 10, 11, 124–8, 216
policy outcomes 180; unanticipated 18–22
policymaking 5, 6; and bounded rationality 13; changing style of 121–4; consensus and coordination

11–12; double squeeze 175; and policy goals 174–5, 182n14; role of state 8–14
positive intervention strategy 83
power approach 10
preceptoral model 23n2
prescription drugs 22
preventative health care 27–8
price adjustment 138n16; policy issues of 133–6, *134*
price control 121–4, 241–2; and cost-shifting 130–3, 136; versus drug franchising 190–1; issues of, drugs 194–6; and medical personnel 195, 196, 202n5; two approaches to 124–8
Price Office 137n11
price-regulating tasks: issues of 126–7; two approaches to 124–8
pricing policy: cost-based price 124, 126; decentralization 122; drugs/pharmaceuticals 211–13; ease of 121–4; and franchise system 176; institutional framework 122; issues, and the re-packaging of health care services 128–30; key actors 217–21; and markets/marketization 122; medical devices 135; production price 126; standards of charges 133, 135; three dimensions of decision-making structure 241–2; two approaches to price-regulating tasks 124–8
principal-agent relationship theory 21, 178
privately managed institutes 41
production price 126
profit-oriented hospitals 5, 35, 39–41
property-rights centered reform 18, 36, 38–41, 43n5, 43n7, 43n9, 54, 56
Provisional Measure of Enterprise Property Right Management 43n7
Provisional Measures of Transactions of State Assets among Enterprises 43n7
Public-Financed Medical Care (PFMC) viii, 31, 62, 64, 69, 76, 76–8, 77, 83, 98, 104, 106, 109, 112, 113, 114, 115, 126, 183n17, 221; control measures 102; enrollees 117n13; establishing 101–3, 115n3; expectation and performance 114; expenditure of 100, 101, 115n1; funding sources 100–1; revenue growth 126; spending control 101; streamlining and rebuilding 99–101
public financing programs, legacies of, during planned economy 99–101

public hospitals 123, 241–2; classification of 58–9, *58*, 61; control of 168; doctors, treatment of 22; and franchise holders 168; government support 243; health care expenditure 85–6; monopoly status 22; reform of 236–7; responsibility of 32–4
public insurance schemes viii, 5, 7, 1682, 183n17, 237, 239, 242–3, 243; and drug markets 221, 227n12, 227n13; enrollees 113; issues of implementation 112–15; re-inventing ix; *see also* individual insurance schemes
public interest 218
public ownership 18
publically managed institutes 41
pure rationality model 9, 23n2, 57, 81, 82

Qian Xinzhong 69n1, 149, 161n3, 161n6, 161n7, 181n2
quasi-foundation 102
quasi-markets 15–16, 68, 242
quid pro quo transactions 35
Quinghai 93n4

rational actor paradigm 11
rationality model 10, 11
Rayner, Derek 69n2
rectification 37, 53, 54, 69n1; campaign 55–6, 69n4; five criteria of 69n3
regional health care planning (RHCP) 66–8, 69
regulated markets 15
Regulations of Rural Cooperative Medical Care (1979) 110
Ren, R. 67
rent-seeking theory 21, 176, 192
Research Office of the State Council 192–3
residential management principle 57–8, 63, 65, 66
resource management 148–52; accountability 150; four categories of 150–1
responsibility system 153
retail prices, ceiling of 194–5
retained revenue 30, 31, 153, 153–4, 155, 159–60, 161n8, 162n11, 175
revenue: generation 35–6, 175; hospitals 192, 202n1; as surplus 155, 162n13
revenue retention system 8, 14, 30, 31, 54, 126, 149, 150, 152, 153–4, 155, 156, 158, 160, 161n8, 162n12, 168

revenue-sharing systems (RSS) 87,
88–9, 89
revenue tools, franchise system 169
reverse pyramid 61, 65, 111, 236
risk-pooling 62, 99, 101–3, 109, 111, 112
Rules of Management of Medical Care
Institutes 40
Rural Cooperative Medical Care
(RCMC) viii, 76, 83, 84, 98, 110, 111
rural health care centers, allocation of
resources 86
Russia 79, 81

SARS (Severe Acute Respiratory
Syndrome) 30, 90
satisficing model 23n2
sequential decision model 13
service charges 31
services, interpretative scheme 104–5
Shangdong Province 199, 200
Shanghai municipality 62, 93n2, 198
side payments 12
Simon, Hebert 10
social security schemes 99–100
social unified funding (SUF) 102, 116n4;
major illnesses 102–3, 116n6; retired
personnel 102, 103, 116n5; three zones
102–3; Zone I SUF program 102, 105,
106, 109; Zone II SUF program 102,
105, 106, 109; Zone III SUF program
103, 105, 106, 109
social utility 92, 125, 156
society: as actor in drug markets 221,
227n12, 227n13; as financial resource
76–7, 79–82, *80*
special item subsidy 77
spending control 101–3; enhanced BMCI
111; MCSPP 108–9; NRCMCI 111;
pilot programs 102
staff organization 57; use of term "staff"
69n8
standards, establishing 33
state 32, 34; characteristics 9; funding
8–9; mandatory power 9, 16; and
market paradigm 12–13; versus
markets 12–13, 235–8; non-
transactional interactions 12–13;
re-engagement of 238–40; role in
BMCI 103–4; role in policymaking
8–14; role of 6; staffing 9; subsidy 7;
use of term 8; *see also* government(s)
State Asset Committee 43n7
State Catalog of Basic Drugs 223,
227n20, 228n20, 228n21

State Chinese Herbal Medicine
Bureau 114
State Council on Health Care Reform
and Development 43n7, 59, 60, 62, 66,
67, 69n6, 112, 133, 137n2, 169, 181n5,
210–11
State Development and Reform
Commission (SDRC) 110, 117n12,
172, 203n9, 203n13
State Food and Drugs Management
Bureau (SFDMB) 195
State General Bureau of Drug
Management (SGBDM) 210, 211
State General Bureau of Labor 69n1,
69n3, 161n1, 181n2
State General Bureau of Pharmacy
Management (SGBPM) 212, 214
State Institutional Reform Commission
70n18, 213
state mandatory catalogs/lists of basic
drugs 223–4, 227n20
state-owned enterprises (SOEs) 59, 69
n.9, 70n10, 77, 99, 100, 113, 126, 160;
drugs/pharmaceuticals 209, 210
State Planning Commission (SPC)
59, 65, 69n4, 70n19, 122–3,
137n4, 193, 202n2, 211–12, 213, 214,
215, 218; and price management
214–15, 226n8
State Price Bureau (SPB) 31, 123, 182n6
State Reform and Development
Commission (SRDC) 212
State Statistical Bureau 85
State Taxation Bureau 182n6
strategic model 13, 23n2
subsidiary of collective units 176
subsidies, hidden 130–1
Sun Huizhu 172
Sun Naqiang 155, 176
Sun Zhigang 110
supplementary enterprise medical care
insurance (SMCI) 107–8, 109
supplementary medical care insurance
(SMC) 106

tax exemptions 16
tax revenue 15–16, 17, 99, 100, 105, 112
Thatcher, Margaret 43n8, 69n2
Thompson, James 20
three types of investments 209
Tian, L. 194
Tianjin 62, 93n2
Trade Union (TU) 160
trade-wide oriented management 66

transaction-oriented management
16–18, *17*, 23, 149, 157; use of term
"transaction" 23n1
treatment upgrading 237

uncertainty approach 178–9
undertaking agreement 153, 158–9,
161n9, 162n17
undertaking system 101
undertaking responsibility system (URS)
8, 31, 86, 149, 152, 153, 154, 158,
161n9, 162n18, 175, 180; and the
franchise system 168–9; issues arising
from 154–7; as output-centered 158
undertaking system (US) 153
UNDP 81
unified funding 62
unified planning system (UPS) 60
unified social funding account (USFA)
104, 105–6, 106, 107, 116n10
unified social funding (USF) 63
unintended consequences 19
United Kingdom 15–16, 68, 69n2
unity of command 55
urban community health centers,
allocation of resources 85–6
Urban Resident Basic Medical Care
Insurance (URBMCI) ix, 34, 84, 98,
109–10, 112, 113, 115, 117n11, 237,
239, 243; accumulated deposit 113–14,
117n14; ceiling 114; disparities with
other insurance schemes 114–15;
implementation 113
USA 81, 88, 219, 226
user charges viii–ix, x, 5, 15, 16, 27, 32,
42, 76, 77, 78, 148, 154, 155, 168, 170,
175, 182n7, 201, 204n16, 238; contribution percentage 79, *80*; medical
devices 147

value for money 191
Vegetable Company of the East City
District, Beijing 102

Wang Bingyi 32, 227n14
Wang Bozhen 128, 197
Wang Dongjin 107
Wang, L. 39
Wang, Ruo 79
Wang Shuming 216
Wang Xiufeng 89, 91–2
Wang Yang 190, 191, 202n2, 211, 222,
227n15
Wang Yanzhong 130–1

Wei Jigang 195–6, 217, 219, 220
welfare 70n10; collective 60; demand 3;
supply 3–4
welfare-oriented policy packages 153,
162n10
Wenhui Daily 156
WHO 81, 223; China's ranking 31, 42n1
wholesale-and-retail (W/R) differential
scheme 189, 192, 194, 197, 201,
202n3, 203n8, 212, 215, 216–17, 222,
227n17, 227n18; abolishing 200,
241; alternatives to 199–201;
implementation of 202; percentages of
199–200, 227n17; zero ratio of 200,
203n15, 241
work unit collectivism 60
work unit insurance 99, 116n10
worthy goods 29
Wu Ming 176, 183n16, 202n3
Wu Qifei 43n9
Wu Ritu 62, 104, 116n9, 117n11
Wuhan 69n7

Xiamen municipality 107
Xie Honggang 55
Xinjiang 93n4
Xizhang (Tibet) 93n4
Xu Bing 176, 183n17
Xu Guanwei 135
Xu Ke 194
Xu Xiulan 82
Xue Bai 219
Xue, Y. 32, 33–4

Yang Hongwei 176
Yearbook of Finance 87
Yin Yungong 137n13
yiyao yangyi (fostering curative services
by [revenue] from drug sales) 171, 191,
192–3
Yu Baorong 122
Yu Fenghua 200
Yu Runji 172
Yu Tezhi 195, 202n5
Yuan Baohua 55, 69n4
Yuan, D. 43n4
Yuan Jie 216–17
Yunnan Province 93n4

Zelikow, Philip 10–11, 12
Zhang Anfa 197
Zhao Lei 219
Zhao Yuxin 85, 86, 221
Zhao Ziyang 55, 56, 69n4

Zhao, D. 33
Zheng Gongcheng 99, 100, 102
Zhenjiang municipality 62, 105, 107
Zhou Liangrong 178, 194–5, 196, 220
Zhou Xuerong 219, 222
Zhu Hengpeng 22

Zhu Hongbiao 124
Zhu, Y. 33
Zone I SUF program 102, 105, 106, 109
Zone II SUF program 102, 105, 106, 109
Zone III SUF program 103, 105,
    106, 109

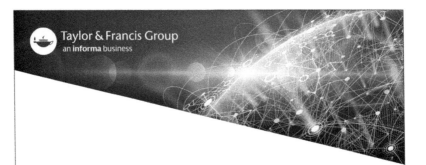